Follow-up Management of the High-Risk Infant

Follow-up Management of the High-Risk Infant

EDITED BY

H. William Taeusch, M.D.
Associate Professor of Pediatrics, Harvard Medical School; Director, Joint Program in Neonatology Infant Follow-up Program, The Children's Hospital, Boston

Michael W. Yogman, M.D.
Assistant Professor of Pediatrics, Harvard Medical School; Director, Infant Health and Development Program, The Children's Hospital, Boston

FOREWORD BY
Mary Ellen Avery, M.D.
Thomas Morgan Rotch Professor of Pediatrics, Harvard Medical School, Boston

INTRODUCTION BY
T. Berry Brazelton, M.D.
Clinical Professor of Pediatrics, Harvard Medical School; Chief of the Child Development Unit, The Children's Hospital, Boston

LITTLE, BROWN AND COMPANY   BOSTON/TORONTO

Library of Congress Catalog Card No. 87-80156

ISBN 0-316-83106-9

Printed in the United States of America

DON

Contents

Contributing Authors

Claudine Amiel-Tison, M.D.
*Associate Professor of Pediatrics, Paris V School of Medicine; Chief,
Department of Pediatrics, Baudelocque Maternity Hospital, Paris*

Janice L. Apol, R.N.C., M.S.
*Research Pediatric Nurse Practitioner, Infant Health and Development
Program, The Children's Hospital, Boston*

Anthony S. Bashir, Ph.D.
*Lecturer, Department of Medicine, Harvard Medical School, Boston; Adjunct
Associate Professor, Division of Special Education and Rehabilitation, Boston
College, Chestnut Hill; Coordinator of Programs in Speech-Language Pathology,
Department of Otolaryngology and Communication Disorders, The Children's
Hospital, Boston*

Mario Becker, M.D.
*Research Fellow, Joint Program in Neonatology and Department of Pediatrics,
Harvard Medical School, Boston*

Leila Beckwith, Ph.D.
*Professor of Pediatrics, University of California, Los Angeles, UCLA School of
Medicine, Los Angeles*

Robert H. Bradley, Ph.D.
*Professor and Director, Center for Child Development and Education,
University of Arkansas at Little Rock; Adjunct Associate Professor, Pediatrics,
University of Arkansas for Medical Sciences, Little Rock*

Elizabeth R. Brown, M.D.
*Associate Professor of Pediatrics, Boston University School of Medicine;
Director of Neonatology, Boston City Hospital, Boston*

Donna M. Bryant, Ph.D.
*Deputy Program Director, Infant Health and Development Program, and
Investigator, Frank Porter Graham Child Development Center, University of
North Carolina at Chapel Hill, Chapel Hill*

Patrick H. Casey, M.D.
Associate Professor of Pediatrics, University of Arkansas for Medical Sciences; Medical Director, Developmental Center, and Director, Infant Health and Development Program, Arkansas Children's Hospital, Little Rock

Allen J. Cherer, M.D.
Fellow, Joint Program in Neonatology, Harvard Medical School, Boston

Linda M. Cohen, M.D., M.P.H.
Pediatrician, Infant Health and Development Program, The Children's Hospital, Boston

Sarale E. Cohen, Ph.D.
Associate Professor in Residence, Department of Pediatrics, Division of Child Development, University of California, Los Angeles, UCLA School of Medicine, Los Angeles

Ann L. Colangelo, R.N.C., B.S.N.
Head Nurse, Neonatal Intensive Care Unit, The Children's Hospital, Boston

F. Sessions Cole, M.D.
Associate Professor of Pediatrics, Washington University School of Medicine; Director, Division of Newborn Medicine, St. Louis Children's Hospital, St. Louis

Michael F. Epstein, M.D.
Associate Professor of Pediatrics, Harvard Medical School; Clinical Director, Joint Program in Neonatology, Beth Israel Hospital, Brigham and Women's Hospital, and The Children's Hospital, Boston

Deborah A. Frank, M.D.
Assistant Professor of Pediatrics, Boston University School of Medicine; Assistant Visiting Physician, Pediatrics, Boston City Hospital, Boston

Stanley I. Greenspan, M.D.
Clinical Professor of Psychiatry and Behavioral Science and Child Health and Development, George Washington University School of Medicine and Health Sciences; Chief, Infant and Child Clinical Development Services Program, Division of Maternal and Child Health, Health Resources and Services Administration, Department of Health and Human Services, Washington, D.C.

Maureen Hack, M.D.
Associate Professor, Pediatrics, Case Western Reserve University School of Medicine; Director, High-Risk Follow-up Program of Pediatrics, Rainbow Babies and Children's Hospital and University Hospitals of Cleveland, Cleveland

Lawrence C. Kaplan, M.D., Sc.M.
Instructor in Pediatrics, Harvard Medical School; Clinical Director, Birth Defects Service, The Children's Hospital, Boston

Daniel J. Kindlon, Ph.D.
*Instructor in Psychology, Department of Psychiatry, Harvard Medical School;
Staff Psychologist, Infant Health and Development Program, The Children's
Hospital and Judge Baker Guidance Center, Boston*

Jane A. Kisielius, R.N., M.S.
Coordinator, Continuing Care Program, The Children's Hospital, Boston

Nancy K. Klein, Ph.D.
*Professor, Specialized Education, Cleveland State University; Clinical Assistant
Professor, Department of Pediatrics, Case Western Reserve University School of
Medicine, Cleveland*

Milton C. Kotelchuck, Ph.D., M.P.H.
*Assistant Professor, Department of Social Medicine and Health Policy, Harvard
Medical School; Research Associate, The Children's Hospital, Boston*

Barbara B. McCauley, M.S.W.
Clinical Social Worker, Private Practice, Arlington, Massachusetts

James E. McCauley, M.S.W.
*Clinical Social Worker, Brighton-Allston Mental Health Clinic, Brighton,
Massachusetts*

Marie C. McCormick, M.D., Sc.D.
*Assistant Professor of Pediatrics, University of Pennsylvania School of Medicine;
Associate Physician, Children's Hospital of Philadelphia, Philadelphia*

Frederick Mandell, M.D.
*Associate Clinical Professor of Pediatrics, Harvard Medical School; Senior
Associate in Medicine, The Children's Hospital, Boston*

Klaus K. Minde, M.D., F.R.C.P.(C)
*Professor, Department of Pediatrics, and Professor and Head, Department of
Psychiatry, Queen's University Faculty of Medicine; Chief of Service,
Department of Psychiatry, Kingston General Hospital, Kingston, Ontario*

Priscilla S. Osborne, R.P.T., M.S.
*Adjunct Clinical Associate Professor, Boston University Sargent College of
Allied Health Professions; Acting Director of Physical Therapy Training,
Developmental Evaluation Clinic, The Children's Hospital, Boston*

Robert A. Petersen, M.D., D.M.Sc.
*Assistant Professor of Ophthalmology, Harvard Medical School; Senior
Associate in Ophthalmology, The Children's Hospital, Boston*

Karen E. Peterson, R.D.
Doctoral Candidate, Department of Nutrition, Harvard School of Public Health; Senior Community Nutritionist, Department of Dietetics and Nutrition, Brigham and Women's Hospital, Boston

Craig T. Ramey, Ph.D.
Research Professor, Departments of Pediatrics and Psychology, University of North Carolina at Chapel Hill School of Medicine; National Program Director, Infant Health and Development Program, and Director of Research, Frank Porter Graham Child Development Center, University of North Carolina at Chapel Hill, Chapel Hill

Patricia N. Rissmiller, D.N.Sc.
Adjunct Assistant Professor, Boston University School of Nursing, Boston

I. Leslie Rubin, M.D.
Instructor in Pediatrics, Harvard Medical School; Assistant in Medicine and Pediatrician, Developmental Evaluation Clinic, The Children's Hospital, Boston

Richard R. Schnell, Ph.D.
Associate in Pediatrics (Psychology), Harvard Medical School; Director of Psychology, Developmental Evaluation Clinic, and Evaluation Coordinator, Infant Health and Development Program, The Children's Hospital, Boston

Martin C. Schultz, Ph.D.
Professor, Communication Disorders and Sciences, Southern Illinois University at Carbondale, Carbondale

Eunice Shishmanian, R.N., M.S.
Director of Nursing Program, Developmental Evaluation Clinic, The Children's Hospital, Boston

Marian Sigman, Ph.D.
Associate Professor of Psychiatry and Psychology, University of California, Los Angeles, UCLA School of Medicine, Los Angeles

Kristine E. Strand, Ed.D.
Adjunct Assistant Professor, Special Education Department, Boston College, Chestnut Hill; Director, Speech-Language-Hearing Department, Kennedy Memorial Hospital for Children, Boston

H. William Taeusch, M.D.
Associate Professor of Pediatrics, Harvard Medical School; Director, Joint Program in Neonatology Infant Follow-up Program, The Children's Hospital, Boston

Toni B. Vento, R.N.C., M.S.
Nurse Coordinator, Neonatal Outreach Program, Joint Program in Neonatology, Beth Israel Hospital, Brigham and Women's Hospital, and The Children's Hospital; formerly Senior Staff Nurse, Neonatal Intensive Care Unit, The Children's Hospital, Boston

Janice Ware, M.Ed.
Doctoral Candidate, Institute for Child Study, University of Maryland, College Park; Coordinator and Psychologist, Infant Follow-up Program, The Children's Hospital, Boston

Kim Wilson
Medical Student, Harvard Medical School, Boston

Paul H. Wise, M.D., M.P.H.
Assistant Professor of Pediatrics, Harvard Medical School; Director, Perinatal Epidemiology, Brigham and Women's Hospital, Boston

Michael W. Yogman, M.D.
Assistant Professor of Pediatrics, Harvard Medical School; Director, Infant Health and Development Program, The Children's Hospital, Boston

Foreword

Follow-up Management of the High-Risk Infant is a collection of essays
and outlines by individuals who are experienced in working with low-
birth-weight infants in the hospital setting and with families and agencies
in the community after discharge. Many topics are of importance to those
who care for this ever-growing group of new citizens. The majority of
these infants fare very well. In some infants, continuing problems include
difficulty with feeding and poor motor coordination; hearing and visual
deficits are found among a small percentage of survivors. Cognitive and
behavioral dysfunctions in some at school age require careful evaluation
and much more research into means of prevention.

Where can we find current approaches to these problems? The illustra-
tive examples and much of the discussion of management issues in this
volume reflect experience in major medical centers in North America in
the 1980s where teams of specialists are available. The reader is given a
number of suggestions and choices. In an evolving awareness of the ongoing special needs of infants, it is appropriate for specialists to conduct
research into the best ways to intervene on behalf of the infant and the environment. It is improbable that approaches outlined in this book could or
should be replicated in many communities; one of the challenges is to
learn which assessments and interventions in the first years of life are useful and which are not. The answers to some of these questions may have
to be deferred until a future edition. Meanwhile, those who share interest
in and concern for the future of low-birth-weight infants will profit from
reading the experiences of those committed to finding some of the answers.

Mary Ellen Avery, M.D.

Preface

Follow-up Management of the High-Risk Infant is a response to the success of the neonatal intensive care unit (NICU) in enabling the survival and discharge of increasing numbers of very low birth weight infants. Some of these infants have chronic problems requiring the involvement of multiple services. For the families, the transition of an infant to home life after an extended hospitalization evokes anxiety compounded by the need to rely on a new network of caretakers. We believe that the aftercare of NICU graduates is assuming an importance equal in many ways to the acute intensive care received by the newborn and the family in the hospital. For those experienced in following children with chronic illness and developmental problems, this perception is old hat; for others, it is a new fad with insufficient evidence to justify another tier of health care professionals for whom the expense is insufficiently justified. In this sense, the attention given to the issues of infant follow-up approximates the attention given to neonatal intensive care in the mid-1960s. At that time, those in the field of neonatology were convinced of the merit of the new approaches for the sick newborn, but it is only within the past five years or so that a favorable cost-benefit ratio for NICUs has been widely accepted.

The current pattern of follow-up care of NICU patients is analogous to the field of neonatal intensive care of the mid-1960s in several other important ways. The approaches in different centers vary widely. The value of the various components of follow-up care is uncertain. Availability of new services (home visiting, physical therapy, home monitoring and oxygen, and early interventions) and new technology (magnetic resonance imaging) and fervent debate over basic principles excite the field. A growing number of disparate professionals are working in the field, with new ideas, new funding, and new articles, sometimes with surprising findings appearing weekly. The area has all the qualities of a new medical frontier.

We work in a large tertiary program in Boston where Beth Israel Hospital, Brigham and Women's Hospital, The Children's Hospital, and Harvard Medical School support programs in perinatology and neonatology involving approximately 12,000 inborn and 400 outborn infants each year. Chapter 2, by Michael F. Epstein, M.D., provides an overview of the acute problems that we see in our nurseries and in our follow-up program. The management of these infants while inpatients has been described in the second edition of *Manual of Neonatal Care*, edited by John P. Cloherty, M.D., and Ann R. Stark, M.D. (Little, Brown, 1985), and our motivation for this book is similar to their motivation for that manual: to provide a guide for managing the specialized yet comprehensive biosocial problems faced by these infants and their families after discharge. Being responsible, in part, for the aftercare of these infants and participating in a large multicenter study involving comprehensive follow-up (the Infant Health and Development Program), we had the opportunity, and saw the need, to ask a variety of international experts for brief outlines of how they handle some of the difficult clinical problems that frequently occur.

The book addresses specific problems and the normal developmental issues of prematurity and their follow-up management. What are the major problems after discharge, and how are they handled? What has been done in a specific area? How does one assess and support parents' strengths, coping, and interaction with their infant? How does one sort familial pathology from acceptable norms of variation? What effective medical and community resources are available? What is the basis for a given approach to management? How does one organize and define a follow-up program? How do the parents and the infant adapt in the years after a high-risk infant graduates from the NICU? These are the types of questions we have tried to address. General pediatricians and other specialists (neurologists, orthopedists, otolaryngologists, ophthalmologists, cardiologists, developmental pediatricians, and radiologists); nurses; early educators; nutritionists; psychologists; occupational, respiratory, speech, and physical therapists; social workers; and audiologists are now frequently involved with the care of NICU graduates who increasingly have NICU-related problems that heretofore were seen less frequently. The book should be of interest to the diverse health professionals caring for these infants.

Some of the experts give differing and even conflicting views on management of similar problems. Disagreement is a sign of a developing field, and we did not (and could not) present a wholly consistent and well-worked-out consensus among experts. Because many of the recommendations in this book are tentative and because of the rapid developments in the field, we anticipate this exciting area will remain a medical frontier for the next decade or so.

H. W. T.
M. W. Y.

Introduction

T. Berry Brazelton

Follow-up Management of the High-Risk Infant summarizes the state of the art in the prevention, treatment, and subsequent follow-up of premature infants. The authors of these chapters point to the dramatically improved outcomes for these fragile babies. In these chapters the authors outline opportunities for prevention of prematurity and support for the subsequent development of premature infants. The amazing contributions of technology to the preservation of the life and future central nervous system (CNS) function of these infants present us with new challenges. The goal for the next decade will be to match the improvements in technologic care of premature infants with opportunities for enhancing the quality of their future lives. As these chapters convey, an intact brain does not necessarily predict an optimal future. The outcome for these babies is heavily correlated to the flexibility of their environments. In no other group of infants is there as high a correlation with the parents' socioeconomic status (SES) (Drillien, 1964; Sigman and Parmelee, 1979). Since SES is correlated with flexibility and resources of families, it is a measure of the parents' ability to adjust to and meet the heavy demands of such difficult infants. This highlights the need for intervention to help already stressed parents adapt to these vulnerable infants.

The remarkable ability of a child to recover from CNS deficits is evidence of plasticity in medicine. Children with known insults and identified defects in CNS tissue seem to be able to compensate for these deficits over time (Neligan et al., 1976; Sigman and Parmelee, 1979). With a defect such as blindness, the child can learn to compensate with increased sensitivity of the other modalities — auditory, tactile, and vestibular. An example of this is the "radar vision" that was marked by heightened sensitivity to auditory, tactile, and vestibular cues in a 14-month-old blind baby, who vocalized as she walked, never ran into tables, and rounded corners of doors by the differences in reverberations as her vocalizations bounced off nearby objects (Als et al., 1979). Since CNS tissue is not thought to be regenerative, the capacity for recovery of function has always been poorly understood.

The redundancy of unassigned pathways in an immature nervous system make it imperative that we start early to assist the fragile baby in attempts to adapt to his or her new environment. We must adapt the environment of the neonatal intensive care unit to the baby as best we can. We have begun to study the organization of the immature infant via two adaptations of the Neonatal Behavioral Assessment Scale (NBAS) (Als et al., 1982; Brazelton, 1984).

With the nine additions to the NBAS (Brazelton, 1984), we are beginning to demonstrate the value of behavioral observations of the premature infant's organization over time, and of the prediction of later outcome which serial assessments of the premature infant's behavioral organization can offer (Als et al., 1982). The nine additional items — quality of alert responsivity, cost of attention, examiner persistence, irritability, robustness, regulatory capacity, state regulation, motor tone, and reinforcement value of infant behavior—measure the infant's capacity to organize and to respond to environmental stimuli and the cost of this response, as well as the degree of effort which the examiner must utilize to organize the infant to respond. These first two (capacity and cost) measure the CNS and autonomic capacity of the infant and predict his or her neurologic intactness. The last is a measure of the demands on the environment which can assist the infant as he or she recovers.

We are aware of the cost to the baby of positive as well as negative responses, and we can now measure this cost by observing the fragile neonate's behavior. Such researchers as Gorski (1983) are monitoring these responses by physiologic measures. Lester and coworkers (1984) have developed a technique for combining behavioral responses and physiologic correlates as state is controlled with the techniques utilized by the NBAS. Even the cry of the baby gives us a way of assessing this cost and even perhaps predicting his or her future recovery (Zeskind and Lester, 1981). We are much closer to an understanding of the internal organization of the fragile baby as well as of what kind of organizational demands the infant will present to his or her environment at discharge. The baby's behavior reflects the capacity for internal organization as well as the quality of the demand for the environment to adapt to him or her.

In other words, there appear to be at least two sources of vulnerability which contribute to the risk of failure in developmental outcome: in the baby's own organizational system and capacity for growth (CNS and autonomic as well as physical), and in the capacity of the environment (usually represented by the parents) to adjust to and nurture the at-risk infant in ways that are appropriate to individual needs. If the interaction between these two is positive, the opportunities are significantly increased for fueling feedback cycles necessary to the baby for developing energy for developmental progress.

We must encourage high-risk nursery personnel to reevaluate the medical care and the environments in which we expect preterm infants to recover and develop. Clinically, we have observed the encouraging positive effects on recovery of such simple interventions as covering the baby's incubator at night to offer a diurnal cycle of light and darkness. We have influenced eating and sucking behaviors by offering infants oral feedings and social interaction contingently (i.e., when they demonstrate they are ready to eat as evidenced by modulated, rhythmic activity rather than waking them according to an imposed schedule). We are convinced that such attention to the needs for diurnal cycles and for responses from the environment which are contingent to the responsiveness of these infants is likely to make a difference in the recovery and in the ultimate CNS organization of such immature infants.

Coincident with the new emphasis on parental bonding to high-risk infants, as propounded by Klaus and Kennell (1976), we have begun to realize that even the behaviors of premature infants have potential for offering rewarding feedback to caregivers. This alone emphasizes the worth of reconceptualizing the behavioral organization of the premature infant. Individual observations before discharge can be translated to parents and can improve their chances for appropriate bonding and interaction.

An understanding of the forces that work toward a child's development is critical to both an understanding of his or her failure and any effort to prevent such failure. There are at least three forces that are constantly at work.

Maturation of the CNS and the autonomic nervous system, which regulate the baby's capacity to control reactions to incoming stimuli, is one of these forces. If the baby is at the mercy of an overreaction of either a motor (Moro or startle) or autonomic reaction (as is seen in an overstressed pulmonary or cardiac system), he or she cannot learn to maintain attention or to react appropriately to a sensory stimulus or to other information necessary to development.

A second force is that of competence within the child, which uses a feedback system relying on the completion of a task that the child *him- or herself* has done. White (1959) called this a "sense of competence," and one sees its power as a source of fuel when a toddler first learns to walk.

The third force is the reinforcement from the environment which feeds the infant's affective and cognitive needs. The feedback cycles necessary for normal affective growth were pointed out by Spitz, later by Harlow in monkeys, and conceptualized as "attachment" by Bowlby (1969). The environmental forces can work powerfully to retard or to enhance the infant's progress. In our laboratory, we are attempting to identify and conceptualize some of the ingredients of these interactive forces as they combine to fuel the child's recovery from severe deficits of prematurity, respiratory distress syndrome, and CNS dysfunction.

The pressures on parents, both internal and external, to succeed with their infant can actually work toward failure. When the feedback systems are not being completed in an expected way, we have been impressed with the power of violations of expectancy in the mother-infant interaction (Tronick et al., 1978).

The ability of the baby to precipitate and encourage the mother's attachment and caregiving behavior must be taken into account from the newborn period (Brazelton, 1961b). With an unresponsive neonate, the feedback mechanisms necessary to fuel mothering behavior are severely impaired. In a series of medicated newborns whose mothers were given obstetric analgesia during labor, the effect on neonatal sucking coupled with the physiologic effect of the medication on the mothers' milk production delayed recovery of weight gain by 36 to 48 hours in a normal group (Brazelton, 1961a). Since this is an observation at a rather gross level, interferences in the interaction, dyssynchrony, and more subtle "lack of fit" in the earliest mother-infant attachment interaction should be carefully sought and observed over time.

The vulnerability of the parent to even mildly distorted cues from the infant can best be understood in the light of a "grief reaction" in the parent (adapted from Lindemann, 1944). Because of the heightened expectations at birth, the opportunity for grieving is enhanced by any minor violation of this expectancy. The very energy that has been mobilized to relate to a baby can turn inward, into grieving, in such cases.

If the parents' resources are turned inward in the grieving process, they become encapsulated and the defenses strengthened to turn the available energy away from the baby. In the period of acute grieving, this self-protective mechanism may be necessary. At the point where the reorganization of the parents' egos has been accomplished, this energy can be made available to the baby for his or her recovery (Greenberg, 1979). It has constantly surprised us that, even in the face of a devastating diagnosis of retardation in the baby, parents can have the energy available to search for and work with the baby's more hopeful, positive behavior. Unless the parents can turn their grieving around, to turn its energy outward in the service of the child's best recovery, it is likely that the parents will remain permanently withdrawn and unavailable to an at-risk child. The job of intervention is to *accept* the negative forces of grieving, but to work to free positive forces for interaction with the child as well. This work can best be done early, by utilizing the best behavior in the child as a demonstration to recapture hope and to encourage reciprocity in the parents.

The dangers of fixation in these defenses and of parents' developing insensitive, inappropriate patterns in dealing with the infant at risk make it critical that we be ready to intervene early in their development together. Time is of the essence. The emotional availability and flexibility of parents of normal infants can be seen as a sign for capturing this availability with the parents of infants at risk as soon as possible. Before fixation can occur, we must be ready to capture and reinforce the positives in the infant's behavior for the parents, and we must be ready to set up a working relationship to help them, with their predictable grief, to work around the violations of expectancy. This energy becomes a force for the baby's recovery—not only as it fuels the parents, but as it serves as an external source of energy for the infant.

We have had an opportunity to understand recovery mechanisms in the neonatal period through the organizational and interactive capabilities of the neonate uncovered by administering the Brazelton Neonatal Behavioral Assessment Scale, and we have been struck with the power of sharing these processes with parents. Sharing the newborn's interactive and state organizational behavior with the parents of normal infants makes a significant difference in their future attachment—both to the infant (Eyler, 1979) and to the caregiver (Als and Brazelton, 1981). With the parents of high-risk infants, this kind of sharing may be even more significant.

The fragile infant's long latency to response, his or her alternating high or low threshold for receiving stimuli, and then his or her tendency to overshoot with an unexpectedly total response or to be overloaded from the cost of such a response all make the infant difficult to work with. When responding, he or she does so with responses that often violate parents' expectancy. In other words, the infant's behavioral responses are so extranormal that they set up the ingredients for a failure in their interaction—both because of the cost of responses to the infant and because of the grief reaction in the parents, which is likely to be engendered by the infant's unexpectedly deviant responses. We feel that if *we* can understand the mechanisms behind the deviant response, the parents can begin to understand them by observing us. By emulating our techniques for eliciting the infant's best behavior, they can begin to understand the infant and to see his or her progress. By harnessing the overloading stimulation and by helping the infant learn containment for him- or herself and achieve homeostasis, they free the infant to begin to interact with his or her environment. The energy for plasticity for recovery comes from two sources: from within, as the infant learns to achieve control and maintain an alert state, in which he or she can then achieve the inner feedback cycle by completing an attentional or motor task which gives a "sense of competence"; and from without, as the infant's parents get to know him or her and begin to understand his or her need for containment and homeostasis, as well as the need for social and motor stimuli that are appropriately and individually geared to his or her capacity to utilize them. We are impressed with the potential energy for recovery and plasticity after identified damage in both the infant and the parents. The timing in early infancy and the sharing quality of the intervention seem to be important aspects of this potential.

We need to develop better and better assessments of infants, of parent-infant interactions, and of the recovery processes involved in optimizing their future. We need more studies to prove the cost-effectiveness of early intervention with these fragile babies. This excellent volume offers us as a baseline the state of the art on which we can build these future investigations.

REFERENCES

Als, H., and Brazelton, T. B. Assessment of behavioral organization in a preterm and a full term infant. *J. Am. Acad. Child Psychiatry* 20 : 239, 1981.

Als, H., Lester, B. M., and Brazelton, T. B. Dynamics of the Behavioral Organization of the Premature Infant. In T. M. Field, A. M. Sostek, S. Goldberg, and H. H. Shuman (eds.), *Infants Born at Risk*. New York: Spectrum, 1979. Pp. 173–192.

Als, H., Lester, B. M., Tronick, E., and Brazelton, T. B. Manual for the Assessment of Preterm Infants' Behavior (APIB). In H. E. Fitzgerald, B. M. Lester, and M. W. Yogman (eds.), *Theory and Research in Behavioral Pediatrics*. New York: Plenum, 1982. Vol. 1.

Bibring, G. L., Dwyer, T. F., and Valenstein, A. F. A study of the psychological processes in pregnancy and of the earliest mother-child relationship. *Psychoanal. Study Child* 16 : 9, 1961.

Bowlby, J. *Attachment* (Attachment and Loss, vol. 1). New York: Basic Books, 1969.

Brazelton, T. B. Psychophysiological reactions in the neonate. No. 1: The value of observation of the newborn. *J. Pediatr.* 58 : 508, 1961a.

Brazelton, T. B. Psychophysiological reactions in the neonate. No. 2: Effects of maternal medication. *J. Pediatr.* 58 : 513, 1961b.

Brazelton, T. B. Neonatal Behavioral Assessment Scale. *Clin. Dev. Med.* No. 50, 1984.

Drillien, C. M. *The Growth and Development of the Prematurely Born Infant*. Baltimore: Williams & Wilkins, 1964.

Eyler, F. Demonstration of premature infants' capabilities to improve maternal attitude and facilitate mother-infant interaction (doctoral dissertation). University of Florida, Gainesville, Fla., 1979.

Garcia-Coll, C., Sepkoski, C., and Lester, B. M. Effects of teenage childbearing on neonatal behavior in Puerto Rico. *Infant Behav. Dev.* 5 : 277, 1982.

Gorski, P. A., Hole, W. T., Leonard, C. H., and Martin, J. A. Direct computer recording of premature infants and nursery care. *Pediatrics* 72 : 198, 1983.

Greenberg, D. Parental reactions to an infant with a birth defect (doctoral dissertation). Smith College School of Social Work, Northampton, Mass., 1979.

Heider, G. M. Vulnerability in infants and young children. *Genet. Psychol. Monogr.* 73 : 1, 1966.

Klaus, M. H., and Kennell, J. H. *Maternal-Infant Bonding*. St. Louis: Mosby, 1976.

Lester, B. M., Hoffman, J., and Brazelton, T. B. The rhythmic structure of mother-infant interaction in term and preterm infants. *Child Dev.* 56 : 15, 1984.

Lester, B. M., and Zeskind, P. S. Brazelton scale and physical size correlates of neonatal cry features. *Infant Behav. Dev.* 4 : 393, 1978.

Lindemann, E. Grief. *Am. J. Psychiatry*, 101 : 141, 1944.

Neligan, G. A., Kolvin, I., Scott, D., and Garside, R. F. *Born Too Soon or Born Too Small* (Spastics International Medical Publications). London: Heinemann, 1976.

Parmelee, A. H., and Michaelis, R. Neurological examination of the newborn. In J. Hellmuth (ed.), *Exceptional Infant: Studies in Abnormalities*. New York: Brunner/Mazel, 1971. Vol. 2.

Sigman, M., and Parmelee, A. H. Longitudinal Evaluation of the Preterm Infant. In T. M. Field, A. M. Sostek, S. Goldberg, and H. H. Shuman (eds.), *Infants Born at Risk*. New York: Spectrum, 1979. Pp. 193–219.

Tronick, E., Als, H., Adamson, L., and Brazelton, T. B. The infant's response to entrapment between contradictory messages in face-to-face interaction. *J. Am. Acad. Child Psychiatry* **17** : 16, 1978.

White, R. W. Motivation reconsidered: The concept of competence. *Psychol. Rev.* **66** : 297, 1959.

Zeskind, P. S., and Lester, B. M. Analysis of cry features in newborns with differential fetal growth. *Child Dev.* **52** : 207, 1981.

1

Basic Principles

NOTICE

The indications and dosages of all drugs in this book have been recommended in the medical literature and conform to the practices of the general medical community. The medications described do not necessarily have specific approval by the Food and Drug Administration for use in the diseases and dosages for which they are recommended. The package insert for each drug should be consulted for use and dosage as approved by the FDA. Because standards for usage change, it is advisable to keep abreast of revised recommendations, particularly those concerning new drugs.

Epidemiology of Prematurity and Goals for Prevention

Milton C. Kotelchuck and Paul H. Wise

I. Introduction

Prematurity is not a randomly distributed phenomenon. It has distinctive epidemiologic patterns, strongly influenced by sociodemographic and socio-economic factors. Socioeconomic factors influence both the underlying biologic risks for prematurity and the access to clinical treatments that can ameliorate risks and lessen subsequent morbidity.

An epidemiologic analysis starts by stratifying birth outcomes into two general components: (1) a distribution of birth weights or gestational ages and (2) a probability of survival (or morbidity) in those specific weight or gestational age categories. Survival rates or most commonly birth-weight-specific mortality (BWSM) has been used to indicate the quality and availability of intensive perinatal services (Paneth et al., 1982; Williams et al., 1982). Birth weight and gestational age distributions, on the other hand, are related to prenatal status and care (Eisner et al., 1979). This distinction has public policy importance in that the poor international standing of the United States in infant mortality relates to an excessive birth rate of low-birth-weight (LBW) infants, and not to BWSM or survival rates. Sweden, for example, has approximately one-half the LBW rate compared to the United States, whereas the BWSM is comparable, or slightly better in the United States (Guyer et al., 1982).

In this chapter, we focus on the epidemiology of prematurity using data from the 1983 Vital Statistics of the United States (National Center for Health Statistics, 1985), the 1980 U.S. National Natality Survey of the National Center for Health Statistics (Health, United States, 1984; Placek, 1984), and the 1985 Institute of Medicine report, *Preventing Low Birth Weight* (Institute of Medicine, 1985). Prematurity status is the obstetric marker used for the analyses presented in this chapter. If unavailable, LBW status is used and assumed to have similar distributions and associations.

II. Rates

Of all U.S. births in 1983, 9.2 percent were premature (less than 37 weeks' gestation), and 1.8 percent were very premature (less than 32 weeks' gestation) (Table 1-1). The LBW (<2,500 g) rate is 6.4 percent, and the very low birth weight (VLBW) (<1,500 g) rate is 1.1 percent. Approximately 3.6 percent of U.S. births are both premature and LBW, and 0.8 percent are very premature and VLBW.

Table 1-1. Prematurity and low-birth-weight status per 1,000 live births*

Birth weight (g)	Gestational age (wk)			Total
	<32	32–36	≥37	
<1,500	8.2	1.7	0.9	10.8
1,500–2,499	4.3	22.8	26.1	53.2
≥2,500	5.1	50.2	844.5	899.8
Total	17.6	74.7	871.5	

*In United States in 1983.
From National Center for Health Statistics. Advanced report of final natality statistics, 1983. *Monthly Vital Statistics Report* Series 34, No. 6[Suppl.]. U.S. Dept. of Health and Human Services publication (PHS) 85-1120. Hyattsville, Md., Sept. 20, 1985.

III. Temporal trends in rates

Although great advances have been made in the past 15 years in reducing infant mortality by improving the survival of LBW infants, little progress has been made in reducing the incidence of prematurity and LBW status. Low-birth-weight rates declined only 11 percent between 1971 and 1981, and VLBW rates have not declined at all (Kessel et al., 1984). Prematurity trends show a similar pattern (Institute of Medicine, 1985). Almost all recent improvements in LBW rates have been for term or very near term infants. The incidence of premature LBW babies has remained relatively stable in the United States in the past decade.

IV. Demographic trends

A. Maternal age

There is a slight U-shaped association of LBW status by maternal age. Women under 20 years and over 35 years are at increased risk for a poor pregnancy outcome, compared with women between 25 and 29 years of age (crude relative risks of 1.62 and 1.21, respectively) (National Center for Health Statistics, 1985). As seen in Table 1-2, however, the maternal age distribution for LBW births is roughly similar to total birth distribution. The relative infrequency of births in women under 20 and over 35 limits their impact. For example, teenage mothers, despite their increased risk for LBW infants, have only 19.2 percent of all LBW babies because they have only 13.7 percent of all U.S. births. The independent impact of maternal chronologic age on poor birth outcomes diminishes substantially when associated factors such as poverty and marital status are taken into account (Institute of Medicine, 1985). Age is a more important factor in determining poor birth outcome in whites than in blacks.

B. Socioeconomic status

The incidence of poor birth outcomes is strongly influenced by the socioeconomic status of the mother. Although not easy to define nor directly indicated on U.S. birth certificates, all measures of socioeconomic status —educational level, family income, race, residency, social class, and occupation—show basically the same pattern: Women of higher socioeco-

Table 1-2. Percentage of total and low-birth-weight neonates by maternal age and race*

Age	All births		White births		Black births	
	Total	LBW	Total	LBW	Total	LBW
<20	13.7	19.2	11.8	16.1	24.2	26.9
20–24	31.9	32.6	31.6	32.0	34.7	34.5
25–29	31.5	27.3	32.9	29.2	24.5	22.7
30–34	17.1	15.0	17.9	16.2	12.1	11.3
35–39	5.0	5.0	5.1	5.4	3.8	3.8
>40	0.7	0.9	0.7	1.0	0.7	0.8
Total		6.8		5.7		12.6

LBW = low birth weight.
*In total population of United States in 1983.
From National Center for Health Statistics. Advanced report of final natality statistics, 1983. *Monthly Vital Statistics Report* Series 34, No. 6[Suppl.]. U.S. Dept. of Health and Human Services publication (PHS) 85-1120. Hyattsville, Md., Sept. 20, 1985.

Table 1-3. Percentage of prematurity and low-birth-weight status by maternal race*

Birth category	Total	White	Black
<1,500 g	1.06	0.84	2.26
<2,500 g	6.34	5.30	13.16
<32 wk	1.75	1.33	3.92
<37 wk	9.12	7.66	16.34
<1,500 g and <32 wk	0.82	0.64	1.73
<2,500 g and <37 wk	3.70	3.01	6.83

*In United States in 1983.
From National Center for Health Statistics. Advanced report of final natality statistics, 1983. *Monthly Vital Statistics Report* Series 34, No. 6[Suppl.]. U.S. Dept. of Health and Human Services publication (PHS) 85-1120. Hyattsville, Md., Sept. 20, 1985.

nomic status have markedly better birth outcomes than women of low socioeconomic status. Poverty conveys a substantial additional risk for poor birth outcomes.

C. Race and ethnicity

Race is widely used as a proxy for socioeconomic status (Muller, 1985). It summarizes a variety of social and economic experiences affecting different groups within our society that includes but goes beyond the family's financial status (Wise et al., 1985). Black women have more than twice the prematurity rate of white women. Blacks give birth to 29.0 percent of all premature infants and 36.2 percent of all very premature infants in the United States, although they represent only 16.2 percent of all births (National Center for Health Statistics, 1985). As seen in Table 1-3, 16.34 percent of black births are premature versus 7.66 percent of white births (a crude relative risk of 2.18). Early prematurity shows an even stronger disparity: 3.92 percent for blacks and 1.33 percent for whites (a crude relative risk of 3.05). Low-birth-weight status shows a similar pattern. There is no evidence that this racial disparity is decreasing, as the rate of reduction in LBW and preterm LBW infants during the 1970s and 1980s has been greater in whites than in blacks (Kessel et al., 1984).

Data for other racial and ethnic groups, including Chinese, Japanese, and American Indians, show LBW rates similar to whites (National Center for Health Statistics, 1985). Rates for Mexican Americans are also reported to be similar to whites while Puerto Ricans have LBW rates midway between whites and blacks (National Center for Health Statistics, 1985). However, the accuracy of these Hispanic estimates can be questioned, since there may be substantial undercounting of the Hispanic populations (Selby et al., 1984).

D. Education

Educational attainment of the mother is a widely used measure of socioeconomic status that is routinely available from U.S. birth certificates. As Table 1-4 indicates, an increase in educational attainment decreases the likelihood of poor birth outcomes (Placek, 1984). In particular, women with less than a twelfth grade education are 77 percent more likely to have a premature infant and 95 percent more likely to have a LBW infant than women with some college education. Women without a high-school diploma seem especially at high risk.

E. Income

Income shows a trend similar to maternal education. Married women with family incomes less than $12,000 are 20 percent more likely to have a premature birth than women with incomes of more than $24,000 (Placek, 1984). Similar income trends are seen for LBW status. A British study reports a 50 percent increase in preterm and a 95 percent increase in LBW status for the poorer social classes IV and V compared to wealthier social classes I and II (Fredrik and Anderson, 1976).

Table 1-4. Prematurity and low-birth-weight status by maternal education and family income*

Education and income	Premature (%)	Low birth weight (%)
Maternal Education (yr)		
<8	14.01	8.53
<12	13.18	9.99
12	10.27	6.90
13–15	7.62	4.96
≥16	7.43	4.99
Family Income		
<$12,000	9.70	6.38
$12,000–24,000	8.32	5.69
>$24,000	8.04	5.55

*In United States in 1980.
From National Natality Survey, National Center for Health Statistics. U.S. Dept. of Health and Human Services, Washington, D.C.

F. Geographic and regional patterns

Prematurity and LBW rates in the United States show wide regional dis-parities. State rates of LBW vary from 4.2 to 7.9 percent for whites and from 11.0 to 15.1 percent for blacks (National Center for Health Statistics, 1985). To a major extent, the variations in state rates reflect the propor-tion of minority and poor populations in that state and, probably to a lesser extent, available preventive health care and social services.

Similarly, local area and within-state analyses also can reveal marked geographic variation in LBW and prematurity rates. These reflect, at the local level, the uneven geographic distribution of poor and minority pop-ulations at increased risk for poor pregnancy outcome and the uneven availability of quality prenatal and obstetric services.

V. Causes of socioeconomic and racial disparities in prematurity and low-birth-weight status

It is easier to document the wide socioeconomic and racial disparities in poor birth outcomes than to understand their causes. The factors responsible for the disparities in the incidence of prematurity can be divided into two broad groups:

Maternal risk: biologic or social factors that convey altered probabilities of a poor birth outcome

Access: factors that augment or limit entrance into programs or treatments that can ameliorate maternal risk factors

A. Maternal risk factors

The Institute of Medicine recently completed a major review of maternal factors that are significantly associated with increased LBW status. Table 1-5, adapted from its report, groups these maternal risk factors (Institute of Medicine, 1985).

A prior poor birth outcome is the single strongest predictor of subse-quent poor birth outcomes. The Collaborative Perinatal Study reported that 24.8 percent of white and 31.2 percent of black women in the United States between 1958 and 1966 had successive LBW deliveries (Niswander and Gordon, 1972). Denmark, with its extremely accurate and comprehensive birth records, reported in 1970 that a woman who had a preterm infant was 3.4 times more likely to deliver her next child prematurely (14% versus 4%). Similarly, a woman who had a LBW infant was 5.5 times more likely to deliver a subsequent LBW infant (16% versus 3%) (Bakketeig et al., 1979). Women with a prior fetal or neonatal death follow a similar pattern. However, because only 57 percent of U.S. births are to multiparous women, obstetric history as a predictor of future out-come is limited.

Multiple pregnancy is probably the strongest obstetric event predicting prematurity. Infants of a multiple birth are 9 times more likely (54.3% ver-sus 6.3%) to be LBW than single infants (National Center for Health Statis-tics, 1980).

Iatrogenic prematurity (immature infants delivered prematurely as the result of medical intervention) accounts for approximately 5 percent of all

Table 1-5. Maternal risk factors for prematurity and low birth weight

Medical Risks Predating Pregnancy
Parity (0 or more than 4)
Low weight for height
Genitourinary anomalies or surgery
Selected diseases such as diabetes or chronic hypertension
Nonimmune status for selected infections such as rubella
Poor obstetric history, including previous low-birth-weight infant, multiple spontaneous
    abortions
Maternal genetic factors (such as low maternal weight at own birth)

Medical Risks Arising During Pregnancy
Multiple pregnancy
Poor weight gain
Short interpregnancy interval
Hypotension
Hypertension, preeclampsia, toxemia
Selected infections such as symptomatic bacteriuria, rubella, and cytomegalovirus
First or second trimester bleeding
Placental problems such as placenta previa, abruptio placentae
Hyperemesis
Oligohydramnios, polyhydramnios
Anemia or abnormal hemoglobin
Isoimmunization
Fetal anomalies
Incompetent cervix
Spontaneous premature rupture of membranes
Iatrogenic prematurity

Behavioral and Environmental Risk
Smoking
Poor nutritional status
Alcohol or other substance abuse
DES exposure and other toxic exposures, including occupational hazards
High altitude

DES = diethylstilbestrol.
From Institute of Medicine, *Preventing Low Birth Weight*. Washington, D.C.: National Academy Press, 1985.

neonatal intensive care unit admissions. Cesarean sections performed to avoid even more serious consequences for the mother and fetus account for much iatrogenic prematurity. However, mistiming of induced labor and elective cesarean sections can result in inappropriate prematurity.

Smoking represents perhaps the most powerful and widely practiced behaviorally related noxious insult to the fetus. Smoking acts principally to retard fetal growth. Approximately one-third of pregnant women smoke, with smoking rates inversely related to family income, especially among whites (Placek, 1984). Smoking one pack per day reduces the birth weight by approximately 200 g and decreases gestation by 1 or 2 days (National Center for Health Statistics, 1980). It is estimated that 20 to

40 percent of LBW babies in the United States are born to women who smoke (Institute of Medicine, 1985).

Poor nutritional status, during and before pregnancy, is also associated with both increased prematurity and LBW (Institute of Medicine, 1985). There is some debate over how powerful a factor this is in the United States, but nutrition supplementation programs such as the Special Supplemental Food Program for Women, Infants and Children (WIC) consistently result in enhanced pregnancy outcomes, especially among women with poorest socioeconomic status (Kotelchuck et al., 1984).

B. Access to ameliorative programs and clinical treatments

Sociodemographic disparities in birth outcomes arise in part because of the inequities in gaining access to effective preventive and therapeutic prenatal interventions. A wide range of barriers exist: financial resources, limitations in availability of physician and health care resources, lack of belief in program efficacy, perceived or actual discrimination, language barriers, and so on. These barriers may be as important as the maternal risk factors in producing the sociodemographic disparities.

There is much debate about the effectiveness of prenatal care (Showstak et al., 1984). To date, most research has principally focused on the frequency, timing, and adequacy of prenatal care and paid little attention to the content of the care. Poorer birth outcomes are consistently reported among women who have no or very late prenatal care (Gortmaker, 1978; Institute of Medicine, 1985; Showstak et al., 1984). However, notably better birth outcomes are not seen for women with earlier or more extensive prenatal care. The Institute of Medicine report (1985) estimates that a woman with inadequate prenatal care has a relative risk of having a LBW infant of 1.56 and 1.35 in the white and black populations, respectively. But because of limited numbers of women with no or late prenatal care (5% total and 9% in the black community), it is estimated that improving prenatal care visitation status alone would reduce LBW incidence by only 3 to 15 percent in the United States.

Utilization of prenatal care is subject to strong sociodemographic determinants. Those least likely to have early and adequate prenatal care are most often young, poor, and minority women. For example, only 62.4 percent of black and 60.0 percent of Hispanic women receive prenatal care in the first trimester, compared to 79.4 percent of white women; similarly, only 53 percent of teenagers start prenatal care in the first trimester (Health, United States, 1984). Thus, moderately efficacious prenatal care is being used least by those who need it most.

Financial barriers are an obstacle to care. In one study, 50 percent of women with no prenatal care mentioned monetary problems as a contributing factor (Institute of Medicine, 1985). Expansion of health care reimbursement programs, such as Medicaid or MediCal, has been shown to increase access to early prenatal care (Norris and Williams, 1984). Recent decreases in the willingness of some obstetricians and gynecologists to accept Medicaid assignment and restrictive changes in federal health care programs are likely to further reduce the possibility of equitable provision of prenatal care services in the United States.

VI. Prediction of prematurity and risk assessment

The assessment of the probability of a poor birth outcome can help determine the most appropriate clinical prenatal and obstetric care. A variety of assessment scales are now being actively evaluated in the United States (Hobel et al., 1978; Creasy et al., 1980). These scales generally calculate a composite risk score based on the summation of weighted maternal risk factors (many of which were noted in the maternal risk and demographic sections). Sociodemographic status, pregnancy history, and smoking status are the most common principal risk factors on all of the scales.

Because of our present inadequate knowledge base about the causes of poor pregnancy outcomes, the ability of these scoring measures to identify women in need of special services remains far from perfect. Of the better instruments, the ability to identify positively women who will deliver prematurely (e.g., the sensitivity) is about 65 percent, but the ability to identify only those at actual risk (e.g., the specificity) is still quite poor. Presently, several low-risk women are identified at risk for each woman who is truly at high risk. Only slightly more than half of the women giving birth to LBW infants in the United States can be identified from existing screening instruments (Institute of Medicine, 1985).

VII. Subsequent mortality and morbidity of premature birth

The socioeconomic and sociodemographic factors associated with prematurity and other poor birth outcomes affect not only the incidence of prematurity but also subsequent mortality and morbidity.

A. Postneonatal mortality

Race and socioeconomic status influence the probability of mortality for premature and LBW neonates over the course of the first year of life. Although overall postneonatal mortality is widely known to be influenced by socioeconomic and sociodemographic experiences, postneonatal mortality as a sequela of prior LBW and prematurity status is even more strongly affected by these circumstances. In the United States in 1980, black moderate-LBW infants (1,500–2,500 g) with no congenital anomalies were almost twice as likely to die in the postneonatal period than white infants with similar birth-weights (relative risk: 1.96), yet black women had similar, if not slightly lower, LBW neonatal mortality rates (Health Policy Project, 1984). Low-birth-weight infants of women with less than a high-school education were almost twice as likely to die in the postneonatal period (relative risk: 1.85) compared with offspring from mothers who had more than a high-school education (Shapiro et al., 1980). The probability of long-term survival of comparable LBW infants is less for women of poorer socioeconomic status relative to white, more affluent women. Morbidity, it can be assumed, follows the same pattern.

B. Illness and hospitalization

While LBW status is perhaps the strongest predictor of subsequent first-year illness and hospitalization, socioeconomic status modifies this association in a predictable manner. In a study of morbidity during the first year of life, black LBW infants with no congenital anomalies had more frequent illnesses than white infants (relative risk: 1.27); similarly, children of women with less than a high-school education had more illnesses than children of women with more than a high-school education (relative risk: 1.82) (Shapiro et al., 1980). Moreover, since these disparities were greater for LBW than normal-birth-weight infants, it suggests that LBW status and socioeconomic status interact to produce increased first-year morbidity. Among children with no congenital anomalies, rehospitalization rates were significantly higher if the mothers were any of the following: black, under 17 years of age, with less than 12 years of education, living alone, or unemployed. For example, 17 percent of the children of women with less than 12 years of education were rehospitalized compared with only 8.7 percent of children of women with more than 12 years of education. Among multivariate predictors were Medicaid or self-payer payment status and then maternal education level under 12 years of schooling (McCormick et al., 1980).

C. Developmental delays

The risk of developmental delay is also related to sociodemographic factors that act to increase the risk of LBW. Low-birth-weight infants of disadvantaged mothers are more likely to fail in school or to have lower intelligence quotients (IQs) than infants of similar birth weight from more advantaged families (Ramey et al., 1978). Escalona (1982) examined the IQs of 119 children who weighed less than 2,250 g at birth with less than 36 weeks' gestation, and belonged to one of three socioeconomic status groups. Through 15 months of age, no socioeconomic status group differences were seen, but by 28 months (and then again at 40 months), significant IQ differences were noted (mean IQ of 74.5 for children of the lowest socioeconomic status, 94.1 for the highest). Poor LBW infants are therefore subject to both biologic and social hazards.

VIII. Goals for prevention

The clinician can play a major role in preventing prematurity and its subsequent morbidity. Even in the absence of a full knowledge of the causes of prematurity, the wide socioeconomic status and racial disparities suggest that there is great opportunity to reduce the frequency of premature births. The primary prevention of prematurity (reducing incidence) is certainly the most desirable way to manage the high-risk infant as well as to reduce the need for secondary prevention (Stubblefield, 1984).

The following are our recommendations for decreasing risk of premature birth:

A. Reduce maternal, fetal, neonatal, and infant risk factors relating to prematurity.
   1. Assess risk status of each woman for the increased likelihood of a poor pregnancy outcome; in particular, target women who have had a premature child as being at high risk in subsequent pregnancies.
   2. Identify risk factors such as nutritional status, immunity status, diabetes, and smoking status during prepregnancy visits.
   3. Identify conditions during pregnancy and prenatal care visits that can

be ameliorated with more focused prenatal care or that require more frequent monitoring (e.g., multiple pregnancy, poor weight gain, hypertension and preeclampsia, and infections).

4. Directly reduce maternal risk factors through provision of office-based medical services: for example, advise patients to limit adverse smoking and drinking behavior; advise patients regarding better nutrition for hypertension and diabetes control and for better weight gain; treat infections; and reduce anxieties or stress.

5. Directly reduce infant risk factors, especially for children of low socioeconomic status born prematurely, by providing office-based pediatric services: for example, give prompt attention to upper respiratory infections, bronchitis, pneumonia, and other acute illnesses; provide nutritional guidance; and enhance awareness of injuries and injury prevention.

B. Enhance access to specialized prenatal care and clinical treatment programs that can reduce the incidence of poor birth outcomes and secondary morbidity.

1. Increase the frequency of prenatal care visits for high-risk women needing greater monitoring.

2. Direct high-risk women into specialized prenatal medical programs and treatments (e.g., diabetes, multiple births).

3. Direct high-risk women into ancillary prenatal care programs that enhance the comprehensiveness of prenatal care (e.g., WIC, exercise programs, smoking reduction workshops).

4. Direct women and their families into social service programs for which they are eligible, such as Medicaid, visiting nurse association programs, food stamps, and public housing, to reduce some of the impacts of poorer socioeconomic status.

5. Direct premature infants into early intervention and other programs that facilitate cognitive, social, and physical development.

6. Increase sensitivity to the health behavior characteristics of different racial and social groups and to the barriers that limit utilization of medical advice.

7. Work with other health professionals to effect public policy and public programs that enhance equality of access to health care services.

IX. Conclusions

Health professionals, both as clinicians and public citizens, have the capacity to lessen the impact of socioeconomic and sociodemographic factors on birth outcomes and subsequent morbidity. Clinically, physicians can both reduce maternal risk factors and facilitate access to programs and treatments known to be effective in improving birth outcomes, especially for high-risk groups who do not routinely have access to quality medical and social services. Public policies and programs, such as social welfare programs, early intervention programs, financial support for prenatal and infant care, and public health risk reduction campaigns, can be developed that foster the implementation of clinical and social strategies to reduce poor birth outcomes. The epidemiologic disparities in the incidence of prematurity and LBW among different subpopulations within the United States suggest that preventive activities, both at clinical and public policy levels, can be efficacious in preventing premature birth.

REFERENCES

Bakketeig, L. S., Hoffman, H. J., and Harley, E. E. The tendency to repeat gestational age and birth weight in successive births. *Am. J. Obstet. Gynecol.* 135 : 1086, 1979.

Creasy, R. K., Gummer, B. A., and Liggins, G. C. System for predicting spontaneous preterm birth. *Obstet. Gynecol.* 55 : 692, 1980.

David, R. J., and Siegel, E. Decline in neonatal mortality, 1968 to 1977; better babies or better care. *Pediatrics* 71 : 531, 1983.

Eisner, V., Brozie, J. W., Pratt, M. W., and Hexter, A. C. The risk of low birth weight. *Am. J. Public Health,* 70 : 887, 1979.

Escalona, S. K. Babies at double hazard: Early development of infants at biologic and social risk. *Pediatrics* 70 : 670, 1982.

Fredrik, J., and Anderson, A. B. M. Factors associated with spontaneous preterm birth. *Br. J. Obstet. Gynaecol.* 83 : 342, 1976.

Gortmaker, S. L. The effects of prenatal care upon the health of the newborn. *Am. J. Public Health* 69 : 653, 1978.

Guyer, B., Wallach, L. E., and Rosen, S. L. Birth weight standardized neonatality mortality rates and the prevention of low birth weight: How does Massachusetts compare with Sweden? *N. Engl. J. Med.* 306 : 1230, 1982.

Hall, M. H., Chng, P. K., and MacGillivray, I. Is routine antenatal care worthwhile? *Lancet* 2 : 78, 1980.

Health Policy Project. *Closing the Gap.* Atlanta, Ga.: The Carter Center of Emory University, 1984.

Health, United States, 1984. U.S. Dept. of Health and Human Services publication (PHS) 84-1232. Government Printing Office, 1984.

Hobel, C. J., Youkeles, L., and Forsythe, A. Prenatal and intrapartum high-risk screening. II. Risk factors reassessed. *Am. J. Obstet. Gynecol.* 135 : 1051, 1978.

Institute of Medicine. *Preventing Low Birth Weight.* Washington, D.C.: National Academy Press, 1985.

Kessel, S. S., Villar, J., Berendes, H. W., and Nugent, R. P. The changing pattern of low birth weight in the United States: 1970 to 1980. *J.A.M.A.* 215 : 1978, 1984.

Kotelchuck, M., Schwartz, J. B., Anderson, M. J., and Finison, K. S. WIC participation and pregnancy outcomes: Massachusetts statewide evaluation project. *Am. J. Public Health* 74 : 1086, 1984.

McCormick, M. C., Shapiro, S., and Starfield, B. H. Rehospitalization in the first year of life for high-risk survivors. *Pediatrics* 66 :991, 1980.

Muller, C. A window on the past: The position of the client in twentieth century public health thought and practice. *Am. J. Public Health* 75 : 470, 1985.

National Center for Health Statistics. Factors associated with low birth weight: United States, 1976. Prepared by S. Taffel. *Vital and Health Statistics,* Series 21, No. 37. U.S. Dept. of Health, Education and Welfare publication (PHS) 80-1915. Government Printing Office, April 1980.

National Center for Health Statistics. Advanced report of final natality statistics, 1983. *Monthly Vital Statistics Report* Series 34, No. 6[Suppl.]. U.S. Dept. of Health and Human Services publication (PHS) 85-1120. Hyattsville, Md., Sept. 20, 1985.

Niswander, K. R., and Gordon, M. *The Women and Their Pregnancies: The Collaborative Perinatal Study of the National Institute of Neurologic Diseases and Stroke.* Philadelphia: Saunders, 1972.

Norris, F. D., and Williams, R. L. Perinatal outcomes among Medicaid recipients in California. *Am. J. Public Health* 74 : 1112, 1984.

Paneth, N., Keily, J. L., Wallenstein, S., et al. Newborn intensive care and neonatal mortality in low birth weight infants: A population study. *N. Engl. J. Med.* 307 : 149, 1982.

Placek, P. Findings from the 1980 National Natality and Fetal Mortality Survey. *U.S. Public Health Reports* 99 : 111, 1984.

Ramey, C. T., Stedman, D. J., Borders-Patterson, A., and Mengel, W. Predicting school failure from information available at birth. *Am. J. Ment. Defic.* 82 : 525, 1978.

Selby, M. L., Lee, E. S., Tuttle, D. M., and Loe, H. D. Validity of the Spanish surname infant mortality rate as a health statistic indicator for Mexican-American population. *Am. J. Public Health* 74 : 988, 1984.

Shapiro, S., McCormick, M. C., Starfield, B. H., et al. Relevance of correlates of infant deaths for significant morbidity at 1 year of age. *Am. J. Obstet. Gynecol.* 136 : 363, 1980.

Showstak, J. A., Budetti, P. P., and Minkler, D. Factors associated with birth weight: An exploration of the roles of prenatal care and length of gestation. *Am. J. Public Health* 74 : 1003, 1984.

Stubblefield, P. G. Causes and Prevention of Preterm Birth: An Overview. In F. Fuchs and P. G. Stubblefield (eds.), *Preterm Birth: Causes, Prevention, and Management.* New York: Macmillan, 1984.

Williams, R. L., and Chen, P. M. Identifying the sources of the recent decline in perinatal mortality rates in California. *N. Engl. J. Med.* 306 : 207, 1982.

Wise, P. H., Kotelchuck, M., Wilson, M. L., and Mills, M. Racial and socioeconomic disparities in childhood mortality in Boston. *N. Engl. J. Med.* 313 : 360, 1985.

2

Major Causes of Neonatal Mortality and Morbidity

Michael F. Epstein

I. Introduction

Chronic problems in infants, for the most part, occur in those who survive after a prolonged and complicated course in neonatal intensive care units (NICUs). The problems that cause chronic morbidity for the most part are related to those leading to neonatal death.

In the twentieth century, we have seen a remarkable reduction in the rate of neonatal deaths in the United States: Neonatal mortality has steadily dropped from 40 to 50 per 1,000 live births between 1900 and 1910 to 7 to 8 per 1,000 live births in the 1980s.

The explanation for this phenomenon must go beyond the crude neonatal mortality figures to examine the two major determinants of this rate—the birth-weight distribution and birth-weight-specific mortality. In general, birth-weight distribution reflects socioeconomic factors that have a notable impact on premature delivery and access to medical care for both the mother and infant. In contrast, birth-weight-specific mortality is largely determined by the availability and quality of medical care for the newborn (i.e., neonatal intensive care). Most analysts agree that the major improvements in neonatal mortality in the last 2 decades reflect improved birth-weight-specific mortality, especially in infants weighing between 1,500 and 2,500 g, and can be attributed to the regionalization and implementation of advances in neonatal intensive care (Gortmaker, et al., 1985). At the same time, there have been few important changes in birth-weight distribution, perhaps reflecting our continued lack of understanding of the basic science underlying parturition and premature labor as well as uncertainty about what components of prenatal care have a salutary effect on the mother and fetus.

Finally, any analysis of neonatal mortality and morbidity must acknowledge the differences in outcome among various groups within the United States. Neonatal mortality among blacks has consistently been 1.5- to 2.5-fold greater than that for whites throughout the twentieth century (McCormick, 1985). This disparity is also evident locally with a neonatal mortality in Boston during 1978 and 1979 of 15.6 per 1,000 live births for blacks and 7.2 per 1,000 live births for whites (Wise et al., 1985).

An understanding of the interaction between social, economic, and medical determinants of perinatal outcome is critical for a meaningful analysis of trends, causality, and public and medical policy decisions; however, a detailed analysis is beyond the scope of this chapter. Rather, I wish to take a cross-sectional look at neonatal morbidity and mortality by examining the re-

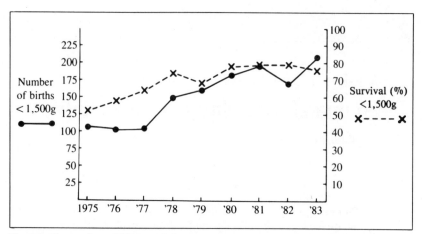

Fig. 2-1. The number of births and the number of survivors (discharged alive from NICU) of very low birth weight infants delivered alive at Brigham and Women's Hospital in Boston for the period 1975 to 1983.

cent experience at a single institution, the Brigham and Women's Hospital (BWH) in Boston, between 1975 and 1983. This 720-bed major teaching hospital of the Harvard Medical School has a 120-bed obstetric service and delivered nearly 9,500 babies in 1985. It is the major maternal referral hospital in central New England. Its 40-bed NICU admits more than 2,000 infants each year. Approximately 1,200 infants stay more than 24 hours, and the remainder return to regular nurseries after observation, diagnostic tests, or brief therapy. Close geographic and professional links to The Children's Hospital, Boston, and the Beth Israel Hospital, Boston, through the Joint Program in Neonatology allow maximum efficiency in the utilization of consultants, surgery, and other specialized services.

II. Neonatal mortality
   Figures 2-1 and 2-2 illustrate the experience in neonatal mortality between 1975 and 1983 at the BWH. During that period, the number of live births increased from 6,052 to 8,210 per year. The neonatal mortality remained relatively static, fluctuating between a high of 11.9 per 1,000 live births in 1979 to a low of 8.4 in 1978. This stability in the crude neonatal mortality looks different when it is adjusted as suggested by Lee and colleagues (1980a) using birthweight distribution as a way of standardizing or normalizing risk. Between 1975 and 1983, the rate of birth of very low birth weight (VLBW) infants (<1,500 g) increased from 17.8 to 25.2 per 1,000 live births. When the crude neonatal mortality is divided by the birth rate of VLBW infants, an index of neonatal outcome standardized for the risk of the population is obtained. The lower this index, the better the outcome. Table 2-1 illustrates how the use of this index produces a more realistic assessment of neonatal outcome over time by indicating that the 41 percent increase in VLBW infants coincides with a 38.7 percent decline in the index. The crude neonatal mortality, in contrast, decreased only 12.7 percent over that period.

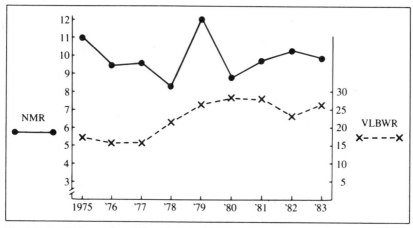

Fig. 2-2. Survival rates for all live births and birth rates for those born weighing less than 1,500 g are shown. *NMR* = number of live births who die in the neonatal intensive care unit/number of live births; *VLBWR* = number of infants under 1,500 g birth weight who are born in the NICU/number of total infants born each year. **(Data from Brigham and Women's Hospital, Boston.)**

Table 2-1. Births and deaths[a]

Year	Total deaths/births	Neonatal mortality[b]	Rate of delivery of VLBW infants[b]	Index
1975	67 : 6054	11.0	17.8	0.62
1983	79 : 8210	9.6	25.2	0.38

VLBW = very low birth weight.
[a]From Brigham and Women's Hospital, Boston, 1975 to 1983.
[b]Per 1,000 live births.

III. Causes of death

Figure 2-3 illustrates the major causes of death in the inborn population at BWH during the years 1982 and 1983. To avoid the problem of uncertain or conflicting assessments of gestational age, extreme prematurity was defined as birth weight of less than 1,000 g. Although some small-for-gestational-age infants of more than 28 weeks' gestation were included in this group and some large 28-week infants were excluded, this group generally included infants of 24 to 28 weeks' gestation. These infants accounted for 1.09 percent of all live-born infants. Yet, despite the more than twofold improvement in survival in recent years (Fig. 2-4), they represented more than 33 percent of the total neonatal mortality. Among the infants weighing less than 1,000 g, acute respiratory insufficiency was the primary cause of death in two-thirds. Intraventricular hemorrhage, asphyxia, sepsis, necrotizing enterocolitis, pulmonary hemorrhage, and bronchopulmonary dysplasia were other important causes of death in this under 1,000 g group. The average age at death was 5 days with a range of 1 to 60 days.

The second major cause of death was fatal congenital anomalies. Table 2-2

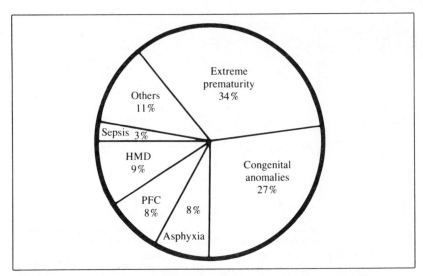

Fig. 2-3. Major causes of neonatal mortality during 1982–1983 in the Joint Program in Neonatology, Boston, are shown as a proportion of total neonatal mortality. *HMD* = hyaline membrane disease; *PFC* = persistent fetal circulation.

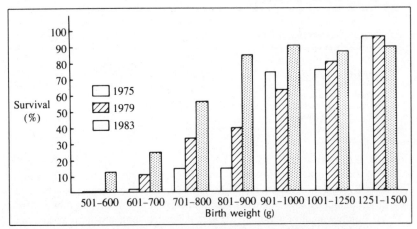

Fig. 2-4. Birth-weight-specific mortality for infants born at Brigham and Women's Hospital and Beth Israel Hospital, Boston, during three time periods.

lists the most common fatal malformations. Cardiac, renal, and central nervous system malformations and fatal chromosomal defects were most frequent, although more than one-third of all fatal anomalies were due to uncommon disorders of unknown etiology. Despite the advent of prenatal ultrasonography, there was no decrease in the percentage of newborn deaths attributable to congenital malformations between 1975 and 1983.

The third leading cause of death in 1982 and 1983 was hyaline membrane disease (used synonymously with respiratory distress syndrome) in infants of

Table 2-2. Lethal congenital anomalies*

Anomaly	Number of infants
Congenital heart disease	
Hypoplastic left-heart syndrome	5
Transposition of great vessels	1
Tetralogy of Fallot	1
Tricuspid atresia	1
Potter's syndrome (aplasia or dysplasia of kidneys)	8
Anencephaly or myelomeningocele	4
Trisomy 11, 13, or 18	5
Multiple complex anomalies of unknown cause	3
Fatal dwarfism	3
Other	12
Total	43

*From Brigham and Women's Hospital, Boston, 1982 to 1983.

birth weight over 1,000 g, followed by asphyxia, persistent pulmonary hypertension, meconium aspiration, nonimmunologic hydrops (alpha thalassemia, endocardial fibroelastosis, idiopathic), and sepsis (group B streptococci, *Escherichia coli, Enterobacter cloaceae, Staphylococcus aureus, Candida*).

Certain diagnoses were remarkable by their absence. No infants died from erythroblastosis fetalis. Infants of diabetic mothers accounted for five deaths, but their neonatal mortality was nearly the same as that of the nondiabetic population. There were no cases of fatal birth trauma, and congenital infections were not fatal in any infant.

IV. Major morbidity

The reasons for morbidity in the NICU in 1982 and 1983 paralleled the major causes of mortality. Prematurity, though accounting for under 8 percent of all BWH deliveries, accounted for over 50 percent of all NICU admissions. Similarly, the major diagnoses were clearly related to prematurity (Williams, 1982). The two most common nonfatal diagnoses were hyaline membrane disease and apnea, both showing an inverse relationship between length of gestation and risk. Intracranial hemorrhage (most frequently located in the germinal matrix adjacent to the ventricles), patent ductus arteriosus, and bronchopulmonary dysplasia were also noted in many of the premature infants with hyaline membrane disease or, more uncommonly, in otherwise healthy premature infants. Necrotizing enterocolitis and neonatal sepsis with or without meningitis were relatively rare but were noted in several infants each year.

An additional area of morbidity in premature infants relates to the more prolonged hospitalization experienced by the very smallest infants. Infants of less than 1,000 g who would have had a 10 to 15 percent survival rate in the 1970s are now surviving at a rate of nearly 70 percent (see Fig. 2-4). An entirely new population of hospitalized patients is therefore created, many of whom stay in the NICU for more than 100 days. One new complication in the care of the premature infant that results from this increase in number of hospital days is nosocomial infection, often with *S. epidermidis*. Recent reports have identified a distinctive syndrome characterized by apnea, temperature instability, and metabolic derangements (Noel, 1984). During 1982 and 1983, the risk of developing blood culture–positive *S. epidermidis* sepsis during hospitalization ranged from less than 1 percent in infants with birth weight of more than 2,000 g to nearly 40 percent in those with birth weight of less than 1,000 g. Although mortality appeared to be the same in infants with and without nosocomial infection, hospital stay was prolonged and exposure to antibiotics, intravenous therapy, and repeat cultures were all increased in the infected group.

Among term infants, the major reasons for admission were to rule out sepsis and to hold for observation. Those infants who needed more prolonged stays had either respiratory problems from meconium aspiration, retained fetal lung liquid, isolated pneumothorax, or pneumonia, or they had sequelae of asphyxia. The sickest term infants were often those with persistent pulmonary hypertension (or persistent fetal circulation [PFC]), and those with severe birth asphyxia and seizures. Infants with PFC continue to have an excessively high mortality. When PFC was identified as a persistent right-to-left shunt by way of a patent ductus arteriosus or foramen ovale accompanied by a postductal arterial PO_2 of less than 100 mm Hg on FIO_2 1.0, mortality during 1982 and 1983 was nearly 50 percent. Despite the use of hyperventilation therapy, vasoactive drugs, and pulmonary artery pressure monitoring, mortality for this condition has not improved in recent years.

Finally, the combination of prematurity, perinatal compromise, anomalies, and invasive therapy and monitoring resulted in a number of infants with chronic medical conditions. Bronchopulmonary dysplasia, retinopathy of prematurity, cognitive and motor handicaps, and other less commonly encountered problems represent the long-term morbidity of a needy few who are discharged from NICUs. Management of these problems represents a new and growing challenge in the field of pediatrics.

REFERENCES

Gortmaker, S., Sobol, A., Clark, C., et al. The survival of very low birth weight infants by level of hospital of birth: A population study of perinatal systems in four states. *Am. J. Obstet. Gynecol.* 152 : 517, 1985.

Kaller, L., et al. Assessment of gestational age: A simplified scoring system. *J. Perinat. Med.* 13 : 135, 1985.

Lee, K. S., Paneth, N., Gartner, L., and Pearlman, M. The very low birth weight rate: Principal predictor of neonatal mortality in industrialized populations. *J. Pediatr.* 97 : 759, 1980a.

Lee, K. S., Paneth, N., Gartner, L. M., et al. Neonatal mortality: An analysis of the recent improvement in the United States. *Am. J. Public Health* 70 : 15, 1980b.

McCormick, M. The contribution of low birth weight to infant mortality and childhood morbidity. *N. Engl. J. Med.* 312 : 82, 1985.

Noel, G., and Edelson, P. J. *Staphylococcus epidermidis* bacteremia in neonates: Further observations and the occurrence of focal infection. *Pediatrics* 74 : 832, 1984.

Williams, R. L., and Chen, P. M. Identifying the sources of the recent decline in perinatal mortality roles in California. *N. Engl. J. Med.* 306 : 207, 1982.

Wise, P. H., Kotelchuck, M., Wilson, M. L., and Mills, M. Racial and socioeconomic disparities in childhood mortality in Boston. *N. Engl. J. Med.* 313 : 360, 1985.

3

Longitudinal Studies of Preterm Infants

Sarale E. Cohen

I. Introduction

The development of preterm infants has been studied for a number of years and is a widely researched topic. Infants born preterm suffer a number of prenatal and perinatal complications, and the neurodevelopmental outcome of these infants is of great concern. Longitudinal study of preterm infants is commonly used to monitor the infant's development, to provide hypotheses concerning underlying causes of brain dysfunction, and to predict and understand developmental problems. Longitudinal studies have been conducted in a number of countries as well as in different hospitals within the same country. A number of studies have concluded that although the group itself generally shows a relatively high rate of children with intellectual, school-related, and behavioral problems, most of the individual children do well (Cohen, 1986; Kopp, 1979). Most studies have focused on group description; however, more meaningful for many clinicians are data directed at predictions for individual children. Some recent reports have addressed the issue of correct identification of outcome for individual children (Cohen, 1983; Hunt, 1982; Siegel, 1982). In the following sections, predicting outcomes for the preterm individual as well as the preterm group is addressed.

II. Purposes of longitudinal studies of preterm infants

Retrospective analyses of children with intellectual and learning problems have reported that a high percentage of the children were born prematurely. To study the effects of being born preterm, prospective longitudinal studies are necessary. Longitudinal studies facilitate monitoring the development of preterm children and make it possible to eliminate confounding variables.

A. Determination of etiologic factors

A primary purpose of longitudinal study, particularly for neonatologists who are involved in critical decisions regarding the care of very sick infants, is to identify and determine the causes of major handicaps. Follow-up of graduates from an individual nursery cannot answer questions about etiology and treatment because in most nurseries there are few cases with major handicaps (e.g., cerebral palsy) and many factors are involved. A follow-up project from a single nursery can be of value in providing monitoring of overall morbidity and mortality and in helping staff morale. To resolve issues of perinatal etiologic factors and critical care, however, large epidemiologic studies involving regions rather than individual centers are required. Further, treatment changes rapidly, and it is necessary to do short-term longitudinal studies with quick feedback to answer applied questions.

B. Documentation and assessment of biologic and social factors
To understand the processes involved in the development of preterm infants, it is essential to design longitudinal studies that carefully document and assess both biologic and social factors. Deficits may show only as the child performs complex learning tasks; therefore, longitudinal study through the school years is recommended. To date most of the long-term longitudinal studies have emphasized intellectual functioning and school achievement. A broad range of social and emotional tasks should be included in assessment protocols to provide data on the functional nature of the child's performance. Neuropsychologic assessment is also suggested, as infant measures have shown preterm infants to be less efficient in their information processing than full-term infants.

C. Early prediction of infants at risk
The purpose of some longitudinal studies is early prediction of infants at risk to select children in need of intervention programs. Most longitudinal studies have found poor prediction from infancy tests to developmental outcome after the second year. Short-term longitudinal studies for 1 or 2 years typically may not answer the questions of the neonatologists or of professionals and parents who require early identification of later deviance.

III. Methodologic problems
Studies must be carefully designed, and the reader must critically analyze the results of studies, as many methodologic problems may distort the conclusions. Changes and advances in perinatal care mandate continued and careful follow-up (Davies, 1984).
Common methodologic problems are as follows:

A. *There is a lack of communality in the reporting of handicap rate.* Idiosyncratic terminology is often employed. It is difficult to equate behaviors across studies; one author may refer to a problem as a minor handicap whereas another may call the same condition major. Incidence rates may be misleading if a control group is not used.

B. *The sample must be described clearly and completely,* including perinatal and demographic characteristics, to evaluate outcome. Preterm infants have diverse medical complications and socioeconomic circumstances. Social factors must be controlled to avoid the confounding social and biologic factors. Further, as developmental outcome measures and low birth weight are independently related to social factors, poor performance may be due to low socioeconomic status.

C. *The year the infant is born and the hospital itself may affect outcome.* Innovations in care can be helpful; however, there is a possibility that technologic advances may lead to new problems (e.g., oxygen use in newborns led to retrolental fibroplasia). Recruitment procedures may also be related to cohort differences, and it is important to know if the infants were born in the hospital or transported to the neonatal intensive care unit (NICU).

D. *The length of time of the follow-up is critical.* Prediction of later problems is better over a short period of time than over a long time interval. Due to the discontinuous nature of development, many changes in behavior occur, and early prediction generally has a high error rate. Therefore, it is prudent to be cautious in basing conclusions on short-term follow-up. Further, some potential problems may involve minor central nervous system dysfunction and may not be apparent until the child is in school and required to do complex tasks.

E. *The type of behavior and the adequacy of the measurement technique must be considered* in designing and evaluating studies. In the past, the primary questions concerned mortality and gross morbidity. The emphasis has broadened, and educational and social problems are of current interest. Physical growth, cognitive development, neurologic behavior, and socioemotional development may have different antecedents and different courses.

F. *Group data without analysis for special subgroups may be misleading* (e.g., hyaline membrane disease [HMD] with and without other complications). Disagreement among research findings may be due to differences in type and range of complications and the difficulty of eliminating confounding factors. These factors include the influence of the long hospitalization that many sick infants experience. The problems of the group need to be defined and identified, and the design and analyses should take into account the severity of the problem.

IV. Factors associated with neurodevelopmental outcome in preterm infants

A. *Biological descriptions* such as birth weight, gestational age, and being small for dates generally do not predict later developmental outcome. It is nonetheless agreed that the smallest infants are the sickest and have the highest incidence of neurologic and developmental problems. Some studies report that birth weight and gestational age are related to later performance (Bennett et al., 1982), probably because these variables are highly related to the occurrence of neurologic problems. When extremely handicapped children are removed from analyses, the relationship of birth weight and gestational age to later intelligence is low.

Recent reports indicate that mortality has decreased since the mid 1970s with the advent of a number of technologic changes in the NICU. Yet the rate of neurodevelopmental morbidity has been constant (Hack et al., 1983). Overall, recent studies show that of the survivors weighing less than 1,500 g, approximately 80 percent are within the normal range (Hack et al., 1983; Stewart et al., 1981). Less favorable outcomes are associated with outborn infants transported to the NICU and severely asphyxiated infants rather than with birth weight.

There is much controversy over the role of the NICU in caring for those infants weighing less than 800 g. Some centers exclude infants weighing less than 750 g from their reports; however, a number of studies are now investigating infants weighing between 500 and 800 g (Bennett, et al., 1983; Buckwald et al., 1984; Kitchen et al., 1983). A recent report detailed the intact survival and favorable outcome at 2 years of an infant weighing 444 g at birth (Pleasure et al., 1984). The major studies reported up to 1984 indicated that between 6 and 35 percent of the survivors were profoundly handicapped, yet in a large number of these very small infants, a high level of cognitive functioning was observed (Bennett et al., 1983; Buckwald et al., 1984; Kitchen et al., 1983). To date, the follow-up studies have been relatively short term.

B. *Early medical complications* have been used as the basis for constituting special subgroups to study the impact of hazardous medical events on neurodevelopmental outcome. The relationship of complications to neonatal mortality and morbidity may be different than the association of these factors with later neurodevelopmental outcome. Once a crisis is past, the long-term effects may not be deleterious.

1. *Hyaline membrane disease* (used synonymously with respiratory distress syndrome) is the major cause of neonatal mortality and morbidity, yet its long-term effect on neurodevelopment in survivors may be minimal (Bennett et al., 1982). Often no data are presented regarding other complications, such as time on ventilator, incidence of hemorrhages, or bronchopulmonary dysplasia, and the outcome may be changed for subsets within this disease category (Mayes and Stahlman, 1982).

2. *Intraventricular hemorrhage* (IVH) is a major complication of preterm infants weighing less than 1,500 g and is estimated to occur in more than 40 percent of these infants. New technologies, such as computerized tomography (CT) scans and ultrasonography, enable the infant to be classified as to the degree of severity of the hemorrhage. Prior to the new technology, only clinical criteria could be used to diagnose IVH. Some studies have reported a high risk of neurodevelopmental defects associated with IVH, particularly grades III and IV, whereas other studies have found few differences (Gaiter, 1982). In one study, the total cohort of infants was evaluated with CT scanning and echoencephalography, and their neurodevelopment was assessed at 6, 12, and 18 months (Scott et al., 1984). Results showed that even low-grade hemorrhages may be associated with a poor developmental outcome. Long-term consequences need to be determined, since most studies to date have been limited to infants. One study reported development at 3½ years for 29 IVH infants who were predominantly infants transported to the NICU and required mechanical ventilation. Of the group, 41 percent had severe educational problems by age 3 (Williamson et al., 1983). This study illustrates that it may be difficult to separate IVH from other complications.

A recent study evaluated the differential outcomes associated with IVH, respiratory distress syndrome, bronchopulmonary dysplasia (BPD), and hydrocephalus secondary to IVH (Landry et al., 1984). Infants were tested at 6, 12, and 24 months of age. The results indicated that IVH was associated with less-favorable intellectual outcomes only when it was accompanied by BPD or progressive hydrocephalus.

3. *Periventricular low density* (PVLD) is also being diagnosed by CT scanning in preterm infants (McCarton-Daum et al., 1983). A group of infants with diffuse PVLD showed deviant developmental scores at 18 months of age. Although the focal and diffuse low densities may have been transient, abnormal neurobehavioral development continued in a high proportion of the group. To date few studies have investigated this problem.

C. *Social factors* are strongly associated with neurodevelopmental outcome even in very small and very sick infants. The confounding of social factors with both preterm birth and neurodevelopmental outcome has made it difficult to establish if poor outcome is a result of the preterm birth and its complications or the unfavorable social circumstances. The group that is disadvantaged both socially and biologically is at "double hazard" and is the lowest-performing group in all studies (Escalona, 1982). There is little evidence that prematurity itself accounts for deleterious neurodevelopmental outcomes. In those children without major brain damage, social factors have been shown to be the most powerful determinants of developmental outcome (Sameroff, 1981). A sharper view of the role of social factors may be seen in studies that measured specific environmental variables (e.g., caregiving, parental attitudes) rather than using broader categories of social class or maternal education. Data on caregiver-child interaction indicated the positive relationship between responsive caregiving in infancy and competence in preterm children, even at age 5 (Cohen and Parmelee, 1983). Responsive caregiving and supportive environments may prevent early deficits for many infants.

V. Prediction of neurodevelopmental outcome
The search continues for single factors, clusters of factors, and risk indices to predict outcome as early in the infant's life as possible.

A. Developmental testing in the first year
The Gesell Developmental Schedules and the Bayley Scales of Infant Development are the most commonly used assessment tools. Preterm infants, as a group, have been shown to have a poorer neurodevelopmental outcome than their full-term counterparts, particularly on motor development.

Studies that have reported correlation coefficients between early measures and functioning at age 5 found modest associations that were significantly lowered if children with very deviant scores (e.g., those with cerebral palsy) were removed from the analysis (Cohen and Parmelee, 1983). Generally, the correlations were too low to predict deviance in individuals. Hunt and colleagues (1982) reported that a high percentage of preterm children showed learning disabilities as measured by clinical ratings given at the time of intellectual assessment. Prediction from early measures was not good. Mild problems in infancy, including mild neurologic dysfunction, were often transient and not significantly associated with later neurodevelopment. Even normal development in infancy did not ensure normal development in childhood. Much shifting is found in most studies; however, repeated testing yielding consistently low development in the early years increases the clinician's ability to predict. Unfortunately, data are rarely reported in this fashion.

B. *Neurological abnormalities* in the first year of life are noted in many longitudinal studies. Although data are reported relating neurologic dysfunction in early infancy to major neurologic handicap in childhood (Knobloch et al., 1982), fewer studies indicate a relationship between early neurologic signs and later "minor" signs in the preterm infant (Drillien et al., 1980). Further, most of the data are presented as group means, whereas the classification for individual children from one period to another is rarely given. Some say that early neurologic deviance is a good predictor of continued deviance (Knobloch et al., 1982). It has been shown that there is a relationship between minor neurologic dysfunction in the first year and later dysfunction in the school years (Drillien et al., 1980). Abnormal neurologic signs noted in the first year, such as variable increase in extensor tone, asymmetries, and marked irritability, were related to poor development later. School-age children who were neurologically abnormal in the first year of life differed from their comparison groups in intelligence, school achievement, and impairment scores. In another study, transient neurologic abnormalities noted in the first year were resolved by age 2 in 40 percent of very low birth weight infants (Hack et al., 1983). The authors concluded that in the vast majority of infants, normalization occurs, although it may take up to 2 or 3 years. No child slipped from normal to abnormal neurologic status; therefore, the absence of neurologic abnormalities was predictive. Some believe that it is hard to diagnose minimal cerebral dysfunction before age 4, as it is apt to be missed. The functional importance of later neurologic signs is not clear at this time.

C. *Perinatal data* did not predict which children developed cerebral palsy by age 2 or which had developmental delay in a study of 252 survivors in two hospitals (Kitchen et al., 1983). Significant correlations were found in both hospitals between perinatal variables and later handicaps, but not one of the correlations was common to both hospitals. Children who as neonates had been transported to the NICU had a higher functional handicap rate (72%), and factors such as delay in mechanical ventilation and inadequate maintenance of the infant's temperature were associated with poor outcome.

D. Risk indices based on more than one measure
Perinatal variables and 3-month neurobehavioral items were used to classify preterm infants into normal, suspect, and normal on 12-month outcome; there was a high rate of correct classification in one study, but prediction was not tried past 1 year (Knobloch et al., 1982). The authors concluded that 1-year functioning cannot be predicted earlier than 3 months because of neurologic immaturity prior to this age.
A risk index based on a combination of reproductive, perinatal, and demographic variables in a multiple regression analysis was used to pre-

dict developmental delay at age 5 (Siegel, 1982). Demographic factors, such as maternal education, were the best single predictor in this study and contributed the most to the risk index. Correct prediction for the preterm group was better for motor performance than for overall cognitive functioning. The addition of the 12-month Bayley score improved prediction to a high level in a small sample. The work needs to be replicated with a new sample before being accepted as a clinical tool. Other research groups have not been as successful in devising a first-year risk index. For example, prediction of delay at 5 years was tested from a combination of first-year measures (neurobehavioral and developmental) that were most associated with IQ scores. Many misclassifications were found, and overall prediction was 73 percent correct (Cohen and Parmelee, 1983).

E. New directions in assessment
   The following new directions may improve prediction in the future.
   1. Research dealing with infant information processing. Assessments of visual and auditory recognition offer modest but significant associations with later development (Cohen, 1986), and current research efforts may develop more discriminating tasks.
   2. Medical technologic advances, such as growth information obtained from ultrasonography.
   3. Neurophysiologic data and power spectral analysis of electroencephalographic records.
   4. Behavioral measures of the infant, such as play, coping, and affect regulation.
   These and other research areas may be useful in predicting the child's later development and providing information regarding the child's functional status.

REFERENCES

Bennett, F. C., Robinson, N. M., and Sells, C. J. Hyaline membrane disease, birth weight, and gestational age. *Am. J. Dis. Child.* 136 : 888, 1982.

Bennett, F. C., Robinson, N. M., and Sells, C. J. Growth and development of infants weighing less than 900 grams at birth. *Pediatrics* 71 : 319, 1983.

Buckwald, S., Zorn, W. A., and Eagan, E. A. Mortality and follow-up data for neonates weighing 500 to 800 grams at birth. *Am. J. Dis. Child.* 138 : 779, 1984.

Cohen, S. E. The Low-birthweight Infant and Learning Disabilities. In M. Lewis (ed.), *Prenatal and Perinatal Factors Relevant to Learning Disabilities.* Champaign, Ill.: University of Illinois Press, 1986.

Cohen, S. E., and Parmelee, A. Prediction of five year Stanford-Binet scores in preterm infants. *Child Dev.* 54 : 1242, 1983.

Davies, P. A. Follow-up of low birthweight children. *Arch. Dis. Child.* 59 : 794, 1984.

Drillien, C. M., Thomson, A. J. M., and Burgoyne, K. Low-birthweight children at early school-age: A longitudinal study. *Dev. Med. Child. Neurol.* 22 : 26, 1980.

Escalona, S. K. Babies at double hazard: Early development of infants at biologic and social risk. *Pediatrics* 70 : 670, 1982.

Gaiter, J. L. The effects of intraventricular hemorrhage on Bayley developmental performance in preterm infants. *Semin. Perinatol.* 6 : 305, 1982.

Hack, M., Caron, B., Rivers, A., and Fanaroff, A. A. The very low birth weight infant: The broader spectrum of morbidity during infancy and early childhood. *J. Dev. Behav. Pediatr.* 4 : 243, 1983.

Hunt, J. V., Tooley, W. H., and Harvin, D. Learning disabilities in children with birth weights <1500 grams. *Semin. Perinatol.* 6 : 280, 1982.

Kitchen, W. H., Yu, V. Y. H., Orgill, A. A., et al. Collaborative study of very-low-birth-weight infants. *Am. J. Dis. Child.* 137 : 555, 1983.

Knobloch, H., Malone, A., Ellison, P. H., et al. Considerations in evaluating changes in outcome for infants weighing less than 1,501 grams. *Pediatrics* 69 : 285, 1982.

Kopp, C. B., and Parmelee, A. H. Prenatal and Perinatal Influences on Infant Behavior. In J. Osofsky (ed.), *Handbook for Infant Development.* New York: Wiley, 1979.

Landry, S. H., Fletcher, J. M., Azarling, C. L., et al. Differential outcomes associated with early medical complications in premature infants. *J. Pediatr. Psychol.* 9 : 385, 1984.

Mayes, L. C., and Stahlman, M. T. Effect of hyaline membrane disease outcome of premature infants. *Am. J. Dis. Child.* 136 : 885, 1982.

McCarton-Daum, C., Danziger, A., Ruff, H., and Vaughan, H. G. Periventricular low density as a predictor of neurobehavioral outcome in very low-birthweight infants. *Dev. Med. Child Neurol.* 25 : 559, 1983.

Pleasure, J. R., Dhand, M., and Kaur, M. What is the low limit of viability? Intact survival of a 444 g infant. *Am. J. Dis. Child.* 138 : 783, 1984.

Ross, G., Schechner, S., Frayer, W. W., and Auld, P. A. M. Perinatal and neurobehavioral predictors of one-year outcome in infants <1500 grams. *Semin. Perinatol.* 6 : 317, 1982.

Sameroff, A. J. Longitudinal Studies of Preterm Infants: A Review of Chapters 17–20. In S. L. Friedman and M. Sigman (eds.), *Preterm Birth and Psychological Development.* New York: Academic, 1981.

Scott, D. T., Ment, L. R., Ehrenkranz, R. A., and Warshaw, J. B. Evidence for late developmental deficits in very low birth weight infants surviving intraventricular hemorrhage. *Childs Brain* 11 : 261, 1984.

Siegel, L. S. Reproductive, perinatal, and environmental variables as predictors of development of preterm (<1500 grams) and full-term children at five years. *Semin. Perinatol.* 6 : 274, 1982.

Stewart, A. L., Reynolds, E. O. R., and Lipscomb, A. P. Outcome for infants of very low birth weight. Survey of world literature. *Lancet* 2 : 1038, 1981.

Williamson, W. D., Desmond, M. M., Wilson, G. S., et al. Survival of low-birth-weight infants with neonatal intraventricular hemorrhage. *Am. J. Dis. Child.* 137 : 1181, 1983.

II

Organizing Follow-up Programs

4

Discharge Planning

Ann L. Colangelo, Toni B. Vento, and H. William Taeusch

I. Introduction

Discharge from the neonatal intensive care unit (NICU) does not mean that recovery is complete. A successful discharge (from NICU to intermediate care or from intermediate care to home) is effected by ensuring that the transition is smooth, with no abrupt decrease in the care of the infant and family. An unsuccessful discharge (usually from the NICU to intermediate care) occurs when an infant is transferred after little preparation—usually when his or her bed is needed for an acutely ill infant. All patients and parents need time, preparation, and medical and emotional support for transitions from one unit to another and from the hospital to home.

Preparing an infant for transfer or discharge can sometimes seem a difficult task for the primary caretakers and an overwhelming one for the family. The family must get to know and adjust to a new system of care with new providers. The parents must assume care for an infant who required the full-fledged support of a complicated NICU only days to weeks earlier. The primary physicians and nurses must conclude the process of NICU care by providing a smooth transition to subsequent caretakers. Discharge planning is the method whereby the needs of the patient and family are identified and a plan of care designed and communicated to subsequent groups and persons caring for the infant and parents. This process allows care to continue without interruption of needed services.

The admission of an infant to an intensive care unit means that that infant and family are at risk. With the belief that one risk situation can trigger others, the importance of careful discharge planning is evident. The continuity of care ensured by discharge planning minimizes fragmentation, repetition, delay, and absence of essential services. It allows NICU personnel to discharge the high-risk infant to a prepared family that is able to provide a nurturing environment. The complexity of the process is indicated in the case histories (see pp. 40–45) and is illustrated by the fact that there are as many as four or five principal caretakers in the NICU involved with the transfer or discharge of a single infant.

II. Process

Discharge planning provides the framework for a successful transfer or discharge. We use a primary team (nurses and NICU physicians) for patient care delivery, and discharge planning is the responsibility of this team. The primary nurse, given his or her accessibility and relationship with the family, is the ideal person to coordinate discharge planning. Discharge planning can be divided into four steps.

A. Assessment

Accurate assessments are the basis for optimal care. The consistency provided by a primary team enables these assessments to be comprehensive and highly individualized. Beginning with admission, the team identifies problems or needs that require special planning, intervention, teaching, or follow-up. This list of needs changes and evolves as the patient and family progress through hospitalization. Prior to discharge, needs of the infant, family, and environment are once again assessed (Table 4-1).

B. Consultation

Using input from peers and other resources refines assessments and supports the efforts of the primary team. Multidisciplinary care conferences are useful forums for the primary team to discuss particular problems, draw out new information and insights, and formulate plans. Consultation sources are

1. Continuing care department: a resource for staff regarding community agencies, services, and programs. This department is invaluable in matching needs to applicable resources. It has a direct role in planning placement in rehabilitation facilities and foster homes.
2. Multidisciplinary consults: any combination of nursing, medical, or social services or other consults for patients with diverse needs. A premature infant with bronchopulmonary dysplasia, an asphyxiated infant with seizures, and an infant of an unmarried, unemployed, 17-year-old mother are examples of infants needing multidisciplinary consults.
3. Community agencies: Agencies that can provide programs or services most specific to the patient's and family's needs. Examples of programs and services are previous health care providers, visiting nurses associations (VNA), social service departments of community hospitals, state welfare agencies, and early intervention programs (EIP).

Table 4-1. Assessment of needs prior to discharge

Infant (Factors and Conditions Requiring Special Follow-up)
Medical issues
  Medications
  Monitors
  Special formulas and diet
  Specialized needs
    Shunts
    Gastrostomy
    Stomas
    Home oxygen therapy
Tests
  PKU and metabolic screen
  Auditory screen
  Ophthalmologic examination
  Radiographs
  Ultrasonography and computed tomographic scans
  Hematocrit and reticulocyte counts
  Theophylline levels

Table 4-1 (continued)

Anticonvulsant levels
Nursing issues: Conditions that require continuing evaluation of serial physical
    examinations
  Physical problems that produce behavioral changes
    Chronic lung disease
    Congenital anomalies
    Premature infant with weak or undeveloped behavior patterns
    Birth asphyxia
  Infant temperament
    Crying
    Poor feeding habits
    Unresponsive
Parents
Demographics
  Age, marital status
  Educational level
  Occupation
Financial implications of care
  Insurance
  Medical assistance
  Plans to return to work
  Maternity
Familial
  Definition of family circle
    Siblings
    Significant others
  Who will be the primary caretakers?
  Who forms the identified support system for this family?
    Extended family
    Neighbors
    Friends
    Clubs
    Community organizations
    Church or synagogue
Transportation: Is it available, reliable, accessible, and adequate?
Social service support
  Are services needed?
  Previous social service involvement with this family
Cultural: What does the culture mean to the individual? How does he or she view the
    health care system?
  Language spoken
  Ethnic issues
    Folk medicines, faith healing, fads, and cults
    Value systems and mores: Are males more "valuable" than females? What is the im-
      portance of a "perfect" child?
    Child-rearing techniques: Who makes the decisions in the family?
Antenatal history: Significant obstetric history (miscarriages, infertility, pregnancy planned)
  Extent of prenatal care
  Participation in prenatal course
Experience
  New parents
  Parents of twins

Table 4-1 (continued)

Previous experience with child requiring lengthy hospitalization or special needs
NICU visiting patterns
  Frequency and length
  Involvement in care
  Attitude (e.g., eager and willing)
  Attentiveness to infant's needs
  Is there positive discussion and attachment to their child's characteristics and personality?
  Do they stroke and hold infant correctly?
Education and teaching: Parental understanding of infant's problems and needs
  What does parent need to know for successful care and nurturing?
  CPR
  Physical assessment skills
  Signs and symptoms of distress
  Whom to call and when
  Behavioral assessment, interaction, and consoling methods
  Use of equipment
  Well-baby care
  Infection control
  Competence of caretaking skills
  Plans for child care
Emotional support
  Family's predominant concerns
  Other stresses on family
  How has present hospitalization affected family dynamics?
  Family's ability and willingness to seek information and resources
  What are the family's coping patterns?
Environment
Heat, water supply, electricity, telephone
How accessible is the home to health facilities?
Have the parents acquired the basic supplies?
  Crib
  Car seat
  Clothes
  Bottles, formula
Modifications for special needs

CPR = cardiopulmonary resuscitation; NICU = neonatal intensive care unit; PKU = phenylketonuria.

C. Implementation

A comprehensive discharge plan should be formulated by the primary team, regardless of whether the infant is transferred to a community hospital or discharged home. For the infant transferring to a community hospital, the discharge plan includes a preliminary assessment of needs and plans that are then added to, implemented, or deleted as the situation warrants. Teaching and referrals initiated at the tertiary center are refined and completed in the community. A mutually trusting and collegial relationship between the two nurseries facilitates this process.

Generally, infants with complex, chronic, long-term problems (e.g., bronchopulmonary dysplasia, multiple congenital anomalies, multisystem failure) are discharged from the tertiary center to home. In this instance, a plan for discharge is formulated, teaching and referrals are done, and the family gradually assumes total care for its infant.

Time and priority must be given to the primary team to allow proper implementation of the following discharge plans:

1. Discharge summary: Discharge summary should include pertinent history, hospital course, and present plan of care.
2. Referrals to community agencies and follow-up services: Referrals may be simple, such as notifying an agency that the infant is in the community, or more complex, such as actually requesting agency involvement prior to NICU discharge.
3. Parent education: Teaching plans are devised and implemented so that parents are competent and confident in caring for their infant.
4. Coordination of support services: The necessary supplies, supports, and services need to be in place with a minimum of providers.
5. Documentation and communication: Plans and their implementation are fully documented in the permanent record. Subsequent health care providers are notified as to the timing of discharge and when their services are to begin.

D. Evaluation of the discharge planning process

Evaluation is a crucial component to the process of discharge planning (Table 4-2). Before and after discharge, the primary team is responsible for ascertaining whether the needed services can be provided by community agencies and whether the services are perceived as supportive to the family.

1. Prior to discharge: Evaluation of the process can be accomplished during multidisciplinary care conferences. At this point, the primary team can investigate whether the available services of a chosen agency will meet the needs of the infant and family (e.g., can the visiting nurse detect signs of congestive heart failure in an infant with bronchopulmonary dysplasia?). If the community agency cannot meet the patient's needs, the team must investigate other agencies to ensure a smooth transition to home care.

    Evaluation of parent teaching is ongoing and accomplished by the primary and associate nurses prior to discharge. Competency of the parents can be determined through repeated demonstrations of care and question and answer sessions. Overnight stays are beneficial to parents' sense of confidence and are best accomplished when the parent and infant can "live" in a family room or isolation room near the NICU. The parent can then assume total responsibility for infant care with the nursing and medical support close by. Passes out of the unit (to the cafeteria, gift shop, or garden) also increase parental independence.

2. After discharge: The primary team continues to evaluate discharge planning through communication with the community agencies, the family, the infant follow-up clinic, and the private pediatrician. All information collected affects future discharge planning for other patients and families. The primary NICU team can serve as troubleshooters for the family after discharge. The team's role at this time is to reinforce teaching, provide emotional support, and direct the family to the prop-

Table 4-2. Intensive follow-up regimen after neonatal intensive care unit discharge

Prior to Discharge: Discharge Planning
Final physical examination and discharge summary
  Head ultrasonography
  Hematocrit, reticulocyte count
  Discharge medications
  Home oxygen, monitors
  CPR training
  24–48 hr continuous care by parents
  Immunizations
ROP check
Hearing check
EIP referral
IFUP referral
VNA referral
Tertiary medical referrals
Referral to other community services (e.g., social service, WIC)
Meetings with primary pediatrician
After Discharge
First week
  NICU nurse phone calls
  VNA
Second week
  Primary pediatrician visit
  IFUP phone call
  NICU phone call
Third week
  EIP visit
  IFUP visit
  NICU calls
  VNA visit
Fourth week
  Primary pediatrician visit
  EIP visit
  Other community services
  Tertiary medical visits

CPR = cardiopulmonary resuscitation; EIP = early intervention program; IFUP = infant follow-up program; NICU = neonatal intensive care unit; ROP = retinopathy of prematurity; VNA = visiting nurse association; WIC = Special Supplemental Nutrition Program for Women, Infants, and Children.

er resources. The goal is to wean the parents from the NICU while increasing support provided by the private pediatrician, community agencies, and infant follow-up clinic (Fig. 4-1).

III. Criteria for discharge from the neonatal intensive care unit
Resolution of acute illnesses and physiologic stability of chronic illnesses are imperative prior to discharge to an intermediate care unit, home, or specialized foster care. Medical criteria for discharge include adequate weight gain and adequate fluid and caloric intake by mouth or nasogastric or gastrostomy tube feedings. The infant must maintain thermal stability outside the warmer or incubator. The infant must maintain respiratory stability (e.g., a stable FIO_2

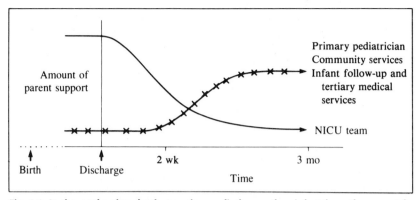

Fig. 4-1. In the weeks after death, transfer, or discharge of an infant from the neonatal intensive care unit *(NICU)*, the NICU staff maintains contact with the family and offers support. During this period, the goals of the NICU staff are to prevent the parents from feeling abandoned and to ascertain that links with community resources are made.

requirement to maintain appropriate PaO_2 levels, both at rest and with activity). Apnea must be controlled or resolved.

Medication levels must be at therapeutic range, side effects documented, and schedules for dosage increases determined. Frequent discharge medications include theophylline, anticonvulsants, digoxin, diuretics, and electrolyte and vitamin supplements.

We ascertain that all consultants' plans, reports, and tests have been completed. We check the need for home monitoring. Finally, we ensure that special needs such as ventriculoperitoneal shunt, tracheostomy, colostomy, gastrostomy, nasal cannula, and hernia repair have been met. Screening tests for many high-risk infants include phenylketonuria (PKU)-metabolic screen, auditory screen, ophthalmologic examination, radiographs, and ultrasonographic examinations.

Communication is paramount but currently is one of the weakest links in the discharge process. A dictated discharge summary with results of recent physical examination, measurements, laboratory values, medication blood levels, and immunizations must be sent to the private pediatrician, community agencies, referral clinics, and infant follow-up clinic (see Fig. 7-2 for a sample discharge form). The private pediatrician or pediatric clinic should be contacted verbally. Follow-up appointments are scheduled for specialty clinics and the infant follow-up program. Finally, prescriptions must be written and filled. A visit with the parents and the NICU staff by outpatient caretakers prior to the infant's discharge from NICU is extremely useful.

IV. Coordination of home services

Coordination of home services is essential to minimize the number of caretakers and agencies without compromising the infant's needs. The following questions must be addressed: What is the extent of skilled medical and nursing care needed by the infant? Does care need to be given throughout the entire day or only during the waking hours? What are the needs of the parents?

A. Supportive services

Often, one agency may be able to provide nursing care, physical therapy, developmental stimulation, and social support. The agencies that we have found most useful include

1. VNAs: nonprofit home health agencies that provide assistance with bedside care, rehabilitation services, and patient education. Fees are usually covered by insurance or Medicaid.
2. Public health nurses: tax-supported health department for patient services at no fee to client.
3. EIPs: community-based service for infants and toddlers who are at risk for developmental delay. The goal is to help the patient achieve optimal developmental level. Fees are no cost, sliding scale, or third-party reimbursement.
4. Respite care: short-term temporary care of handicapped children so families can meet emergency needs, fulfill vacation plans, obtain reprieve, or provide an alternative to institutionalization. Respite care is often provided through state departments of mental health, social service, or public health.
5. Parent support groups.
6. Regional departments of social services.

B. Financial aid

Parents often need information concerning financial aid available after discharge of their infant. The programs we use frequently are

1. Special Supplemental Nutrition Program for Women, Infants, and Children (WIC): federally funded supplemental food program for pregnant and postpartal women, infants, and children less than 5 years old. Families of low or moderate income who are at nutritional risk are eligible.
2. Supplemental security income (SSI): federally and state funded program providing a guaranteed income to blind, disabled, and elderly persons. Eligibility includes low income and disability that will last at least 1 year.
3. Aid to Families with Dependent Children (AFDC): minimum income for unemployed, single-parent families through state departments of public welfare.
4. Medicaid: provides payment for health services for low-income families or families with overwhelming medical costs. Medicaid is available through state departments of public welfare.

C. Specialized care

When an infant requires specialized care that the parent cannot provide at home, it is necessary to consider referral to another institution. The following placements are examples of specialized alternatives:

1. Rehabilitation hospitals may be beneficial when parents need time to learn skills to meet infant's needs. The goal of rehabilitation is to increase the parents' or family's skill and functional abilities in preparation for discharge.
2. Chronic care hospitals provide long-term care to patients with ongoing medical and nursing needs or an unstable medical status.

3. Pediatric nursing homes provide care for severely handicapped or retarded children between ages of 3 months and 21 years.
4. Specialized foster care provides care for infant in a home setting when
the parent(s) cannot meet the child's medical needs at home. Foster
care homes are supervised through the department of social services.
5. Hospice programs provide supportive and palliative care in a family-
centered environment when death is imminent.

V. Needs of parents
The parents must be emotionally ready for their child's discharge from the
NICU. This need is addressed by conscientious planning by the primary team.
Parental involvement and practice are invaluable; for instance, overnight stays
at the NICU prior to discharge offer the parents an opportunity to assume re-
sponsibility while support is readily available.

A contract between the parents and health care team often increases parents'
success. Mutually agreed upon plans increase parental compliance by defin-
ing realistic expectations for them within a time span that is appropriate for
their learning styles. Education for parents should include the following:

A. Training in cardiopulmonary resuscitation (CPR) should be provided prior
to discharge for parents whose infant is discharged on home oxygen therapy or who has respiratory impairment (i.e., apnea, seizures, neurologic disease, airway obstruction). A staff nurse meets with the parents to review
techniques of resuscitation and provide practice time on an infant manne-
quin. The goal is to prepare the parents to recognize early signs of distress,
to function competently in an emergency, and to call appropriate community resources for help. This approach is comparable to those described by
Lund and Lefrak (1982) and Rehm (1983).

B. Physical assessment skills such as respiratory, cardiac, and neurologic.

C. Signs and symptoms of distress.

D. Instruction, administration, and desired effects and side effects of medication.

E. Special needs such as use of nasal cannula, stoma care, dressing changes,
suctioning, and feeding techniques.

F. Behavioral assessment skills and interaction and consoling methods.

G. Use of equipment such as low-flow FIO_2 meter, portable oxygen tanks, air
concentrators, suction machines, and cardiac and apnea monitors.

H. Well-baby care such as bathing, dressing, taking a temperature, and positioning.

I. Emotional support of parents: Prior to discharge, meetings with family and
team members can be used to prepare parents for discharge by acknowl-

edging their fears and concerns, providing realistic expectations for them, and reinforcing support systems that have been set up. It is often helpful to the family if the team gives sanction to the use of respite care after discharge.

J. Siblings: Sibling rivalry should be recognized and discussed with the family. Identifying strategies and coping mechanisms with the family may decrease anxiety caused by this normal behavior. By providing realistic expectations for the parents and siblings, the primary team facilitates family adaptation.

K. Infection control: Minimizing the infant's exposure to communicable disease at home must be discussed with parents. Parents need to know how common diseases are spread, why their infant is at risk of compromise from such diseases, and how to avoid exposure.

L. Emergencies: In case of an emergency, parents must know whom to call day or night. They need to know circumstances that warrant notifying a physician. Providing the telephone numbers of police, ambulance, and fire department, and the location of the nearest hospital is important.

M. Environmental needs: The basic environmental needs of the infant are addressed with the parents, and if concern exists about their adequacy, a home visit may be necessary to check on heat, food, hot water, electricity, access to telephone, and transportation to medical services. Needed minimal supplies for the infant must be on hand (e.g., crib, car seat, clothes, bottles, formula) as evidence of parental competence.

N. Medical equipment: It is most beneficial if the medical equipment company assumes 24-hour responsibility for any medical equipment in the home by way of a service contract. Repair and maintenance of equipment are therefore ensured.

CASE HISTORY 1
  I. Background
    Baby M was a 2,400 g 35-week-gestation infant born after a first pregnancy to a 17-year-old mother. Prenatal care was minimal. Baby M's NICU hospitalization was marked by prolonged ventilator support secondary to hyaline membrane disease (HMD). After 2 weeks of therapy, Baby M was extubated and weaned to a nasal cannula at 0.5 liter per minute flow, 50% oxygen. His chest radiograph showed chronic changes consistent with bronchopulmonary dysplasia (BPD), and he was treated with diuretics. Weight gain was adequate on 24 cal per oz of formula.
    The NICU staff was concerned that Ms. M might not be able to meet the needs of her infant. She had difficulty keeping appointments, visited infrequently, and had unrealistic expectations about the care her baby required. Ms. M lived with her parents, siblings, and one friend; she was not employed and did not attend school. Her medical expenses were covered by Medicaid.

II. Assessment of needs

Discharge plans were initiated when Baby M was weaned to oxygen administered by a nasal cannula and it was apparent that he would require home oxygen therapy. Communication with the pediatrician revealed that the community hospital was inexperienced in providing care for infants with BPD and subsequently was uncomfortable with discharge planning and teaching for this infant and family. Therefore, the decision was made to discharge Baby M from the NICU to home. The following needs were identified and documented by the primary team:

A. Needs of infant
1. Medical issues: home oxygen therapy, medications, and increased caloric requirements for growth
2. Nursing issues: frequent evaluation for signs and symptoms of congestive heart failure and respiratory distress; teaching and support for mother
3. Screening tests: developmental examination, phenylketonuria (PKU) screening, and ophthalmologic examination prior to discharge
4. Communication: imperative for primary team to have ongoing, extensive collaboration around special needs with private pediatrician as well as infant follow-up clinic for long-term BPD management

B. Needs of parent
1. Education: Ms. M was required to learn the following aspects of infant care prior to discharge and demonstrate competence in each area: well-baby care, physical and behavioral assessment, signs and symptoms of respiratory distress, special needs (i.e., administration of oxygen and medication, use of nasal cannula and portable tanks, preparation of formula, use of home equipment, infection control, and how to handle emergencies (CPR, identify whom to call and when).
2. Psychosocial support: In view of Ms. M's psychosocial status and the complexity of her needs, a multidisciplinary approach was most beneficial. Ms. M was referred to the NICU social worker. Family meetings between the primary team and Ms. M served to establish realistic expectations of Ms. M's behavior as well as Baby M's status and prognosis and to identify available support systems for Ms. M.
3. Environmental assessment: Transportation (from home to the NICU) was assessed and found to be a major problem for Ms. M. At home Ms. M had a crib, clothes, bottles, and car seat. Prior to discharge, a medical equipment company was needed to deliver the oxygen tanks and nasal cannulas. A telephone was readily available.

III. Consults

To facilitate comprehensive discharge planning, the primary team used multidisciplinary staff members as consults.

A. Social service

The NICU social worker was instrumental in obtaining financial assistance for transportation. She also explored financial aid programs for Ms. M and provided social support as needed.

B. Community health nurse-specialist (continuing care department)
The continuing care nurse offered assistance with referrals to a local visiting nurse association and medical equipment company.

IV. Implementation
Teaching Ms. M to care for her infant was difficult because of her infrequent visits. The primary team, Ms. M, and the maternal grandmother contracted for a minimum number of required 8- and 24-hour visits during which teaching would be accomplished. Discharge was dependent on the family's completing the required visits and demonstrating competence in parental behaviors. Content was divided into three phases to accommodate Ms. M's learning style, and teaching was done by the primary and associate nurses.

The first phase consisted of well-baby care, diagnosis of BPD and reasons for distress, signs and symptoms of distress (physical and behavioral), and interventions to alleviate distress. The second phase focused on administration of medications, medication side effects, formula preparation, use and care of nasal cannula, use of equipment (oxygen tanks and blender), and CPR.

Finally, in the third phase, Ms. M assumed partial in-hospital care of her baby using the primary nurse as a support. The primary nurse was available to validate Ms. M's and the grandmother's competence in meeting the infant's special needs.

V. Referrals
Necessary community services were identified by the primary team during the multidisciplinary care conference. Referrals to the following community agencies were deemed crucial to the long-term care of Baby M and Ms. M:

A. Visiting nurse association
Nursing evaluation was needed daily at first and then later weekly. The visiting nurse also made a predischarge home assessment 1 week prior to hospital discharge.

B. Early intervention program
The EIP program involved developmental evaluation and planning. Frequency of visits was determined by the case worker after initial evaluation.

C. Special Supplemental Nutrition Program for Women, Infants, and Children
The WIC program supplemented income for nutritional expenses to cover cost of special formulas and nutritional supplements.

D. Medical equipment company
The medical equipment company delivered oxygen tanks to Ms. M's home 2 days prior to Baby M's discharge, assessed home environment for safety, and taught Ms. M to use the portable tanks. A therapist was scheduled to visit weekly to change and service equipment.

E. Private pediatrician
Extensive communication between the NICU and pediatrician was neces-

sary for smooth transition of services for Baby M's special needs. An appointment was made with a private pediatrician for 1 week after discharge.

F. Infant follow-up program
A physician met with the mother prior to discharge to explain the services of the follow-up clinic and to schedule the first appointment for 1 week after discharge. Services provided included oxygen management, physical assessment, medication regulation, and developmental monitoring.

VI. Follow-up after discharge
The primary nurse contacted Ms. M and the visiting nurse weekly, then biweekly, for Baby M's first few months at home. The attending neonatologist contacted the private pediatrician on a similar schedule. The infant follow-up clinic provided the NICU staff with summary letters of all appointments. The discharge process was evaluated via communication with the referral agencies and mother 2 weeks after discharge and then monthly during this time.

VII. Outcome
At 2 years, Baby M is active, relatively nonverbal, and actively "negative" according to his mother. He has had no hospitalizations and has been off home oxygen for 14 months. He is not involved with an EIP (his mother's preference). (The mother has a 7-month-old born at 36 weeks' gestation with moderate RDS with no BPD.)

CASE HISTORY 2

I. Background
Baby G was born weighing 740 g after 26 to 27 weeks' gestation. She required mechanical ventilation for a moderate course of hyaline membrane disease, further complicated by pulmonary interstitial emphysema and a patent ductus arteriosus. A grade IV intraventricular hemorrhage produced marked hydrocephalus, ultimately requiring a ventriculoperitoneal (VP) shunt for management. Her parents were married, in their thirties, responsible, and extremely committed to their child.

II. Assessment of needs
With the placement of a VP shunt, Baby G's acute problems were resolved, and the focus of her care was shifted to discharge. Because of her size (1,200 g) and the need for further revision of her shunt, it was decided that Baby G would be discharged to an intermediate care nursery. The following list of needs was compiled by the primary team:

A. Needs of infant
1. Growth: Baby G required supplemental calories in the form of fortified breast milk to accommodate her increased metabolic needs for growth. Once her weight gain was substantial, she would begin weaning to breast feedings. Thermal regulation required the use of an incubator to minimize the number of calories needed for heat production.
2. Neurologic: Because of her small size, Baby G could be fitted with on-

ly a valveless VP shunt. (Recently, smaller shunt valves for tiny infants have become available.) She had to remain flat until her ventricular system adjusted to the shunt, and then her head could be elevated 10 to 15 degrees. Close observation was necessary to detect complications of injection or shunt malfunction.
3. Screening: The following tests and examinations were carried out for Baby G: eye examination, auditory-evoked potentials, periodic head ultrasonography, PKU and metabolic screen, and developmental and neurologic examinations.

B. Needs of parents
Baby G was a much-desired and planned-for baby. Her parents dealt with the emotional difficulties of her premature birth and hospitalization by reading about her specific problems, involving themselves in her physical care, and actively requesting information and meetings with her caretakers. Family meetings between the parents and the primary team were held approximately every 10 days. The parents were able to discuss their concerns, and the primary team was able to assess Mr. and Ms. G's understanding of their infant's problems and their ability to adapt. From these meetings, a list of teaching needs was devised, which included needs and development of premature infants, hydrocephalus, and VP shunts.

III. Consults

A. Multidisciplinary meeting
A meeting of parents, primary team workers, and neurosurgical professionals was scheduled prior to discharge. The parents were given information about future care, prognosis, and follow-up in familiar surroundings.

B. Community health nurse-specialist
A consultation was made by the community health nurse-specialist who identified appropriate VNA and EIP referrals.

C. Pediatricians
As transfer became imminent, Mr. and Mrs. G. interviewed several pediatricians for Baby G's final discharge.

IV. Implementation
Consistent, informal explanations of care and development of premature infants had been given to the parents throughout hospitalization. Near the time of discharge, these explanations were repeated and given special emphasis. Special sessions were arranged for the primary nurse to teach Mr. and Mrs. G about hydrocephalus and shunt care.

A coordinating call was made to the community hospital about a week prior to transfer. Baby G's history, course, and current problems were reported to the staff, and a primary nurse was identified. To ease transition, the parents were encouraged to visit the community hospital and meet the new staff. Referrals to the VNA and EIP were discussed by the primary nurses at both hospitals, and it was decided that the community hospital would make the VNA referral.

Because the parents had been investigating EIPs, we facilitated their independence by identifying other resources in their community and encouraging them to make their own choice. The primary physician at the NICU coordinated medical follow-up with the private pediatrician and the neurology clinic. Discharge summaries were written and follow-up was planned by both physicians and nurses. These accompanied Baby G and her chart on transfer. Telephone calls to the community hospital after transfer revealed that Baby G and her parents had settled in and care was progressing as planned.

V. Outcome

At age 2, Baby G is active, verbal, and walks and runs with ease. She is small and has mild generalized hypotonia and moderate myopia requiring glasses. Her parents are doing well. Her mother is now a leader in activities supporting parents of NICU graduates.

REFERENCES

Ahman, E. (ed.). *Home Care for the High Risk Infant: A Holistic Guide to Using Technology.* Rockville, Md.: Aspen, 1986.

Cagan, J., and Meier, P. A discharge planning tool for use with families of high-risk infants. *J.O.G.N. Nurs.* 8 : 146, 1979.

Glassanos, M. R. Infants who are oxygen dependent: Sending them home. *Matern. Child Nurs. J.* 5 : 42, 1980.

Hartsell, M. B., and Ward, J. H. Selecting equipment vendors for children on home care. *Matern. Child Nurs. J.* 10 : 26, 1985.

Hurt, H. Continuing care of the high-risk infant. *Clin. Perinatol.* 11 : 3, 1984.

Julian, K. C., and Young, C. M. Comprehensive health care for the high-risk infant and family: Follow-up of the high-risk family. *Neonatal Network* 2 : 32, 1983.

Koops, B. L., Abman, S. H., and Accurso, F. J. Outpatient management and follow-up of bronchopulmonary dysplasia. *Clin. Perinatol.* 11 : 101, 1984.

Lund, C., and Lefrak, L. Discharge planning for infants in the intensive care nursery. *Perinatol. Neonatol.* 6 : 49, 1982.

Rehm, R. S. Teaching cardiopulmonary resuscitation to parents. *Matern. Child Nurs. J.* 8 : 411, 1983.

Strong, C. The tiniest newborns. *Hastings Cent. Rep.* 1983. Pp. 4–19.

5

Community Resources

Jane A. Kisielius and Janice L. Apol

I. Introduction

The key elements in successful discharge planning are that health professionals recognize the ongoing nursing, medical, social, and emotional needs of infants and their families and design a plan that continues quality care after discharge. Discharge planning poses many challenges to the primary health team. In neonatology we are faced with infants who require ongoing, sophisticated, highly technologic care for extended periods. The long-term needs of these infants cover a broad range. There are those infants who may require minimal or routine follow-up care as well as those who need an intense array of community health resources based on nursing, medical, social, and environmental factors.

We see the following components as essential in effective discharge planning and utilization of community resources:

A. *Assess* the medical, social, cultural, and environmental needs of the infant and his or her family. Assessment is key to any workable discharge plan and appropriate community referral.

B. *Begin discharge planning early.* Discharge planning begins when the infant is admitted to the hospital and is an ongoing process. It is important to remember that appropriate resource selection and coordination take considerable effort and time.

C. *Use a multidisciplinary approach.* Each member of the health care team can offer valuable input and recommendations based on his or her area of expertise.

D. *Consult with the hospital's continuing care program or designated discharge planning unit.* The continuing care program is designed to assist primary team members with discharge planning efforts. This program's staff will have current information on available community resources and the mechanisms of access.

E. *Routinely offer resources to families.* Make the family aware of available resources and use their input in discharge planning. Family members are most often the best judges of what will and will not work for them. Resources should be described in a nonjudgmental manner.

F. *Design discharge plans that most efficiently meet patient and family needs while avoiding duplication.*

G. *Be aware of timing.* It may be necessary for a resource to be in place at discharge (e.g., private-duty nursing), or it may not be needed for several weeks after discharge (e.g., early intervention program [EIP]).

H. *Be flexible.* Plans often change or require revision several times before discharge.

I. *Make sure the discharge plan is well documented and communicated.*

What resources are available for the high-risk infant and family? How does a primary caretaker select the most appropriate services from a large and changing group of community health resources? In this chapter we summarize the community services available in Massachusetts used most frequently after discharge of a high-risk infant (Table 5-1).

Although resources vary somewhat from state to state, the categories of services described in this chapter can be found nationwide.

II. Home-based skilled services

A. Visiting nurse association and certified home health agencies
Visiting nurse associations (VNA) and other certified home health agencies provide skilled care in a patient's home on an intermittent basis. Both private nonprofit and proprietary agencies provide this level of care. Services vary depending on the patient's and family's needs and include nursing visits, physical therapy, home health aid assistance, occupational therapy, and social work. Visits can be made daily (sometimes twice a day), usually lasting 1 hour.

1. Referral process
Referral to a VNA or certified home health agency can be initiated by phone at least 48 hours prior to discharge. Phone referral is followed by a written patient care referral form. (Directories are available in most states that list home health agencies.)

It may be beneficial to invite the community health nurse from the specified agency to the hospital to meet the patient and family prior to discharge to learn about the specific infant's needs directly. In complex situations this predischarge meeting greatly assists the smooth transition from hospital to home.

2. Families who may benefit
Families with infants who require continuing skilled assessment and intervention after hospital discharge will benefit from intermittent home health services (e.g., infants with continuing nursing and medical problems resulting from conditions such as bronchopulmonary dysplasia, tracheoesophageal fistula, necrotizing enterocolitis, congenital cardiac defects, multiple congenital anomalies, neurologic problems, or prematurity).

Services may also be useful for parents who would benefit from being

Table 5-1. Community resources in Massachusetts for the high-risk infant

Home-based skilled services
  Visiting nurse association/certified home health agencies
  Coordinated home health care
  Private duty nursing
  Public health agencies
  Early intervention programs
  Hospice programs
  Respite care
  Home health equipment companies
Alternatives to home care
  Rehabilitation hospitals
  Specialized foster care
  Chronic care hospitals
  Pediatric nursing homes
Financial, medical, and support services
  Insurance/Medicaid
  Supplemental security income
  Massachusetts Commission for the Blind
  Department of public health
  WIC program
  Department of social services
  Department of public welfare
  Department of mental health
  Office for Children
  Parent support services
Hospital-based infant follow-up programs

WIC = Special Supplemental Nutrition Program for Women, Infants, and Children.

taught about issues related to home management of their infant such as anxious parents with limited support systems; single, first-time, or adolescent parents; those with limited cognitive ability; those with complex social history; or those whose infant had an extended hospital stay.
3. Cost and reimbursement
   Care is provided on a fee-for-service basis that is usually covered by medical insurance or Medicaid.

B. Coordinated home health care
   Coordinated home health care (CHHC) is a program that is available through Blue Cross agencies throughout the country and in Massachusetts through specified VNAs located throughout the state. The goal of the program is to enable an infant to receive hospital services in the home. It may allow an infant to go home sooner as well as prevent repeated hospital admissions. It benefits an infant who needs frequent or extensive home health services. Services include

   Intermittent nursing care
   Physical therapy
   Respiratory therapy
   Speech therapy

Occupational therapy
Nutritional guidance
Medical social worker services
Home health aid services
Diagnostic services including laboratory tests and x-ray examinations
Prescription drugs
Medical and surgical supplies including intravenous solutions, dress-
ings, and oxygen
Transportation (professional ambulance or chair car)

1. Referral process
   A referral is made by telephone to the VNA with a CHHC contract and
   followed by a written patient care referral form. The patient must be visited at home within 72 hours of discharge from the hospital.
2. Families who may benefit
   Coordinated home health care services may benefit families with infants who require *close monitoring or assessment* of a nursing or medical problem.
   Examples include infants requiring frequent monitoring and adjusting
   of medications, nutritional management, and other problems resulting
   from multiple system involvement.
3. Cost and reimbursement
   If an infant qualifies medically and is covered under a specific Blue
   Cross policy (i.e., Prolonged Illness or Master Medical), home services
   are reimbursed 100 percent; under Major Medical Plan, reimbursement is 80 percent.

C. Private-duty nursing
   Private-duty nursing (PDN) at home provides nurses through home health
   agencies to families caring for infants who require frequent skilled intervention on a 24-hour basis. Home health agencies provide home nursing
   services on an hourly basis or by shifts. Identifying consistent, trained pediatric staff through these agencies requires advanced planning and screening. It is best to consult with the hospital's continuing care program before
   agency selection.
   1. Referral process
      Referral should be initiated by phone at least 1 week prior to discharge
      to establish adequate staff. The agency's representative may come to the
      hospital to review the infant's total care plan.
   2. Families who may benefit
      Private-duty nursing services may benefit a family with an infant who
      requires skilled intervention every 3 hours or more frequently, such as
      an infant with a tracheostomy requiring frequent suctioning, an infant
      requiring close observation, or an infant requiring multiple medications
      or frequent medication adjustment.
      These services may also benefit a family with an infant who has multi-
      system involvement or a complex feeding regimen, such as one requir-
      ing nasogastric tube feedings, gastrostomy tube feedings, or constant
      enteral infusion.

The amount of PDN requested is based on the frequency of required intervention and the parents' ability to manage the infant's care realistically on a 24-hour basis.

3. Cost and reimbursement

Reimbursement through medical insurance is *not automatic* and needs to be explored on an individual basis.

D. Public health agencies

Public health agencies are tax-supported health departments at the city, county, or state level of government. Public health nurses are employed by health departments (or the board of health) to provide home visits, clinic services, school health programs, treatment and control of communicable diseases, and health education and promotion.

A public health nurse does not provide hands-on care and visits an average of once a week.

1. Referral process

The referral process is initiated by telephone, 24 to 48 hours prior to discharge, followed by a completed patient care referral form.

2. Families who may benefit

Public health agencies may benefit families who require services such as well-child care teaching including environmental safety, home nursing assessment prior to discharge to plan more accurately for ongoing needs, reinforcement of teaching of care, assistance with medical compliance, assessment of parent-child interaction, or assistance with control of communicable diseases (e.g., tuberculosis testing).

3. Cost and reimbursement

There is no direct fee for service to the patient.

E. Early intervention programs

Early intervention programs are community-based and provide services for infants and children from birth to 3 years old who have identified handicapping conditions or who are at risk for developmental delays owing to biologic or environmental factors.

The goal of EIPs is to assist a child to reach his or her highest possible level of development. Parental involvement and the home environment are recognized as crucial factors in the child's attaining full potential. Parents are active participants in the ongoing process of assessment, planning, and implementation of their child's program. Thus, the process encourages and supports the parents' independence in advocating and planning for their child's special needs.

Services include, but are not limited to, developmental screening and evaluation, parent-infant education, speech therapy, occupational therapy, physical therapy, nursing, social work, and psychologic services. These services can be provided in a wide variety of settings including the child's home (especially during the first year with high-risk infants), nurseries or day care centers, and specialized centers offering these services.

1. Referral process

Referrals to EIPs can be initiated by a parent or a member of the health care team. The referral is initiated by telephone contact to the designated program, followed by written nursing, medical, and social information. The hospital's continuing care program can assist you in locating EIPs. In addition, the state department of public health or mental health can assist in locating programs.

Referral to EIPs should be considered during the discharge planning process for every high-risk infant. Referrals can be made directly from the nursery. For some infants, services can begin prior to discharge.

2. Families who may benefit

Children in three broad categories of risk should be considered for EIPs: established risk, biologic risk, and environmental risk.

Established risk includes infants or children whose diagnosed medical disorders are strongly associated with developmental delays (e.g., Down's syndrome, hydrocephaly, cerebral palsy, hearing and vision impairments, and other congenital anomalies).

Biologic risk includes infants and children with a history of prenatal, neonatal, or early developmental events suggestive of insult(s) to the developing central nervous system (e.g., prematurity, abnormal neurologic findings, or behavior such as inconsolable crying, sleep disturbances, feeding difficulties).

Environmental risk includes infants or children who are at high risk for delayed development because of limited early environmental experience (e.g., families with adolescent parents, parental psychologic or physical illness, or parental substance abuse).

Some families may benefit from having a period to get settled or an adjustment period after discharge from the nursery. In these situations a referral to an EIP can be made prior to discharge by the primary nurse, and at a later time the parents or the program can activate actual involvement in the program's services.

Some infants who meet the high-risk criteria for EIPs may not need the full services available. In these instances, the infant can be referred for developmental monitoring, parent support, or both. The EIP staff and the parents can then decide when and if any additional services are needed.

3. Cost and reimbursement

Fees for service vary from no cost, to sliding scale, to third-party reimbursement.

F. Hospice programs

Hospice programs offer a family-centered approach to palliative and supportive care, enabling the patient and family to maintain the highest quality of life when a cure is no longer considered possible and death is probable in a short time.

The goals of the hospice are to help the dying patient achieve maximum freedom from physical and emotional pain, to keep him or her functioning at a maximum level so he or she can live as fully as possible until death comes, and to meet any special needs of the patient and family members that arise from the stresses associated with the final stages of illness, dying, and bereavement.

Five forms of hospice care have evolved: home care services, hospice teams in hospitals, palliative care units in hospitals, hospices with hospital affiliations, and free-standing hospices.

Most hospice programs in Massachusetts are home based; that is, support services are arranged to help the patient and family at home. Home support services include nursing visits, home health aid assistance, homemaker assistance, PDN, and hospice volunteers. Hospice volunteers have completed a training course that focuses on the issues of death and dying and methods of helping families during their stages of grieving and bereavement. They contract with families to spend up to 10 hours each week in ways most helpful to that family (e.g., companion for the patient, listener for a family member).

Currently, a number of VNAs offer hospice care as part of their services.

1. Referral process

   The hospital continuing care program or state hospice association can be of assistance in locating a hospice program. Referral is made by telephone contact followed by a completed patient care referral form.

2. Families who may benefit

   Hospice services may benefit families caring for terminally ill infants with problems such as trisomy 13, severe congenital heart defects, or severe congenital anomalies.

3. Cost and reimbursement

   Most skilled services are reimbursed by third-party payers. Volunteer and paraprofessional services are based on a sliding scale or are provided at no charge to the family.

G. Respite care

   Respite care is the provision of short-term care for infants and children in or out of the home to allow the family to meet emergency needs, fulfill vacation plans, obtain routine reprieve, or provide an alternative to institutionalization. Families of infants with special medical problems and needs are eligible to receive respite services in the state of Massachusetts (and other states as well).

   In Massachusetts, respite care is funded through the departments of mental health, public health, and social services. Services are limited, averaging 10 days every 6 months. Different levels of care are provided based on need (i.e., unskilled to skilled care requiring trained to professional personnel). Respite care can be used for infants on apnea monitors as well as infants with multisystem involvement. In other areas of the country, respite services may be provided through a special bureau for handicapped children or department of mental health. For information, contact the local department of public health or department of special education.

   1. Referral process

      The hospital's continuing care program will assist in proper agency selection. These agencies can also be contacted directly.

   2. Families who may benefit

      Respite care may benefit any family with an infant who has a special medical problem requiring trained or professional caretakers. Some examples include an infant on an apnea monitor, an infant requiring a special feeding regimen such as a nasogastric or gastrostomy tube, and an infant with a compromised respiratory status such as those on oxygen therapy or with a tracheostomy.

3. Cost and reimbursement

At present in Massachusetts, respite services are provided to families free of charge. In other states, there may be fees for services based on a sliding scale.

H. Home health equipment companies

Numerous home health equipment companies nationwide provide a full range of equipment to families in their homes. Proper selection of a company qualified to meet the needs of the high-risk neonate is crucial. Qualified companies should perform the following functions:

1. Provide specialized equipment with trained personnel.
2. Set up equipment and educate family prior to and after discharge from hospital.
3. Provide frequent home visits from professionals.
4. Provide 24-hour on-call availability to assist families with any problem (e.g., malfunctioning equipment).
5. Be responsive to family's ongoing needs.
6. Provide equipment suitable for infants and children.
7. Be able to handle all third-party billing.

Available services and equipment include home respiratory therapy such as oxygen (portable and in-home), suction machines and catheters, ventilators, cardiac/apnea monitors, oxygen mist tents, and compressors-nebulizers; total parenteral nutrition supplies and equipment; enteral supplies such as infusion pumps; home intravenous antibiotic therapy; and durable medical equipment such as special wheelchairs and carriages.

The hospital's continuing care program is able to assist in ordering necessary home equipment and providing current information on available resources.

III. Alternatives to home care

A. Rehabilitation hospitals

Pediatric rehabilitation offers an alternative for the high-risk infant with multisystem involvement who requires ongoing hospitalization. When the acute medical problems have stabilized, a rehabilitation hospital concentrates on fostering maximum growth and development of the infant and contributes to the family's ability to provide ongoing care. This transitional setting is able to allot more time for continued family teaching, addressing parents' needs, and providing intensive developmental intervention than is a busy neonatal intensive care unit (NICU) environment. It is possible for a discharge plan to consist of letting the infant have short leaves away from the hospital before the family assumes total responsibility of care, thereby increasing the family's level of confidence and abilities.

1. Referral process

Currently there are several rehabilitation hospitals with pediatric programs in Massachusetts. Hospital continuing care programs assist with the referral process. A liaison nurse from the rehabilitation hospital reviews each infant's situation with the primary team and family. The information is then presented to the rehabilitation hospital's admissions committee, which decides if the admission is appropriate.

2. Families who may benefit
A rehabilitation hospital may benefit families with infants who have specialized medical needs requiring a transitional setting before discharge home. Infants requiring prolonged hospitalization due to conditions such as a bronchopulmonary dysplasia or other respiratory problems (i.e., infants with a tracheostomy), neurologic deficits, fluid and electrolyte imbalance, compromised nutritional status, cardiac defects, and other problems causing multiple system involvement. This transition enables extended teaching periods for the family, further stabilization of the infant's condition, rescheduling of required interventions, and the infant's continued growth and development through the provision of intensive therapies.

3. Cost and reimbursement
Financial clearance is obtained prior to admission. Rehabilitation hospitalization is usually covered by third-party payers and Medicaid.

B. Specialized foster care
Specialized foster care provides care by paraprofessionals in a home setting for infants and children who have medical needs that cannot be met in their parents' homes.

Specialized foster care homes are recruited and supervised through area offices of the department of social services or department of mental health. Parents who place an infant in specialized home care must agree to voluntary custody of their infant with the department of mental health or department of social services. This arrangement provides necessary care for the infant through Medicaid and, if eligible, supplemental security income (SSI). Visiting privileges for the parents are prearranged, and the parents have the option to remove their infant from the specialized home after giving the department of social services (or the specific agency) 72-hour notice.

1. Referral process
   a. A family is identified as a suitable candidate.
   b. The family meets with primary caretakers, social worker, and hospital continuing care program. Alternatives are presented to the family, and their questions are answered.
   c. The continuing care nurse or social worker contacts area department of social services office.
   d. The family is interviewed at department of social services office by an intake worker.
   e. A home finder is assigned to locate a specialized foster care family.
   f. A case worker is assigned to work with the family to complete the process for placement (i.e., applying for SSI, signing voluntary custody papers).
   g. Specialized foster care parents and biologic parents meet with the

case worker to work out visiting times.
- h. Specialized foster care parents receive training.
- i. Patient is discharged to specialized foster care family.
- j. A referral is made to any additional community agencies that are needed (e.g., EIP, VNA).
2. Families who may benefit
Specialized foster care may benefit families in which the home environment is incompatible with the infant's disease process or in which the parents are intellectually, emotionally, physically, or socially impaired and are either unable or unwilling to provide care for the infant.
3. Cost and reimbursement
Funding for specialized foster care is provided by the state agency that arranges the placement. A child who is placed becomes eligible for Medicaid and SSI to meet medical expenses.

C. Chronic care hospitals
Chronic care hospitals provide long-term care to patients who require continued medical and nursing management because of an unstable medical status. According to public health regulations, the patient must require at least 4 hours of skilled nursing services per day and physician intervention at least once a week.
1. Referral process
Two chronic care hospitals in Massachusetts accept infants. The process for referral varies with each facility. The hospital continuing care program can assist with hospital identification and referral.
2. Families who may benefit
A chronic care hospital may benefit families whose infants require nasopharyngeal suctioning at least once per nursing shift or continuous intubation or mechanical ventilation (few facilities accept ventilator patients). Infants with life-threatening arrhythmias or electrolyte imbalance (some facilities accept hyperalimentation) are also considered. These hospitals might also benefit families with infants having seizures at least 3 times a week, infants with multiple medical problems, infants who are on steroids and are being monitored, and infants with refractory heart failure.
3. Cost and reimbursement
Reimbursement is available through third-party payers.

D. Pediatric nursing homes
Pediatric nursing homes care for severely retarded or brain-damaged multihandicapped persons between the ages of 3 months and 21 years. There are four pediatric nursing homes in Massachusetts. These institutions are licensed by the department of public health. The hospital continuing care staff is available to assist in assessing the appropriate level of nursing home care and to initiate the application to the medical review team at the department of public health, which certifies an infant for nursing home placement.
1. Referral process
- a. Identify the infant's need for continuous skilled care by a physician and primary nurse.

   b. Consult with hospital care staff.
   c. Continuing care staff and primary health team review options with
      the family members, who then make the decision that their infant
      cannot be cared for at home and requires appropriate level of nurs-
      ing care.
   d. Application is made by the hospital to the medical review team at
      the department of public health for certification for nursing home
      care. The medical review team will notify the hospital, nursing
      home, and family of their decision.
   e. The hospital continuing care staff will contact the nursing home to
      initiate the referral process. The nursing home will review the infant
      for admission and notify hospital of transfer date.
   f. On transfer of the infant to the nursing home, a completed patient
      care referral form and medical discharge summary are sent with the
      infant.
2. Families who may benefit
   A pediatric nursing home may benefit families with an infant who is severely neurologically damaged and requires continuous skilled nursing
   care.
3. Cost and reimbursement
   In Massachusetts, pediatric nursing homes are reimbursed through the
   Medicaid system. In most other states, pediatric nursing homes are also
   state funded.

IV. Financial, medical, and support services

   A. Insurance
      Insurance coverage of families with high-risk infants should be routinely
      explored. Some policies may only cover 80 percent of in-hospital costs,
      which leaves the family with an overwhelming balance, especially after a
      long NICU stay. Determining what insurance benefits a family has is also
      instrumental in trying to plan for continuing care after discharge.
         A contact person at the subscriber's place of employment who can iden-
      tify specific benefits should be contacted. Presently, there are insurance
      companies that have developed their own individual case management
      (ICM) programs. Individual case management programs offer a system for
      assessing individual patients and planning alternative treatments for eligi-
      ble patients needing prolonged care. For example, in the acute setting, a
      suggested resource such as rehabilitation hospitalization or extended
      home care services, which may not normally be covered under the
      patient's insurance plan, may be approved with ICM. The insurance team
      works closely with the discharge planning staff and primary health team to
      review cases. On approval, all legitimate costs are provided for. Compa-
      nies with case management programs include Blue Cross, Prudential, and
      Aetna.
         When necessary, families should be encouraged to apply for supple-
      mental assistance through state programs such as Medicaid and SSI. In
      some states funding is available through special bureaus for handicapped
      children.

B. Supplemental security income

Supplemental security income is a federally and state-funded program providing a guaranteed minimum income to blind, disabled, and elderly persons. Families receive a monthly check and are automatically eligible for Medicaid in Massachusetts. Supplemental security income is available to blind and disabled children as well as adults.

To be eligible for SSI, a child and his or her parents must have low income and resources, and the child must have a serious disability or a combination of lesser disabilities that have lasted, or will last for, 1 year or result in death. In Massachusetts, income guidelines and SSI information can be obtained from the Public Health Department, Case Management Services Unit.

If a child is hospitalized for more than 1 calendar month, a family may apply regardless of its income. The child is then considered to be living out of his or her home. The advantage is that if the child is eligible, the family receives a small monthly stipend and automatically receives Medicaid for the child in Massachusetts. This greatly benefits a family whose hospital insurance covers only 80 percent, as Medicaid will assist with the balance. The SSI benefit continues as long as the infant is hospitalized.

The Social Security Administration is responsible for deciding whether a child's disability qualifies him or her for SSI. A child can meet the SSI disability standard in three ways:

1. The child has a so-called listed impairment.
2. The child has an impairment that is equivalent to a listed impairment.
3. The child has two or more impairments that together are as disabling as a listed impairment.

The standard for determining a disability in the two last instances is whether the child's impairment substantially interferes with growth and development. The meaning of this standard is still undergoing change, but the following comments should be useful.

The Social Security Administration attaches some importance to learning and behavioral problems such as dyslexia, hyperactivity, or a poor self-concept. Other minor physical, mental, or developmental problems are also important when found in conjunction with more serious impairments. Any data on the child's developmental milestones should be included in a disability report. For patients who do not have listed impairments, nonmedical evidence is usually necessary to prove impaired growth and development. Examples of infants qualified for SSI are those with severe prematurity, bronchopulmonary dysplasia, multisystem involvement, cardiac defects, neurologic involvement, myelodysplasia, and developmental delay.

C. Massachusetts Commission for the Blind

The Massachusetts Commission for the Blind (MCB)* focuses on enhancing the economic and personal independence of blind persons by provid-

*Massachusetts Commission for the Blind, 110 Tremont Street, Boston, Massachusetts, 02108, (617-727-7520).

ing financial and medical assistance as well as specialized social and rehabilitation services. The MCB serves persons of all ages.

Services available through MCB for a person who has met the criteria
that establish him or her as legally blind include

Rehabilitation program
Vocational rehabilitation
Legal assistance
Individual and family counseling
Homemaker services
Housing services
Recreation services
Aids and appliances
Children's services
Talking book program
Medical assistance
Respite services

The MCB can advise and follow a family through the application process. In other states, services for the blind can be located by contacting the
local bureau of handicapped children's services.

D. Massachusetts Public Health Department: Family Health Services Division
Family Health Services Division provides preventive and therapeutic
health care services to families in Massachusetts. Family Health Services
programs fall into two categories: Services for Handicapped Children
(SHC) and Maternal and Child Health Services Program.
1. Services for Handicapped Children offers services providing or arrang-
ing for early identification of disabilities, treatment, surgery, appliances,
and genetic counseling. Following are descriptions of the five units
through which these services are provided.
a. Clinic Unit
A regional statewide clinic program provides diagnostic and treatment services for children who have one or more of the following:
cerebral palsy; developmental delay; myelodysplasia; oral-facial
plastic surgery; scoliosis; or cardiac, neurologic, or orthopedic disabilities. Nonregional clinics at major medical centers cover epilepsy,
cystic fibrosis, seizures, hemophilia, and inborn errors of metabolism. Nursing, physical therapy, social work, and nutrition counseling are provided.
In addition to direct services, financial assistance for certain services and equipment is also provided, based on a family's size, annual income, medical expenditures, and health insurance coverage.
b. The Community Services Unit provides a comprehensive range of
community-based support services to families to enable them to
care for their multi-handicapped child at home. Programs supported
through this unit offer educational and therapeutic services (EIP, developmental day program), home nursing or child care, respite care
training programs, and residential care in pediatric nursing homes.

   c. The medical review team is a multidisciplinary group of profession-
      als that determines the eligibility of a child for services; children are
      referred to the team by hospitals, school systems, and social agen-
      cies. Eligibility for services is based on medical and nursing care
      needs as well as on social factors.
   d. The Genetic Unit offers comprehensive screening, diagnosis, and
      counseling services through a statewide network of Family Health
      Services clinics and private medical centers to residents of Massa-
      chusetts who are at risk for hereditary disorders.
   e. The Case Management Service Unit* provides a case manager for
      any child with a handicapping condition. The case manager coordi-
      nates service providers, writes an individual service plan, and pro-
      vides technical assistance to parents who are interested in locating
      additional services as well as in advocating for their child. In addi-
      tion, they can be helpful to parents in an appeals process (Chapter
      766 [Massachusetts's Program for Special Education Services for
      Children] SSI).
2. Maternal and Child Health Services Program
   a. Perinatal Unit serves as a resource center to consumer and health
      care providers in areas of pregnancy, childbirth, and newborn care.
   b. Primary Care Unit provides health care to high-risk, low-income
      mothers and their children.
   c. Services to School-Age Children Unit monitors hearing and vision
      screening, adolescent health programs, and psychotropic drug and
      poison control programs.
   d. Women, Infants, and Children Unit (WIC) receives funding from the
      Federal Maternal Child Health Block Grant, which is administered in
      Massachusetts by the Public Health Department. The WIC program is
      a prevention-orientation program that provides nutritional assess-
      ment, counseling, and supplemental food to clients in the following
      categories: pregnant women, non-breast-feeding women, breast-
      feeding women, infants, and children up to 5 years of age. Families
      who are eligible for WIC must meet the income guidelines, be con-
      sidered a nutritional risk (e.g., iron deficiency, low birth weight, in-
      adequate weight gain), have a medical referral form completed by a
      health care provider outlining the infant's medical history, and par-
      ticipate in reevaluation and recertification in the program every 6
      months. The WIC program has higher income guidelines than any
      other federal program, and families should be encouraged to apply.

E. Department of social services
   The department of social services provides protective and community services to children at risk for neglect or abuse (or both) and their families.
   This department has a regional and area office structure similar to that of
   other state agencies. Each office has a protective services unit and a community services unit.

*CMSU:DPH Boston, 39 Boylston Street, 6th Floor, Boston, Massachusetts, 02116, (617-727-0747).

The protective services unit is responsible for investigating all formal reports of child abuse and neglect, in accordance with individual state laws. When these requests are reported to the department of social services, a family-home assessment is initiated. A treatment plan is then developed. For social services guidelines for reporting actual or suspected child abuse or neglect, contact the local social services office.

The community services unit provides temporary home services to families in stressful situations. Some of these services include babysitting, homemaking, and respite care. Services such as foster care and respite care can be arranged outside of a child's home. Respite care in the home is available to developmentally disabled children and adults who periodically need brief services to support the family's effort to provide care at home. For information regarding referral for community services, contact the hospital continuing care program or department of social services.

Developmental disability has been defined by U.S. public law 95-602 as a severe, chronic disability that is

1. Attributable to a mental or physical impairment or combination of mental and physical impairments.
2. Manifested before age 22.
3. Likely to continue indefinitely.
4. The cause of substantial functional limitations in three or more of the following areas of major life activity: self-care, receptive and expressive language, learning, mobility, self-direction, capacity for independent living, and economic self-sufficiency.
5. Reflective of the person's need for a sequence of special, interdisciplinary treatments, or other services that are of lifelong or extended duration and need to be individually planned and coordinated.

F. Department of public welfare

The department of public welfare serves poor, elderly, and disabled residents through area offices. These programs exist nationwide. However, services may vary from state to state. Programs administered by the department include:

1. Aid to Families with Dependent Children (AFDC): minimum income for unemployed, single-parent families.
2. Food stamps: a supplemental program for families whose income is at or near poverty level. Food stamps may be used to purchase only food (no paper products, cigarettes, alcohol, etc.).
3. Medicaid: pays for health services for residents eligible because of income and assets level, overwhelming medical care costs, or acceptance to the SSI program.
4. Job training: the newest program in Massachusetts is the Employment and Training Program (ET), which provides training and education, supported work experiences, job search assistance through employment security, and career counseling and assessment.

G. Department of mental health

The department of mental health serves the state's mentally ill and mentally retarded residents through a variety of services administered by central, regional, and area offices. In Massachusetts, each region of the Mental Health Department has a state hospital and a state school; each of the 40 areas offers a mental health clinic as well as respite, case management, and advocacy services for eligible clients. In keeping with the federal mandate of the early 1970s to deinstitutionalize state psychiatric hospitals and state schools for the mentally impaired, the department has as its primary goal consumer-client advocacy, working toward increased normalization for each client.

The department of mental health provides respite care to families with infants who are neurologically impaired.

H. Massachusetts Office for Children
The Massachusetts Office for Children (OFC), created in the early 1970s, is a state department within the Human Services Executive Office that serves as a statewide information, referral, and advocacy system for children. In addition, OFC coordinates and monitors all Massachusetts public and private services for children.

The OFC has regional and area offices. Each area office is assisted by its Council for Children. Council membership is voluntary and includes both consumers and providers of children's services. Together staff and council members are responsible for establishing an information and referral system, and advocating for area children.

The OFC is responsible for setting the standards for licensing and approving day care programs (family- and center-based), group care facilities, and foster care and adoption agencies. Area offices are able to provide a list of approved day care alternatives on request.

I. Parent support services
Giving birth to a high-risk infant requiring NICU care is a crisis experience. During the infant's hospitalization, parents deal with many emotions ranging from fear and guilt to joy. Parents need the support of all professionals who care for their infant, but there are times when parents need the support of another parent—a peer who has been through what they are experiencing. As the infant's condition improves and the family moves toward discharge to the community hospital and eventually home, these needs for support remain and must be addressed.

As with any referral or resource, parental readiness must be assessed and considered. Use of any resource must be an individual family decision, and respect for and support of that decision are essential. Referral to parent support services can simply be informational: giving the parents the necessary information about available services and how to use them, allowing them to initiate as they feel comfortable.

There are a variety of parent support services available through hospitals as well as community-based groups. Some offer education and support around specific parenting issues such as premature infants, teenage parenthood, twins, and breast-feeding. Others offer a wider base of parent education and support. We include a number of groups that are specific to the needs of families of high-risk infants. Some are valuable resources for identifying other agencies that may be helpful to a particular family. Some of the parent support services listed in this chapter are specific to the Boston area, but exemplify services in other regions. These can be used as resources along with the national groups that are included.

1. NICU: Parent Support, Inc. (formerly Project WELCOME Parent Group) is a parent-led, professionally supported program that provides support and education to families of NICU babies.* It offers a variety of services to parents of high-risk infants.
   a. Parent-to-parent telephone support around a variety of issues: before, during, or after discharge from the NICU; while a child is enrolled in EIPs, and getting pregnant again.
   b. Education programs offered according to parental needs.
   c. Resources: where to get breast pumps, clothes for premature infants, reading materials, and information; other available resources and how to use them (e.g., professional counseling, EIPs, and parent support groups).
   d. A newsletter for parents written by parents and professionals.
   e. Outreach training program: Outreach parents are parents of NICU graduates who are available for telephone support calls.

2. Parent Care/Parents of Premature and High-Risk Infants International, Inc.,† is a national group that offers information, referrals, and other services to families, parent support groups, and professionals concerned with infants who require special care at birth. Some specific services include
   a. Support for families of critically ill infants
   b. Encouragement of communication between parents and professionals
   c. Support for parents as they begin support groups
   d. Support for and facilitation of networking and communication between various parent support groups and organizations involved with high-risk infants
   e. Enhancement of public awareness of the issues and concerns of families of premature and high-risk infants

3. Federation for Children with Special Needs‡ provides information about and assistance around referrals needed for children with a variety of special needs.
   a. They provide training and support for parents around advocacy issues in both the educational and medical systems.
   b. They publish a newsletter that addresses issues for parents of children with special needs.
   c. They offer parent support through their member organizations. These groups are divided according to the child's special needs (i.e., cardiac problems, spina bifida, hearing or visual impairments, cerebral palsy).

*NICU: Parent Support, Inc., 84 Hinckley Road, Milton, Massachusetts, 02186.
†Parent Care, National Headquarters, University of Utah Medical Center, Room 211210, 80 North Medical Drive, Salt Lake City, Utah, 84132, (801-581-7052).
‡The Federation for Children with Special Needs is located in Massachusetts as well as in 45 other states. Further information can be obtained by calling the Massachusetts chapter at (617) 482-2915.

d. They also provide information on eligibility for and obtaining re-spite care.
4. SKIP, Inc. Sick Kids need Involved People* is a national organization composed of parents and professionals from a variety of disciplines who serve as a support, educational, and resource group for parents who have made the decision to initiate intensive home care for their hospitalized child. By supporting a family's efforts, SKIP desires to pro-mote optimal health and development for the medically fragile child within the normal environment of his or her home. SKIP has a number of chapters throughout the country in various stages of development.
5. United Cerebral Palsy† (UCP) offers a variety of services to families with children who have developmental delays or have been diag-nosed with cerebral palsy. Some of the services, which vary among programs, include
   a. Information and referral
   b. Program services for infants and children (as well as people of all ages)
   c. Advocacy roles within the education system
   d. Respite services
   e. Parent support services
6. Easter Seal Society‡ is a national organization with chapters located throughout the country that provides a variety of services to persons with physical disabilities. Local chapters should be contacted for spe-cific information on the services they provide. Services include
   a. Information on and referral to existing community resources
   b. Specific rehabilitation programs for a variety of age groups (e.g., preschool swimming program)
   c. Equipment loan program
   d. Home health care services
7. Mothers of twin groups typically provide peer support for parents around the many issues of parenting twins. Many mother of twins groups also have equipment exchange or resell programs. These groups can be located by contacting the local VNA or community health nursing department.
8. Nursing mothers groups include La Leche League and the Nursing Mothers Council. These groups provide information and support for breast-feeding mothers as well as information on where to rent breast pumps. Nursing mothers groups can be located by contacting the lo-cal VNA or community health nursing department.
9. Coping with the Overall Pregnancy/Parenting Experience§ (COPE) is a United Way agency that provides counseling, support groups, educa-tion, training, information, and referral services in the greater Boston area. These services are provided by trained professionals, including

---

*SKIP, Inc., National Headquarters, 216 Newport Drive, Severna Park, Maryland, 21146, (301-647-0164).
†For further information about local chapters, the telephone number of the national office is (212) 481-6300.
‡The telephone number of the Massachusetts chapter is (617) 482-3370.
§COPE, 37 Clarendon Street, Boston, Massachusetts, 02116, (617-357-5588).

social workers, nurses, psychologists, and psychiatrists. This program also includes an extensive parenting preparation program and staffs a counseling and parent education project at Boston City Hospital.

Fees for services are covered by third-party insurance and Medicaid and a sliding fee schedule for counseling services.

10. Social service organizations. In addition to departments of social services, numerous private nonprofit social service agencies provide services to families with high-risk infants. Services vary from agency to agency but generally include family counseling, mental health services, work with single parents, juvenile delinquents, foster care and specialized foster care, adoption, and child protective services to children at risk for neglect, abuse, or both.

Agency listings appear in the yellow pages of the telephone book under the Social Service Agencies heading. Examples of agencies in the greater Boston area are Boston Children's Service, Catholic Charitable Bureau, and Jewish Family Services.

11. Associations for retarded citizens throughout the country assist families and individuals who are affected by mental retardation. Agencies exist on the national, state, and local levels. The primary functions of associations for retarded citizens are advocacy, information, and referral. Several agencies on the state and local levels provide direct services including respite, group homes, and workshops for mentally retarded clients.

The agency is a good resource to assist families of and individuals who are mentally retarded obtain the services they require.

V. Hospital-based infant follow-up programs

Hospital-based IFUPs offer continued assistance and support services for NICU graduates and their families by providing an interdisciplinary clinic after discharge. These programs are designed to collaborate with and to complement the care provided by the primary health care provider and other community-based services.

Services provided by an IFUP typically include periodic assessment of the health and development of the infant or child; identification of areas in which abnormalities may exist; medical, neurologic, or psychological, also, referrals to appropriate community resources or services (e.g., EIPs) and overall support and education for the parents around the issues of caring for their high-risk infant.

The IFUP has an interdisciplinary team that usually includes professionals from the fields of nursing, social work, psychology, physical therapy, developmental pediatrics, and neonatology.

A. Referral process

The referral process varies with each program. Many IFUPs have a nurse coordinator who begins the process in the NICU in conjunction with the infant's primary care team. The nurse coordinator is included in the discharge planning of NICU care to facilitate contacts and referrals between the NICU and IFUP.

Parents are also included in the referral process at an appropriate point prior to discharge. The specifics of the program are discussed with them, and an appointment is made for between 2 and 6 weeks after discharge.

B. Criteria for referral

Specific criteria to select infants for follow-up vary from program to program. Common eligibility criteria include neurologic problems, sociofamilial problems, chronic disease, very low birth weight, anomalies, and research protocols.

Communication between IFUPs, community agencies (EIPs and VNA), primary care providers, and NICUs is essential. This occurs through phone contact, written progress reports, or case conferences with the various service providers.

VI. Conclusion

Discharge planning is a challenging and integral part of patient care. Designing an effective discharge plan takes time, patience, skill, and creativity—especially as caring for high-risk infants becomes increasingly sophisticated in both the hospital and the community. This challenge includes not only becoming more familiar with the many needs of high-risk infants and their families but also knowing how to use the myriad of resources available in the community effectively.

Discharge planning serves as the vehicle for meeting patients' continuing care needs. The process begins at the time of admission and is a result of a continuous assessment of both family strengths and needs. Through communication and collaboration the health care team uses the data gathered and designs an individualized plan that matches identified needs with the most appropriate community resources.

All families, regardless of socioeconomic status, are entitled to information about available community resources and assistance with access and use of these services. Discharge planning is a multidisciplinary effort, with the family at the center of the process. Health care professionals should not isolate themselves in accomplishing this task but use the expertise of all involved team members to develop an individualized plan that provides ongoing care without fragmentation or interruption.

REFERENCES

Gikow, F., Anderson, E., Bigelow, L., et al. The continuing care nurse. *Nursing Outlook* 33 : 195, 1985.

Mack, S. *After Neonatal Intensive Care: Helping Parents Deal with Ongoing Issues.* Boston: Wheelock College, Project WELCOME, 1983.

Mayer, R. *Access to Developmental Services for NICU Graduates: A State of the Art Paper of New England.* Boston: Wheelock College, Project WELCOME, 1983.

McKeehan, K. *Continuing Care: A Multidisciplinary Approach to Discharge Planning.* St. Louis: Mosby, 1981.

Mintzer, D., Als, H., Tronick, E., Brazelton, T. B. Parenting an infant with a birth defect: The regulation of self-esteem zero to three. *Bull. Natl. Center Clin. Infant Programs* 5 : 1, 1985.

Porter, S. *Organizing Support Programs for Parents of Premature Infants.* Boston: Wheelock College, Project WELCOME, 1983.

Porter, S., and Flemings, M. *The Early Years: A Guide for Parents of Premature Infants.* Boston: Wheelock College, Project WELCOME, 1983.

Stein, R. Home care: A challenging opportunity. *Report on ACCH Conference.* May 1984. Pp. 2–8.

Primary Care for the Neonatal Intensive Care Unit Graduate

Linda M. Cohen and H. William Taeusch

I. Introduction

Pediatric primary care for the healthy full-term infant is designed to promote and support normal growth and development through preventive practices such as immunizations, early diagnosis and treatment of disease, anticipation of age-appropriate behaviors and problems, and education of parents.

Primary care for the low-birth-weight premature infant is this and more. (Low birth weight is 1,000–1,500 g; very low birth weight [micro premie] is <1,000 g.) Pediatric providers caring for these infants, aware of the neonatal course and familiar with the potential sequelae of prematurity, should anticipate common problems such as failure to thrive, anemia, hearing and vision defects, neurodevelopmental lags, and effects of chronic lung disease. Parents of premature infants are especially concerned about long-lasting effects of the early birth and neonatal course. For the child who needs subspecialty care, the primary-care pediatrician functions as the coordinator of a team: referring, consulting, interpreting, and in general, ensuring comprehensive care. A supportive provider who can provide answers to the inevitable questions, such as, "Is my child normal?" and "What can we expect?" is important.

II. Schedule of visits

The schedule of visits for premature infants follows the guidelines outlined by the American Academy of Pediatrics, with modifications for individual problems. Soon after discharge from the neonatal intensive care unit (NICU), early and frequent visits may be necessary to monitor growth, weight gain, and parental and infant adjustment and to review with parents questions about the perinatal events. Once the infant demonstrates satisfactory out-of-hospital stability, the need for follow-up is determined by the presence of acute and chronic conditions. The 2,000 g infant with no problems may need only routine pediatric care, whereas the infant on home oxygen therapy for bronchopulmonary dysplasia with an increased rate of head growth may need biweekly visits. Routine well-baby care recommendations (adapted from the American Academy of Pediatrics, 1981) are shown in Table 6-1. Additional items appropriate for NICU graduates are starred.

III. General infection risk

Concern for increased risk of infection continues for some infants after discharge from the NICU. Infants with surgical procedures (e.g., gastrostomy

Table 6-1. Guidelines for health supervision

Procedure	Age										
	1 Mo	2 Mo	4 Mo	6 Mo	9 Mo	12 Mo	15 Mo	18 Mo	24 Mo	3 Yr	4 Yr
Initial and interval history					At all visits						
Measurements											
Height and weight					At all visits						
Head circumference	+	+	+	+	+	+					
Blood pressure	*	*		*		*		*		+	+
Sensory screen[a]											
Vision	+[c]	+	+[b]	+	+	+	+	+	+	+[b]	
Hearing	+[c]	+	+[b]	+	+	+	+	+	+	+[b]	+
Development and behavior assessment					At all visits						
Physical examination					At all visits						
Laboratory procedures											
Metabolic screening	+										
Immunization		+	+	+			+	+	+		
Tuberculosis test						+			+		
Hematocrit		*	*	*		+			+		
Fep Pb[c]						+					
Urinalysis										+	
Anticipatory guidance					At all visits						
Dental referral										+	

+ = to be performed; * = checks specific for neonatal intensive care unit graduates.
[a]Formalized testing if in high-risk group.
[b]Formalized testing.
[c]Repeat every 6–12 months, depending on risk.
Adapted from the American Academy of Pediatrics, Committee on Practice and Ambulatory Medicine, 1981.

and ventricular shunts) are at increased risk for site-specific infections. Very low birth weight infants may have diminished immune responses for an indefinite period after hospital discharge. Infants with chronic lung disease are vulnerable to repeat episodes of bronchiolitis and cor pulmonale during the first year of life. Generally, we recommend that NICU graduates be kept from crowds and persons with known or evident infections during the first year of life. The advent of center-based early intervention programs available in the second and third years of life for high-risk infants probably conveys an enhanced, but often tolerable, increased risk of respiratory and gastrointestinal infection. Day care homes carry less infectious risk than do larger day care centers (Bartlett et. al., 1985). Adjustment of immunization schedules and common-sense infection control precautions in the home or center are reasonable steps that may offset risk. Some infectious disease risks are worth taking, when we contrast today's attitudes with those of our predecessors:

"Are there any valid objections to kissing infants?" There are many serious objections. Tuberculosis, diphtheria, and many other grave diseases may be communicated in this way. . . . Infants should be kissed, if at all, upon the cheek or the forehead, but the less, even of this, the better. (Holt, 1927)

	DPT	Polio	TB test	Measles	Mumps	Rubella	HIB	Tetanus-diphtheria
2 months	✔	✔						
4 months	✔	✔						
6 months	✔							
1 year			✔					
15 months				✔	✔	✔		
1½ years	✔	✔						
2 years							✔	
4–6 years	✔	✔						
14–16 years								✔

Fig. 6-1. Schedule of immunizations. This chart, available from the American Academy of Pediatrics, allows parents to keep track of their children's immunizations.
DPT = diphtheria-pertussis-tetanus vaccine; *HIB* = *Haemophilus influenzae* type B; *TB* = tuberculosis.

IV. Immunizations

A recommended schedule of immunizations for children 2 months to 16 years of age is shown in Fig. 6-1.

A. Diphtheria-pertussis-tetanus and polio

Diphtheria-pertussis-tetanus (DPT) and polio vaccines may be administered to most premature infants on the same schedule as full-term infants, according to the chronologic age, without consideration of the degree of prematurity. Premature infants demonstrate immune responses to the vaccines similar to full-term infants (Bernbaum et al., 1985). Modification of the schedule should be considered, however, in patients with neurologic illness, poor weight gain, unstable health, acute illness, or decreased muscle mass at injection sites. Pertussis should be withheld from any infant who has a possible or evolving neurologic illness. In practice we usually give the first DPT and oral polio vaccine about 1 month after discharge from the NICU. The sickest and smallest infants may by then be 6 months' chronologic age.

B. Pneumococcal immunization

Current recommendations are for a 0.5-ml dose of the 23 strain pneumococcal vaccine, polyvalent, in high-risk children at 2 years of age. Children having (1) sickle cell disease, (2) functional or anatomic asplenia, (3) nephrotic syndrome, or (4) selected malignancies are candidates for the vaccine. Infants with chronic lung or heart disease or with intracranial shunts may benefit as well, but specific data are absent. Antibody responses appear to be low and for the most part unsustained when pneumococcal immunization is given before 2 years of age. Nonetheless, an infant with chronic lung disease enrolled in a day care center is a reasonable candidate for immunization (American Academy of Pediatrics, Committee on Infectious Diseases, 1985).

C. Immunization for *Haemophilus influenzae* type B
One single immunization at 24 months of age is currently recommended for all children. The Centers for Disease Control (CDC) (and the American Academy of Pediatrics [AAP]) recommend immunization at 18 months for infants at special risk, such as those in day care, but because clinical efficacy in preventing infection in this younger age group is uncertain, reimmunization is recommended after 24 months. The *Haemophilus influenzae* type B (HIB) vaccine is insufficiently immunogenic for protection of infants less than 18 months of age. Incidence of notable HIB disease in the United States is estimated at 1 per 200 children under 5 years of age. It is not known whether the incidence is higher and the degree of protection lower in premature infants. Reactions to the vaccine are local in approximately one-half the infants. High fevers are rare, and nonfatal anaphylaxis occurred once in 58,000 children immunized (Peltola et al., 1984).

D. Hepatitis immunization
Current recommendations are for infants born to mothers who are positive for hepatitis B surface antigen (HB_s Ag) to receive 0.5 ml hepatitis B immune globulin within 12 hours of birth. Thereafter, they should receive hepatitis B vaccine (0.5 ml; 10 μg) in the first week and again at 1 and 6 months of age. Mothers who have antigenemia may excrete virus in breast milk, creating an ill-defined but probably increased risk of infection for the infant (Centers for Disease Control, 1984; Dienstag, 1984; Wang et al., 1984).

E. Influenza vaccine
We recommend that infants with chronic lung disease or symptomatic heart disease receive killed split virus influenza vaccine during the early fall. Children between 6 and 35 months should receive two doses (0.25 ml) more than 4 weeks apart unless they have been previously immunized with influenza vaccine, in which case a single dose suffices. Those with immediate hypersensitivity to egg antigens should not receive this vaccine. These recommendations are current for fall 1985 and should be verified before implementation and for sites other than New England.

V. Vitamin and mineral deficiencies
Preterm infants are at high risk for certain mineral and vitamin deficiencies because, deprived of the last few weeks to months of gestation, they have not accumulated adequate stores. The earlier the birth, the more rapid the postnatal growth rate and nutritional requirements, so these infants quickly outgrow what stores they have. In addition, premature infants have poor absorption of certain vitamins, and because of their ability to tolerate only limited amounts of fluids, their overall intake may be low. See Chap. 16 for a full discussion of the nutritional needs of the low-birth-weight infant.

A. Vitamins A, B, C, and D

The AAP recommends that low-birth-weight infants routinely receive daily multivitamin preparations with vitamins A, D, C, and B. Vitamin D requirements of 500 IU per day (400 IU in vitamin preparations and 100 IU in formula or breast milk) are suitable for most premature infants, although some seem to need much higher doses of vitamin D as well as calcium and phosphorus to prevent osteopenia and rickets. Follow-up blood tests including alkaline phosphatase, calcium, and phosphorus and assessment of bone mineralization by radiography are necessary to monitor the adequacy of supplementation in very low birth weight infants during the first months of life (Hillman et al., 1985).

B. Iron

Most low-birth-weight infants supplemented with 2 to 3 mg/kg/day of elemental iron as ferrous sulfate will avoid iron deficiency. Full feedings of standard formulas with iron (12 mg/liter) give approximately 1 mg/kg/day of elemental iron. Additional iron can be given separately or in conjunction with multivitamin drops. Iron-fortified cereal contains 3.6 mg of elemental iron per tbsp. The timing of the iron supplementation is controversial. It can be given shortly after birth if vitamin E intake is adequate or given 2 to 3 months after birth when the iron stores are being depleted. Iron supplements are continued for 6 to 12 months. The hematocrit and reticulocyte count should be routinely measured at 4- to 6-week intervals for the first 6 months of life. In practice we generally stop vitamin E and start iron supplements when premature infants exceed 2,000 g. Common iron supplements are

Fer-In-Sol drops: each 0.6-ml dose provides 15 mg elemental iron
Fer-In-Sol Syrup: each 5-ml dose provides 18 mg elemental iron
Feosol elixir: each 5-ml dose provides 44 mg elemental iron

C. Vitamin E (tocopherol)

Although the administration of vitamin E to infants in NICUs for the prevention of bronchopulmonary dysplasia and retrolental fibroplasia remains controversial, many pediatricians were convinced by the reports of Oski (1967) and others that treating very low birth weight infants with vitamin E would diminish hemolytic anemia associated with vitamin E deficiency. The hemolysis was exacerbated by iron and unesterified fatty acid intake. In more recent studies (Gross, 1985), infants weighing less than 1,500 g at birth were not benefited by vitamin E supplements when indicators of hemolysis were evaluated. These infants were on feedings with low iron content and high E–linoleic acid ratios. We conclude from these and other data that after discharge of very low birth weight infants, there is no need for routine use of vitamin E supplements.

D. Folate

The minimum daily requirement for folate is estimated to be 40 to 50 μg per day for full-term infants in the first 6 months of life. Although very low birth weight infants may need supplemental folate during the first weeks to months of life, its routine use in premature infants after discharge is rarely indicated.

E. Fluoride

Guidelines for use of fluoride do not exist for premature infants. We generally recommend 0.25 mg fluoride per day after 6 months of age if the local water supply or bottled water has a fluoride content of less than 0.3 parts per million. (This information is available from local health departments.) Fluoride is not transmitted in breast milk, so infants who are exclusively breast-fed without water or other supplements for 4 to 6 months should receive daily fluoride drops, beginning sometime in the first 6 weeks and continuing until another source of fluoride is given.

VI. Common problems

A. Hearing

Premature infants are at high risk for hearing loss either because of factors responsible for the premature birth (e.g., congenital infection, maternal disease, congenital anomaly) or from events that follow the birth (e.g., asphyxia and birth trauma, hyperbilirubinemia, neonatal infection, ototoxic drugs). In the United States, very low birth weight infants are at 30 times greater risk for hearing impairment than full-term infants: 1 : 1,500 versus 1 : 50.

Infants who meet the criteria for neonatal hearing screening are frequently tested before they are discharged home. Infants who fail an initial hearing screening should be retested. All infants should be tested during routine pediatric follow-up by observing their behavioral responses to auditory stimuli; infants who repeatedly fail to respond are referred for more formalized testing.

Criteria for neonatal hearing screening include

1. Family history of childhood hearing loss
2. Rubella, cytomegalovirus, toxoplasmosis, or herpes simplex during pregnancy
3. Birth weight less than 1,800 g
4. Neonatal meningitis
5. Congenital malformations of the head, such as cleft palate, abnormal pinna, or abnormal skull shape
6. Ototoxic drug (gentamicin or kanamycin) given to newborn for a full course of treatment
7. Hyperbilirubinemia over 20 mg per dl or an exchange transfusion
8. Severe asphyxia

B. Otitis media

Some pediatricians believe that infants who have had prolonged nasopharyngeal intubation have increased problems with recurrent otitis media. However, whether this is true or whether premature infants as a group have more than the usual incidence of otitis media (one to two episodes in the first 2 years of life) is not clear. Recurrent or chronic otitis media in infants discharged from NICUs is as problematic as it is for those who have not had perinatal problems, and management is the same (Lim, 1985).

C. Eyes

The most widely accepted risk factors for retinopathy of prematurity (ROP) include the degree of prematurity, duration of oxygen therapy (more so than the oxygen concentrations), neonatal infection, and apnea. Recently, light as commonly found in the standard NICU, has been implicated as a risk factor (Glass et al., 1985). The incidence of ROP is closely correlated with birth weight: 38 to 54 percent if less than 1,000 g, 5 to 15 percent if between 1,000 and 1,500 g, and 0.6 to 3.0 percent if more than 1,500 g. Guidelines for ophthalmologic screening of the premature infant include

Birth weight less than 1,500 g
Gestational age less than 32 weeks
Oxygen therapy more than 4 hours
Mechanical ventilation
In utero transfusion
Exchange transfusion in premature infants

In the pediatrician's office, an infant's visual acuity can be assessed by simple clinical observations and knowledge of development. Visual fixation can be demonstrated in most newborn and premature infants at 40 weeks' corrected age. (Corrected age is chronologic age minus the number of weeks of prematurity.) Infants can follow intermittently when the stimulus is a human face. If, at 3 to 4 months' corrected age, an infant cannot fixate and follow, referral to an ophthalmologist is indicated. Intermittent strabismus is frequent during the first 6 months; persistent deviations are reason to refer at any age.

D. Development

During well-child visits, infant development is assessed informally by history and observation and formally by specific developmental tests. Corrected age is used by custom in evaluating development until 2 years of age. The frequently used Denver Developmental Screening Test was not originally developed for evaluation of premature infants and will identify many age-appropriate children as delayed (false-positive) when plotted against chronologic age. We use it as a rough guide to remind us of age-specific developmental milestones (Elleman et al., 1985).

E. Breast-feeding

Many mothers decide to breast- or bottle-feed prior to the birth of their infant. After delivery of a premature infant, mothers may be uninformed of the advantages and disadvantages of breast versus bottle. Well-informed pediatricians and nurses can help a mother through what may be weeks to months of an NICU hospitalization during which the infant may be unable to breast-feed. The muscular strength and ability to coordinate sucking, swallowing, and breathing are not well developed before 32 to 34 weeks' gestation. Mothers who want to breast-feed infants less than 30 weeks' gestation should be encouraged to pump so the milk can be used for gavage feeding. The infant can be put to breast as soon as vigor and temperature stability allow, initially 1 to 2 times per day and by gavage the rest of the time with breast milk or formula.

The method of feeding and the timetable should be individualized according to the gestational age, clinical state, birth weight, and mother's wishes. Strong feelings exist in the minds of many caretakers about the need for breast-feeding, and care should be taken to address the mother's needs (not the caretaker's needs) during periods of high stress. A mother must be supported in her decision, whether it is to breast-feed or bottle-feed. Questions and problems with either breast- or bottle-feeding may continue to arise after discharge from the hospital and should be continually addressed during pediatric visits.

Preterm human milk differs from full-term milk: Protein, fat, sodium, chloride, and vitamins A and E are increased, and lactose and vitamin C are decreased.

F. Hypertension

Measuring an infant's blood pressure with a standard sphygmomanometer is difficult at best and often impossible. Several studies attribute hypertension in premature and sick infants to umbilical artery lines. One study of hypertension screening of premature infants seen in follow-up visits identified 8.9 percent (7 infants) with systolic blood pressures considered hypertensive (113 mm Hg = 95th percentile) (Sheftel et al., 1983). Three were found to have specific causes including neuroblastoma, coarctation of the aorta, and ureteropelvic junction obstruction; the other four were considered idiopathic. No differences were noted between the hypertensive and normotensive groups regarding many obstetric, maternal, or perinatal factors. Another report documented a high incidence of hypertension in premature infants with chronic lung disease and recommended close monitoring of blood pressure in follow-up of these infants (Abman et al., 1984). We measure blood pressure two or three times in the first year using a Dinemap* automated blood pressure device.

G. Inguinal hernias

Rescoria and Grosfeld (1984) recently studied complications of inguinal hernia repair in 100 infants less than 2 months of age. Of these, 31 had incarceration, 22 of which were reducible preoperatively. Eight of the 100 infants had postoperative complications, including infection, hematoma, apnea, cardiac arrest, and recurrence. Rescoria and Grosfeld recommend elective repair of inguinal hernias of very low birth weight infants just before hospital discharge when weight is greater than 2,200 g. They prefer early repair because of the 31 percent incidence of incarceration and 9 percent incidence of bowel obstruction in this selected sample.

*Critikon, P.O. Box 22800, Tampa, Florida, 33630.

Many physicians report success using only sedation and local anesthetic during repair, especially in infants who have chronic lung disease. Others (Steward, 1982) have reported an approximate 30 percent incidence of apnea or other pulmonary complication following hernia repair in premature infants after general anesthesia. Some authors recommend control of the inguinal hernia with yarn trusses until the infant can tolerate surgery. Unfortunately, in our institution, the yarn truss is now a lost art.

H. Undescended testicles (cryptorchism)
    Undescended testicles are more frequent in premature infants than in full-term infants. Whether premature infants have a greater prevalence of undescended testicles at 2 to 3 years of age is unknown. In the United States, surgery (orchiopexy) is recommended when the child is around 2 years of age.

I. Umbilical hernias
    Umbilical hernias occur most frequently in preterm black infants. Taping a coin over the hernia is of no benefit. We do not recommend repair until after the age of 2 years, and then primarily for cosmetic reasons. Incarceration has occurred in umbilical hernias but is extremely rare.

J. Hemangiomas
    Two major groups of vascular lesions in infancy have been described by Finn, Glowacki, and Mulliken (1983): hemangiomas that grow quickly in the first months of life and regress over the next years and vascular malformations that grow in proportion to the infant, are usually present at birth, and fail to involute. Raised hemangiomas are about twice as common in girls than in boys and are more frequent in premature infants than in term infants. Most authorities believe that surgery is necessary only for a small percentage of children with lesions and usually should be considered for static lesions (if lesions are in nonvital areas) after the age of 5. Involution, if it occurs before 5 years of age, is usually complete and not associated with scarring. Glucocorticoids to hasten regression are now rarely used. Carbon dioxide laser surgery is a useful recent development for surgical repair of hemangiomas; its indications are currently not well defined.

K. Crying and colic
    Colic—intermittent, recurrent, inconsolable crying of nonorganic origin during the first 3 months of life—occurs equally in full-term and premature infants. However, the onset for premature infants is delayed until several weeks after the expected delivery date. There appear to be no identifiable risk factors. The effect of aminophylline for apnea of prematurity may account for irritability in some premature infants, but this has not been systematically studied. Treatment for colic varies with the supposed cause and with the provider. Parents should be encouraged to look for explanations for irritability in their infants and to soothe, cuddle, gently rock, and carry them. When attempts to calm the infant are unsuccessful, it may be that the well-intentioned adults are contributing to an already overloaded, overstimulated infant. In this situation, or when the

parents are "beyond" themselves, the infant may need to be left alone for a period of time (Schmitt, 1985).

L. Acquired immune deficiency syndrome
Fourteen percent of children up to 13 years of age with acquired immune deficiency syndrome (AIDS) are nonhemophiliac transfusion–associated cases. Since many premature infants have received multiple small-dose transfusions of plasma and blood and its components during a NICU stay, they are at a small but definite risk for acquiring the virus. Because of a long period between infection and development of AIDS (7 years or more), physicians caring for children who were born prematurely must consider this diagnosis in certain clinical situations. Systematic screening of donors for human T-cell lymphotrophic virus (HTLV-III) and lymphadenopathy-associated virus (LAV) antibodies since March 1982 for blood and spring 1985 for plasma greatly reduces the potential for transmission of the virus through transfusion. Routine screening for children at risk is not recommended but should be considered if these children have any of the following: (1) failure to thrive, (2) recurrent persistent thrush, (3) chronic interstitial pneumonia, (4) hepatosplenomegaly, (5) chronic diarrhea, (6) lymphadenopathy, or (7) recurrent severe bacterial infection. Many parents of preterm infants who had transfusions have fears of their children developing AIDS, which may be expressed in cloaked terms or multiple concerns. Asking the parents, "What is your worst fear?" and addressing the real underlying issue may relieve both parent and provider.

VII. Repeat premature birth
A major national goal is to decrease the steady rate of premature births. Recent reports review the epidemiology of the problem. Although the precise risks of repeat prematurity are not known, one study found that if a woman's first child was premature, 17.2 percent of the second births and 28.4 percent of the third births were also premature (Bakketeig and Hoffman, 1981). In general, women who have had one premature infant after premature rupture of the membranes or premature labor have an approximate 10 to 20 percent chance of recurrence. In our follow-up program, we routinely recommend that women who have had a premature infant consult with a perinatologist prior to becoming pregnant again, the goal being to formulate a plan to forestall the birth of a repeat premature infant. We are aware that the efficacy of this approach is uncertain, and if this plan were generalized, there are too few perinatologists to meet the need. The key elements in such a plan are listed as follows:

A. Planning before conception, including perinatology consultation, birth spacing, and genitourinary examination

B. Nutrition and habit counseling (drugs, alcohol, smoking)

C. Careful dating of pregnancy onset

D. First-trimester fetal ultrasonographic examination

   E. Maternal alpha-fetoprotein screening

   F. Frequent routine obstetric visits with repeat examinations assessing cervical competence

   G. In-depth education of mother in signs and symptoms of premature labor

   H. Assessment of placental and fetal integrity and growth by ultrasonographic examination early in third trimester

   I. Collaborative management among obstetrician, perinatologist, ultrasonographer, pediatrician, and neonatologist

   J. Delivery of high-risk infant in perinatal center with intramural NICU

VIII. Circumcision
   There is no clear-cut medical justification for routine circumcision of newborn infants. We recommend that parents leave the final decision to the one possessed of the foreskin in question. For infants who have survived up to 3 months in an NICU, after weeks of tracheal intubation, chest tubes, blood lettings, and spinal taps, a circumcision without anesthetic seems unnecessarily cruel. One recent study found that uncircumcised male infants had a twentyfold greater incidence of urinary tract infections than circumcised male infants (Wiswell et al., 1985). This finding needs confirmation and further analysis before justifying circumcisions on this basis.

IX. Car seats
   Car seats in general are not well designed for infants less than 7 lb. An infant prone to positional apnea and who has poor motor tone may have breathing difficulty when placed in a poorly fitting car seat. Nonetheless, infants held in a parent's arms are especially vulnerable in an accident. Bull and Stroup (1985) list several brands of infant car seats that are appropriate for smaller infants (e.g., Questor Dyn-o-mite and Cosco-Peterson First Ride). They do not recommend (for small infants) seats with lap pads or shields. Car seats can be adapted for premature infants by using rolled towels on the sides and under the legs.

X. Supplies and reading
   Manufacturers now realize that special clothes and supplies are needed for preterm infants. Many such products were developed initially by industrious parents. There are several good books with bibliographies and resource lists for groups, equipment, and reading material for special needs infants, for example, *The Premature Baby Book* (Harrison, 1983), *Born Early* (Avery and Litwack, 1983), *Born Too Soon: Preterm Birth and Early Development* (Goldberg and DiVitto, 1983), *Premature Babies: A Handbook for Parents* (Nance, 1982), and *The Premie Parents' Handbook* (Lieberman and Sheagren, 1984).

REFERENCES
   Abman, S. H., Warady, B. A., Lum, G. M., and Koops, B. L. Systemic hypertension in infants with bronchopulmonary dysplasia. *J. Pediatr.* 104 : 928, 1984.

American Academy of Pediatrics. *Report of the Committee on Infectious Diseases* (20th ed.). American Academy of Pediatrics, 1986.

American Academy of Pediatrics. Care of the uncircumcised penis.

American Academy of Pediatrics, Committee on Infectious Diseases. Recommendations for using pneumococcal vaccine in children. *Pediatrics* 75 : 1153, 1985.

American Academy of Pediatrics, Committee on Nutrition. Soy protein formulas: Recommendations for use in infant feeding. *Pediatrics* 72 : 359, 1983.

American Academy of Pediatrics, Committee on Nutrition. Nutritional needs of low-birthweight infants. *Pediatrics* 75 : 976, 1985.

Anderson, G. H. Human milk feeding. *Pediatr. Clin. North Am.* 32 : 335, 1985.

Avery, M. E., and Litwack, G. *Born Early.* Boston: Little, Brown, 1983.

Bakketeig, L. S., and Hoffman, H. J. Epidemiology of Preterm Birth: Results from a Longitudinal Study of Births in Norway. In M. A. Elder and C. H. Hendricks (eds.), *Preterm Labor.* Stoneham, Mass.: Butterworths, 1981. Pp. 17–46.

Bartlett, A., Moore, M., Gary, W., et al. Diarrhea in infant-toddler day care. Number comparison of day care homes and households. *J. Pediatr.* 107 : 503, 1985.

Berger, L. R., and Schaefer, A. R. The premature infant goes home. Guidelines for primary care. *Am. J. Dis. Child.* 139 : 200, 1985.

Bernbaum, J. C., Anolik, R., Polin, R. A., et al. Development of the premature infant's host defense system and its relationship to immunizations. *Clin. Perinatol.* 11 : 73, 1984.

Bernbaum, J. C., Daft, A., Anolik, R., et al. Response of preterm infants to diphtheria-tetanus-pertussis immunizations. *J. Pediatr.* 107 : 184, 1985.

Boocock, G. R., and Todd, P. J. Inguinal hernias are common in preterm infants. *Arch. Dis. Child.* 60 : 669, 1985.

Bull, M. J., and Stroup, K. B. Premature infants in car seats. *Pediatrics* 75 : 336, 1985.

Centers for Disease Control. Postexposure prophylaxis of hepatitis B: Recommendations of the immunization practices advisory committee. *Ann. Intern. Med.* 101 : 351, 1984.

Child Day Care Infectious Disease Study Group. Infectious diseases in child day care centers. *J. Pediatr.* 105 : 683, 1984.

Child Day Care Infectious Disease Study Group. Considerations of infectious diseases in day care centers. *Pediatr. Infect. Dis.* 4 : 124, 1985.

CO_2 laser in pediatric surgery. *J. Pediatr. Surg.* 19 : 248, 1984.

Cochi, S. L., Broome, C. V., and Hightower, A. W. Immunization of US children with *Hemophilus influenzae* type B polysaccharide vaccine: A cost-effectiveness model of strategy assessment. *J.A.M.A.* 253 : 521, 1985.

Dienstag, J. L. Hepatitis B vaccine in health care personnel: Safety, immunogenicity, and indicators of efficacy. *Ann. Intern. Med.* 101 : 34, 1984.

Elliman, A. M., Bryan, E. M., Elliman, A. D., et al. Denver Developmental Screening Test and preterm infants. *Arch. Dis. Child.* 60 : 20, 1985.

Eviatar, L. Evaluation of hearing in the high-risk infant. *Clin. Perinatol.* 11 : 153, 1984.

Finn, M. C., Glowacki, J., and Mulliken, J. B. Congenital vascular lesions: Clinical application of a new classification. *J. Pediatr. Surg.* 18 : 894, 1983.

Forsyth, B., McCarthy, P., and Leventhal, J. Problems of early infancy, formula changes, and mothers' beliefs about their infants. *J. Pediatr.* 106 : 1012, 1985.

Fuchs, F., and Stubblefield, P. *Preterm Birth.* New York: Macmillan, 1984.

Glass, P., Avery, G. B., Subramanian, K. N., et al. Effect of bright light in the hospital nursery on the incidence of retinopathy of prematurity. *N. Engl. J. Med.* 313 : 401, 1985.

Goldberg, S., and DiVitto, B. *Born Too Soon: Preterm Birth and Early Development.* New York: Freeman, 1983.

Groff, D. B., Hirikati, S., Pietsch, J. B., et al. Inguinal hernias in premature infants operated on before discharge from the neonatal intensive care unit. *Arch. Surg.* 120 : 962, 1985.

Gross, S. J., and Gabriel, E. G. Vitamin E status in preterm infants fed human milk or infant formula. *J. Pediatr.* 106 : 635, 1985.

Harrison, H. *The Premature Baby Book.* New York: St. Martin's, 1983.

Henig, R. M., and Fletcher, A. *Your Premature Baby*. New York: Rawson, 1983.

Hillman, C., Hoff, W., Salmons, S., et al. Mineral homeostasis in very premature infants: Serial evaluation of serum 25-hydroxyvitamin D, serum minerals, and bone mineralization. *J. Pediatr.* 106 : 970, 1985.

Holt, E. *A Catechism for the Use of Mothers' and Children's Nurses* (13th ed.). New York: Appleton, 1927.

Hurt, H. Continuing care of the high-risk infant. *Clin. Perinatol.* 11 : 3, 1984.

Inglefinger, J. *Pediatric Hypertension*. Philadelphia: Saunders, 1982.

Institute of Medicine of the National Academy of Sciences, Committee to study the prevention of LBW. *Preventing Low Birth Weight*. Washington, D.C.: National Academy Press, 1985.

Kitchen, W. H., Ryan, M. M., Rickards, A. L., and Lissenden, J. V. *Premature Babies*. Emmaus, Penn.: Rodale, 1983.

Lieberman, A., and Sheagren, T. *The Premie Parents' Handbook*. New York: Dutton, 1984.

Lim, D. (ed.). Recent advances in otitis media with effusion: Report of research conference. *Ann. Otol. Rhinol. Laryngol.* 94: [Suppl. 116] part 3, 1985.

Ludington-Hoe, S. M. What can newborns really see? *Am. J. Nurs.* 9 : 1286, 1983.

Mandell, F., and Yogman, M. Developmental aspects of well child office visits. *Dev. Behav. Pediatr.* 3 : 118, 1982.

Margileth, A. M. Hemangiomas: A before-and-after look. *Contemp. Pediatr.* 3 : 14, 1986.

Meyer, J., and Thaler, M. Colic in low birth weight infants. *Am. J. Dis. Child.* 122 : 25, 1971.

Nance, S. *Premature Babies: A Handbook for Parents*. Berkeley, Calif.: Arbor House, 1982.

Neifert, M., and Seacat, J. Contemporary breast-feeding management. *Clin. Perinatol.* 12 : 319, 1985.

Olds, D. L., Henderson, C. R., Tatelbaum, R., and Chamberlin, R. Improving the delivery of prenatal care and outcomes of pregnancy: A randomized trial of nurse home visitation. *Pediatrics* 77 : 16, 1986.

Oski, F. A. Vitamin E deficiency: A previously unrecognized cause of hemolytic anemia in the premature infant. *J. Pediatr.* 70 : 211, 1967.

Peevyl, K. J., Speed, F. A., and Hoff, C. J. Epidemiology of inguinal hernia in preterm neonates. *Pediatrics* 77 : 246, 1986.

Peltola, H., Hayhty, H., and Virtanes, M. Prevention of *Hemophilus influenzae* type B bacteremic infections with the capsular polysaccharide vaccine. *N. Engl. J. Med.* 310 : 1561, 1984.

Porat, R. Care of the infant with ROP. *Clin. Perinatol.* 11 : 123, 1984.

Redo, S. F. *Principles of Surgery in the First Six Months*. Hagerstown, Md.: Harper & Row, 1976.

Redshaw, M., Rivers, R., and Rosenblatt, D. *Born Too Early: Special Care for Your Preterm Infant*. New York: Oxford University Press, 1985.

Rescoria, F. J., and Grosfeld, J. L. Inguinal hernia repair in the perinatal period and early infancy: Clinical considerations. *J. Pediatr. Surg.* 19 : 832, 1984.

Riordan, J., and Nicholas, F. H. Breastfeeding and self-care. *J. Perinatol.* 5 : 30, 1985.

Schmitt, B. D. Colic: Excessive crying in newborns. *Clin. Perinatol.* 12 : 441, 1985.

Sheftel, D. N., Hustead, V., and Friedman, A. Hypertension screening in the follow-up of premature infants. *Pediatrics* 71 : 763, 1983.

Shojania, A. M. Folic acid and vitamin B_{12} deficiency in pregnancy and in the neonatal period. *Clin. Perinatol.* 11 : 433, 1984.

Special Care Magazine: For Parents of High Risk Infants. Petaluma, Calif.: Neonatal Network Publishers.

Steward, D. J. Preterm infants are more prone to complications following minor surgery than are term infants. *Anesthesiology* 56 : 304, 1982.

Symposium on developmental and behavioral issues in perinatology. *Clin. Perinatol.* 12 : 307, 1985.

Task Force on Prevention of Low Birth Weight and Infant Mortality. *Closing the Gaps: Strate-*

gies for Improving the Health of Massachusetts Infants. Report to the Massachusetts Public Health Department. Privately printed, May 1985.

Taubman, B. Clinical trial of the treatment of colic by modification of parent-infant interaction. *Pediatrics* 74 : 998, 1984.

Trause, M. A., Hilliard, J. K., Malek, V. R., and Kramer, L. I. Successful lactation in mothers of preterms. *J. Perinatol.* 5 : 22, 1985.

von Hofsten, C. Eye-hand coordination in the newborn. *Dev. Psychology* 18 : 450, 1982.

Wallerstein, E. *Circumcision: An American Health Fallacy.* New York: Springer, 1980.

Wiswell, T. E., Smith, F. R., and Bass, J. R. Decreased incidence of urinary tract infections in circumcised male infants. *Pediatrics.* 75 : 901, 1985.

Wong, V. C. W., Ip, H. M., Reesink, H. W., et al. Prevention of the HB_sAg carrier state in newborn infants of mothers who are chronic carriers of HB_sAg and HB_eAg by administration of HBV and HBIG. *Lancet* 1 : 921, 1984.

Mechanics of Follow-up Clinics

H. William Taeusch and Janice Ware

I. Introduction

Follow-up assessment and care for graduates of neonatal intensive care units (NICUs) are a new frontier of pediatrics. Large numbers of infants are being discharged with new diagnoses for which pediatricians have not been trained (e.g., chronic lung disease of prematurity and intraventricular hemorrhage [IVH]). "Old" diseases thought to be a thing of the past, such as retrolental fibroplasia (retinopathy of prematurity), have an increasing prevalence.

Our neonatology program has a renewed interest in follow-up care for several reasons. It seems immoral to us to spend upward of $1,000 per day on the inpatient care of a premature infant and then to abnegate responsibility abruptly when the parents take the infant home (Hack, 1986). There is clear evidence that recovery from the events of premature birth takes place during the months, even years, after discharge. Caretakers in the general community are insufficiently trained and experienced in the special risks, assessments, and care required by these infants and parents during the first years of life.

In this age of too many doctors and excessive health care costs, we are reluctant to contribute yet another layer of health care. An infant follow-up program (IFUP) in an urban setting associated with a tertiary medical center can be viewed as a hard-to-justify expense and a redundancy in the face of other tertiary services. Nonetheless, forces from the areas of teaching, service, and research continue to push in favor of programs such as these.

II. Goals

A. Service

The IFUP coordinates tertiary services for NICU graduates at highest risk. For example, a 19-year-old mother may need help in coordinating cardiology, ophthalmology, and social service appointments. Parents can be helped to distinguish major from minor problems. An IFUP can serve as a safety net to help families to avoid errors of omission from lack of knowledge (e.g., how to avoid a repeat premature birth). The IFUP emphasis on development addresses the major question of most parents of a high-risk infant: "Will my infant be all right?" The IFUP link with neonatology directs attention to specific problems relating to the neonatal period, for example, hearing and retinopathy screening. The follow-up staff provides a force for improved discharge planning from the NICU by providing a viewpoint from "the other side of the fence." All of these functions are best viewed as adjuncts to primary pediatricians, other tertiary services, and early intervention programs. Finally, the service function of an IFUP is best justified if its focus is on those at highest risk.

In more specific terms, follow-up programs should meet a variety of needs.

1. Infant

   The IFUP identifies the extent of disabilities associated with fetal and neonatal diseases to create strategies for maximal recovery. Assessment of development and family nurturing capabilities must be geared to the special needs of NICU graduates, and these assessments are usually more detailed than assessments for normal newborns. Direct links with the NICU guarantees implementation of discharge medication and planning. Appropriate consultation and referral is easily and often informally carried out in the setting of an IFUP.

   One of the biggest lessons learned from follow-up is that risk does not equal injury, injury does not equal damage, and even a precise description of damage does not allow a precise prediction about recovery or outcome. This point is illustrated by our changing thinking about IVH:

   a. Early 1970s: Infants with the clinical diagnosis of IVH perhaps should not be supported on ventilators because of the potential for severe developmental impairments.

   b. Mid 1970s: Clinical diagnosis of IVH when assessed by newer imaging techniques is often wrong. Computed tomographic (CT) scans and ultrasonography indicate adverse outcome with severe IVH and presence or absence of hydrocephalus.

   c. Early 1980s: Infants with severe IVH and shunted hydrocephalus may have far better outcome than predicted, depending on care received in the first 2 years (after NICU discharge).

2. Parents

   After discharge of their infant from the NICU is often the first time that the parents can think about more than whether their infant will live or die that day. They want the best information about how to care for their infant and about the consequences of perinatal conditions for later life.

3. Pediatrician

   The pediatrician needs advice and information that he or she cannot readily obtain in an office setting. Legible, specific test results received soon after the follow-up program visit are most useful. The pediatrician needs the support of the NICU and follow-up program in the continuing care of the infant. The follow-up program should not overstep its consulting role by subverting the pediatrician. Visits should be carefully coordinated to spread the support that parents receive and to avoid redundancy (e.g., two or three visits within the same week).

4. Community service

   Community service agencies need concise and factual medical information about the status of the infant with well-thought-through requests, recommendations, and assessment plans. Key, consistent, and accessible personnel familiar with the infant should be identified for future contact.

5. House staff

The house staff should be encouraged to participate in providing follow-up care for NICU families after discharge in an organized and supervised manner, yet the follow-up care of the infants should not rest solely with the house staff, because of their heavy in-service time demands. Feedback to the house staff from the IFUP program in the form of letters on the current status of their former patients and intermittent teaching sessions on various aspects of care of NICU graduates are key and underdeveloped aspects of current pediatric training.

6. NICU nurses

Year-in, year-out work in the stressful environment of an NICU can distort the nurse's vision of the meaning of this narrow segment of time in a family's life. One of the great needs of those who work in the NICU is for information, specifically and generally, about the outcome of their patients. This information provides additional meaning for their work. The IFUP can meet these needs by providing copies of medical reports on former NICU patients as well as data summaries of NICU graduates grouped by disease, treatment techniques, and year of birth.

B. Education

Perinatologists and neonatologists are dealing with new diseases and new approaches to old problems that continue after infants are discharged from NICUs. Nurses, house officers, fellows, psychologists, physical therapists, social workers, and others find the IFUP an excellent training ground. An IFUP should have a component of outreach so that those involved with primary care can gain familiarity with the new diseases and ways to treat and prevent them.

C. Research

The IFUP is easiest to justify in terms of research. Neonatologists fear problems such as those that occurred after exposure to diethylstilbestrol, sulfonamides, and thalidomide in utero or oxygen after birth. Recent studies of infants after exposure to glucocorticoids and indomethacin have documented the reassurance possible by follow-up research. Prevention of repeat premature birth and explorations of efficacy of early intervention are currently exciting applied-research frontiers in the area of follow-up. An invaluable service of the IFUP is maintaining contact with high-risk infants for potential follow-up studies (e.g., those with shunted hydrocephalus or those who received new or unusual drugs). The study of development (cognition, vision, language, emotional, behavioral) in a normal population that was dramatically immature at birth should allow important new insights into regulators of infant development.

III. Patient selection

In our follow-up program, patient selection is dictated by our wish to provide service only for those at high risk and by limited staff in the follow-up clinic.

A. Very low birth weight infants (<1,250 g birth weight)

B. Infants with specific neurologic problems
   1. All grades of IVH
   2. Seizures related to IVH or asphyxia
   3. Asphyxia requiring ventilator treatment
   4. Hearing and vision problems

C. Infants with chronic lung disease

D. Infants from the NICU with complex sociofamilial situations

E. Infants on specific study protocols
   With more than 12,000 infants born per year in the nurseries for which the Joint Program in Neonatology, Boston, is responsible, we estimate that approximately 350 infants per year (about one-third of our NICU discharges with length of stay >24 hours) meet the criteria for these special follow-up needs. The breakdown of new patients according to entry criteria is

<1250 g	36%*
Bronchopulmonary dysplasia	22%
Neurologic abnormality	32%
Research	30%
Other	20%

   In our program a variety of infants in special categories, (e.g., meningomyelocele, chromosomal defects, phenylketonuria defects [PKU]), are seen in other specific clinics or programs.

IV. Patient flow
   Staff from our follow-up program spend about 3 hours per week in each of our three nurseries identifying the patients who meet intake criteria and consulting on available follow-up services. They generate a master file referral form and request that an infant follow-up clinic referral form (Figs. 7-1 and 7-2) and a dictated discharge summary be sent to the follow-up program office. (The master referral form is encoded on an IBM PC microcomputer using Ashton-Tate's Database III Program.) The IFUP nurse is responsible for calling the parents in the first several weeks after discharge. A postdischarge IFUP visit is set up at that time.

V. Clinic visits
   Most families are seen between 2 and 6 weeks after discharge. A neonatologist sees the family at this visit for several purposes:

   To ensure that discharge plans are understood and are being implemented

*Individual patients may be allocated to one or more categories.

Fig. 7-1. Master file referral form from the Joint Program in Neonatology *(JPN)*, completed for each JPN discharge referred to infant follow-up program *(IFUP)*. *BI* = Beth Israel Hospital; *BPD* = bronchopulmonary dysplasia; *BWH* = Brigham and Women's Hospital; *DEC* = Developmental Evaluation Clinic; *ICH* = intracranial hemorrhage; *NEC* = necrotizing enterocolitis; *PDA* = patent ductus arteriosus; *PFC* = persistent fetal circulation; *PT* = physical therapy; *RDS* = respiratory distress syndrome; *ROP* = retinopathy of prematurity; *TCH* = The Children's Hospital.

```
I. Contact information          Data code number  |_|_|_|_|        (1)
Last name                       |_|_|_|_|_|_|_|_|_|_|_|_|_|_|      (2)
First name                      |_|_|_|_|_|_|_|_|_|_|_|_|_|_|      (3)
Primary caretaker                                 |_|_|           (4)
     MO = Mother
     FA  = Father
     EX  = Extended family
     FO  = Foster care
     O   = Other
Caretaker's name                |_|_|_|_|_|_|_|_|_|_|_|_|_|_|_|    (5)
Mailing address                 |_|_|_|_|_|_|_|_|_|_|_|_|_|_|_|    (6)
City                          ·|_|_|_|_|_|_|_|_|_|_|_|_|_|_|_|     (7)
State |_|_|                              Zip |_|_|_|_|_|         (8–9)
Home phone                      |_|_|_|-|_|_|_|-|_|_|_|_|        (10)
Insurance                                        |_|_|_|_|       (11)
     BCBS    = Blue Cross/Blue Shield
     CHAM    = Champus
     COMM    = Commercial
     HCHP    = Harvard Community Health Plan
     MEDI    = Medicaid
     MEDC    = Medicare
     OHMO    = Other health maintenance organization
     SELF    = Self-pay
Primary pediatrician  |_____|         (12)
     Address       |_|_|_|_|_|_|_|_|_|_|_|_|_|_|_|_|_|_|_|_|      (13)
     City          |_|_|_|_|_|_|_|_|_|_|_|_|_|_|_|_|_|_|_|_|      (14)
     State |_|_|                          Zip |_|_|_|_|_|_|   (15–16)
II. Infant follow-up criteria information (0 = no, 1 = yes)
     1. <1250                                      |_|           (17)
     2. Neurologic                                 |_|           (18)
     3. BPD                                         |_|           (19)
     4. Research project                           |_|           (20)
          Specify:              |_____|               (21)
     5. Other (indicate all):                      |_|           (22)
          Social concerns                          |_|           (23)
          Parental desire                          |_|           (24)
          Other, specify       |_____|               (25)

III. Natal data
     A. Birth data
          1. Birthdate (M, D, Y)   |_|_|/|_|_|/|_|_|            (26)
          2. Gestational age (weeks)          |_|_|             (27)
          3. Birthweight (grams)            |_|_|_|_|           (28)
          4. Sex                               |_|              (29)
               1 = Male
               2 = Female
          5. Maternal age                    |_|_|              (30)
          6. Birth hospital       |_____|            (31)
```

Fig. 7-1 (continued)

```
        7. JPN nurseries—list all (0 = no, 1 = yes)
           (a) TCH                                        |___|      (32)
           (b) BWH                                        |___|      (33)
           (c) BI                                         |___|      (34)
        8. Date of discharge              |__|_/_|__/_|__|            (35)
        9. Discharged where?                              |___|      (36)
           1 = Home
           2 = Level II, specify      |_____|            (37)
     B. Risk data
        1. Major diagnoses (0 = no, 1 = yes)
           (a) Apnea                                      |__|       (38)
               (1) Home monitor                           |__|       (39)
               (2) Theophylline                           |__|       (40)
           (b) Asphyxia                                   |__|       (41)
           (c) BPD                                        |__|       (42)
               Home on $O_2$?                             |__|       (43)
           (d) ICH                                        |__|       (44)
               (1) Grade I, II, III, IV, or ?            |__|       (45)
               (2) Shunt (0 = no, 1 = yes)               |__|       (46)
           (e) NEC                                        |__|       (47)
           (f) PDA                                        |__|       (48)
               (1) Indomethacin (0 = no, 1 = yes)        |__|       (49)
               (2) Surgery (0 = no, 1 = yes)             |__|       (50)
           (g) PFC                                        |__|       (51)
           (h) ROP                                        |__|       (52)
               Grade 1, 2, 3, 4, or ?                    |__|       (53)
           (i) RDS                                        |__|       (54)
        2. $FiO_2$ on day 28                           |__|__|__|    (55)
        3. # Vent days                                |__|__|__|    (56)

IV. Contact and scheduling information
     A. Contact information
        1. Referral contact made? (0 = no, 1 = yes)      |__|       (57)
        2. Date referral contact made      |__|_/_|__/_|__|          (58)
        3. How made?                                      |__|       (59)
           1 = Letter
           2 = Phone
        4. Appt. made? (0 = no, 1 = yes, 2 = recontact)   |__|       (60)
           (a) If yes, date                |__|_/_|__/_|__|          (61)
           (b) If no, specify reason                      |__|       (62)
               1 = Parental disinterest
               2 = Lack of funds or insurance
               3 = Does not meet criteria
               4 = Other, specify |_____|               (63)
           (c) If recontact, specify date  |__|_/_|__/_|__|          (64)
     B. Scheduling information
        1. Date last vision test           |__|_/_|__/_|__|          (65)
        2. Date last hearing test          |__|_/_|__/_|__|          (66)
        3. Specialty evals this visit (0 = no, 1 = yes, ? = not sure)
           (a) Psychology                                 |__|       (67)
           (b) PT                                         |__|       (68)
           (c) Refer to DEC ?                             |__|       (69)
V. Comments _____

VI. Form completed by  _____  Date  _____
    Infant follow-up program
```

Fig. 7-2. Infant follow-up clinic discharge form from the Joint Program in Neonatology.
AGA = average for gestational age; *BPD* = bronchopulmonary dysplasia; *CPAP* = continuous positive airway pressure; *GI* = gastrointestinal; *IVH* = intraventricular hemorrhage; *LGA* = large for gestational age; *LMP* = last menstrual period; *NICU* = neonatal intensive care unit; *PDA* = patent ductus arteriosus; *RDS* = respiratory distress syndrome; *SGA* = small for gestational age.

Referral criteria (circle) 1. < 1250 g   2. BPD   3. Neuro
           4. Study   5. Other _____

Infant's name _____ Chart # _____ Hospital _____
Mother's name _____ Address _____ Tel. # _____
Para _____ Maternal age _____
Gravida _____

Sex   M   F
Birth date (M/D/Y)   ____/____/____
Birth weight (g)   _____
Weight at discharge (g)   _____
Birth length (cm)   _____
Discharge length (cm)   _____
Head circumference (cm at birth)   _____
Head circumference (cm at discharge)   _____
Apgar   1 _____ 5 _____
LMP (M/D/Y)   ____/____/____
Gestational age   By wk __ By exam __
                              AGA/SGA/LGA (circle)
Multiple birth (sequence #/total)   _____ / _____
Cesarean section (Y/N ?emergency ?elective)   _____
Number of days in nursery   ICU_____Total_____
Date of discharge/transfer (specify home or list which
   hospital)   _____
Number of days parenteral alimentation   _____
Discharge hematocrit/retics (date)   Hct ____ Retics ____
                              Date ___ / ___ / ___
                  Patient's name   _____
Resuscitation at delivery (Y/N/type)   _____
Birth trauma (Y/N/type)   _____
Was this pregnancy complicated (Y/N/why?)   _____
Retinopathy of prematurity (ROP) (Y/N)   ____Date of last exam
                              ____/____/____
Retrolental fibroplasia (RLF) (Y/N)   ____Date of last exam
                              ____/____/____
   Grades: I
            II
            III
            IV
            V
   Right eye (grade)   _____
   Left eye (grade)   _____
RDS (Y/N/note mild, moderate, or severe)   _____
Other lung disease (Y/N/specify)   _____
Air leak(s) (Y/N) (describe)   _____
BPD (Y/N)   _____
PDA (Y/N/specify treatment: diuretics, indomethacin,
   surgery)   _____
Cyanosis and/or congestive cardiac failure (Y/N)   _____
   If yes, specify use of digoxin or diuretics   _____

Fig. 7-2 (continued)

Congenital heart malformation (Y/N/specify) _____
Cardiac/pulmonary arrest requiring resuscitation (Y/N) _____
Hypotension/shock (Y/N) _____
IVH (Y/N) _____
   If yes, grade?
         I
         II
         III
         IV _____
   Severity (mild, moderate, severe) _____
   How confirmed _____
Seizures (Y/N/specify suspected or confirmed) _____
Meningitis (Y/N/specify suspected or positive culture) _____
Asphyxia (Y/N) _____
   If yes, specify perinatal or neonatal _____
   If yes, specify severity (mild, moderate, severe) _____
Other (i.e., rare neurologic disease; specify) _____
Necrotizing enterocolitis (Y/N/suspected) _____
   If yes, ?surgery (Y/N) _____
Other GI condition (include malformations or anomalies) _____
Renal (failure or specify other) _____
Other infections (Y/N/note confirmed, suspected, or type) _____
   Sepsis _____
   Urinary tract infection _____
   Other _____
Highest bilirubin: Total _____
             Indirect _____
                        Date _____/_____/_____
Polycythemia (Y/N) _____
Hypoglycemia (<25) (Y/N) _____
Hyperglycemia (Y/N) _____
Hyponatremia (Y/N) _____
Hypernatremia (>150) (Y/N) _____
Other (specify) _____

Treatments
Phototherapy (Y/N) _____
Exchange transfusion(s) (Y/N) _____
Ventilatory support (Y/N) _____
   If yes, specify
      # of days on ventilator _____
      # days CPAP _____
      Total days on O_2 _____
      # of days O_2 >40% _____
Chest tube(s) (Y/N) _____
Umbilical artery catheter (Y/N) _____
Central venous catheter (Y/N) _____
Surgery (Y/N/specify) _____
Medications
   New, unusual, or experimental (specify) _____
   Vasoactive drugs (specify) _____
   Theophylline/caffeine (Y/N) _____
   Discharge medications (specify) _____
_____
_____

Fig. 7-2 (continued)

```
Hearing exam (Y/N/specify type of test)      _____
  If yes, specify date                       _____/_____/_____
  Results                                    _____
Home on monitor (Y/N)                        _____
Home on oxygen (Y/N)                         _____
Discharge diagnoses (list)                   _____
                                             _____
                                             _____
                                             _____

Date of discharge                            _____/_____/_____
Names and titles of NICU staff who know infant
  well and desire feedback                   _____
                                             _____
                                             _____
                                             _____
Follow-up appointment plans                  _____
                                             _____
Primary pediatrician                         _____
  Address                                    _____
  Telephone #                                _____-_____-_____
Specify R.N./M.D. to see in follow-up clinic _____
Comments:


Person completing form   _____
```

To respond to unresolved questions or concerns about events that took
   place during the fetal and perinatal period
To assess problems occurring since discharge
To plan for the coordinated use of resources for the next months

Families are then seen according to their individual plan, but at the minimum, they are seen at 6 months' corrected age by a nurse or physician (or
both) skilled in perinatal and developmental pediatrics, then at 1, 2, and 3
years' corrected age by the same professional and an infant psychologist.
(Corrected age is chronologic age minus the number of weeks of prematurity.) Physical therapists consult frequently, especially in the first year, to diagnose, recommend treatments, and monitor progress. Virtually all of the infants meeting our criteria for referral are referred to community-based early
intervention programs.
   A typical visit at 1 year corrected age for a former 900 g premature infant
with a history of grade II IVH, mild chronic lung disease, and necrotizing enterocolitis includes

Routine pediatric history and examination, including growth and nutrition-
   al assessments
Bayley examination by an infant psychologist
A check by a physical therapist if tone abnormalities persist

We ensure that routine hearing and vision checks have been done and that
other consultations and research needs have been met (e.g., neurologic ex-

Fig. 7-3. Every-visit data-coding form from the Joint Program in Neonatology (JPN) to be completed during every infant follow-up program (IFUP) visit. BPD = bronchopulmonary dysplasia; DEC = Developmental Evaluation Clinic; DOB = date of birth; NICU = neonatal intensive care unit; ROP = retinopathy of prematurity; TCH = The Children's Hospital.

```
 1. Last name  |_____|   (1)
 2. First name |_____|   (2)
 3. DOB                                        |___/___/___|        (3)
 4. Date of this visit                         |___/___/___|        (4)
 5. Reason for IFUP visit (indicate all)
      <1,250|___|            Neuro|___|         BPD|___|
      Research project, specify |_____|  Other, specify |_____|  (5-9)
 6. TCH #                           |___ ___-___ ___-___ ___|        (10)
 7. Height (cm)                              |__|__|__|"|__|         (11)
 8. Weight (kg)                              |__|__|__|"|__|         (12)
 9. Head circumference (cm)                  |__|__|__|"|__|         (13)
10. Maternal race                                        |__|       (14)
      1 = Caucasian   3 = Hispanic
      2 = Black       4 = Other, specify |_____|        (15)
11. Last grade mother completed in school                |__|       (16)
      1 = Less than 9th grade        3 = High school graduate
      2 = 9th through 12th grade     4 = Completed some college
                                     5 = College degree or more
12. ROP: Date last exam                       |__|/__|/__|          (17)
      Result (1 = normal, 2 = abnormal, 3 = suspect)      |__|       (18)
13. Hearing: Date last exam                   |__|/__|/__|          (19)
      Result (1 = normal, 2 = abnormal, 3 = suspect       |__|       (20)
14. # Hospitalizations since NICU discharge              |__|__|    (21)
15. Exam outcomes (1 = normal, 2 = abnormal, 3 = suspect)
      A. Developmental assessment                        |__|       (22)
      B. Pediatric exam                                  |__|       (23)
      C. Neurologic assessment                           |__|       (24)
      D. Behavior/temperament                            |__|       (25)
      E. Maternal-infant interaction                     |__|       (26)
      F. Major social problems                           |__|       (27)
      G. Language                                        |__|       (28)
      H. Gross motor                                     |__|       (29)
      I. Fine motor                                      |__|       (30)
      J. Psychologic exam                                |__|       (31)
         1. Mental age (months)                |__|__|"|__|         (32)
         2. Psychologist |_____|            (33)
      K. Physical therapist |_____|             (34)
16. List current major diagnoses  A. |_____|            (35)
                                  B. |_____|            (36)
                                  C. |_____|            (37)
17. List today's lab tests        A. |_____|            (38)
                                  B. |_____|            (39)
                                  C. |_____|            (40)
18. Date of next IFUP appointment             |__|/__|/__|          (41)
19. Clinic site of this visit (1 = JPN, 2 = DEC)         |__|       (42)
20. Total charge for this visit             $ |__|__|__|            (43)
21. MD/RN signature |_____|          (44)
```

amination or serial pulmonary function testing for infants with chronic lung disease). A letter with our findings is addressed to the primary pediatrician with copies to parents and all consultants and support services. Data forms (Figs. 7-3 and 7-4) are filled in at every visit, and selected items are entered on the cumulative Database III record. Color-coded and age-specific forms have been found useful in several large follow-up studies. Our IFUP is relatively new and currently represents a bare-bones approach. Older IFUPs offer an expanded range of services, research, and training opportunities (Sell, 1986).

VI. Consultants

The follow-up program should be contiguous to other ambulatory clinics such as surgery, neurology, genetics, pulmonary, psychiatry, special needs, orthopedic, neurosurgery, and cardiology. Consultation should be readily accessible and enhance service, teaching, and research in these areas.

VII. Fees

Patients are charged according to a sliding scale depending on the number of professionals seen, regardless of the length of visit. The range of clinic visit charges is from $40 to 160. Blue Cross/Blue Shield and most other private insurers often pay 80 percent of the charge; Medicaid pays 100 percent. Coverage varies and depends on the policies of the individual insurer. Pre-paid health care plans usually refuse to pay. In this case, if the parents are unable to pay, they are not charged. All research patients are underwritten.

VIII. Staffing and budget

A minimal yearly budget for an IFUP serving a delivery base of about 12,000 infants per year as previously described is $94,000. This budget is broken down as follows:

   25 percent of full-time equivalent salary for (FTE) director
   25 percent FTE for associate director or trainee
   100 percent FTE for secretary and data coordinator
   50 percent FTE for registered nurse or nurse practitioner
   50 percent for FTE physical therapist
   50 percent for FTE psychologist
   Fellows, advisory group, and consultants from relevant divisions
   Equipment and supplies
   Computer hardware and software (data entry by clinic personnel)
   Total is $94,000 per year; approximately $200 per patient visit equals direct costs

Because charges frequently do not cover costs, the inpatient neonatology charges and research studies are justifiable sources of income. We and others hypothesize that an active IFUP shortens both initial hospital stay and rehospitalization rates for this high-risk group; recent data support this assumption.

Fig. 7-4. Every-visit infant follow-up form from the Joint Program in Neonatology, to be completed during every infant follow-up program *(IFUP)* visit. *ABD* = abdomen; *BP* = blood pressure; *BPD* = bronchopulmonary dysplasia; *COR* = cor pulmonale; *DOB* = date of birth; *DPT* = diphtheria-pertussis-tetanus vaccine; *DTR* = deep tendon reflexes; *EENT* = ear, nose, and throat; *EIP* = early intervention program; *FE* = iron supplements; *GI* = gastrointestinal; *GU* = genitourinary; *HT* = hematocrit; *MS* = musculoskeletal; *ROP* = retinopathy of prematurity; *TNR* = tonic neck reflex; *VITS* = vitamins; *VNA* = visiting nurse association; * = datum to be encoded.

*1. Date of IFUP visit _____ / _____ / _____
2. Reason for IFUP visit
      <1250 _____ BPD _____ Neuro _____ Other (specify)_____
3. DOB _____ / _____ / _____
4. Chronologic age (to closest month) _____
5. Corrected age (to closest month) _____
6. IFUP visit #_____ 7. Date last IFUP visit _____ / _____ / _____
8. Parent concerns/problems:

  * A. Receiving community services? (EIP, VNA, etc.) _____
                 Yes = 1   No = 2
    Specify program/s and relevant details

    Contact person/s _____
    B. List specialists following child (include primary care pediatrician)

9. Interim health history:

  * A. #Hospitalizations since level II/III discharge
    B. Recent hospitalizations:
      (1) Hospital _____
            Date _____ / _____ / _____ Diagnosis _____
            Length of stay (# of days)_____
      (2) Hospital _____
            Date _____ / _____ / _____ Diagnosis _____
            Length of stay (# of days)_____
  * C. Date of most recent ROP check _____ / _____ / _____
       Result of test _____
           1 = Normal
           2 = Abnormal
           3 = Suspect
           4 = Not done
           5 = Don't know if done
           6 = To be scheduled
  * D. Date of most recent hearing test _____ / _____ / _____
       Result of test (code using vision codes 1–6 above) _____
    E. Other tests completed (including x-rays), list: _____

Fig. 7-4 (continued)

10. Review of systems/nursing assessment
    A. Feeding assessment
       (1) Breast-feeding? (> 50% of feeds)   Yes   No
       (2) Formula amounts/24 hours _____
       (3) Other foods _____
       (4) Vits (in addition to formula)   Yes   No
       (5) Fe (in addition to formula)   Yes   No
       (6) Nutritional adequacy _____
           1 = Adequate
           2 = Slow, gradual progress
           3 = Inadequate
       (7) Feeding skill development (code same as above) _____
       (8) Mother needs assistance with feeding   Yes   No
    B. Other systems
       (1) Neuro/dev/landmarks (specify milestones achieved):
           *Speech and language (age with 5 words) _____
           *Head control (age head in vertical plane for 30 secs _____ (months)
           *Sitting (age when sits 30 secs w/out support) _____
           *Walking (5 steps w/out support) _____
       (2) Behavior/habits:
           a. Temperament assessment _____
              1 = Easy
              2 = Difficult
              3 = Slow-to-warm-up
              4 = Other _____
           b. Developmental habits of concern (e.g., nail biting, sleep problems, encopresis)
       (3) Adaptive behaviors (e.g., occupies self, follows simple directions, self-feeding) _____
       (4) Family situation_____
       (5) Cardiovascular system _____
       (6) Pulm _____
       (7) Elimination/GI _____
       (8) Endo/growth _____
       (9) Musculoskeletal _____
       (10) Immune/infect _____
       (11) Heme_____Recent Hct?_____
       (12) Trauma/surg _____
       (13) Immunizations: DPT_____Sabin_____Mumps_____
       (14) Allergy _____
    C. Prescription medications?   Yes   No
       Drug _____ Dose _____ Frequency _____
       Drug _____ Dose _____ Frequency _____
       Drug _____ Dose _____ Frequency _____
    D. Physical exam results
       *(1) Weight in g (to one decimal place) _____
       *(2) Height in cm (to one decimal place) _____
       *(3) Head circum. in cm (to one decimal place) _____
       (4) Resting respiratory rate _____
           After pull to sit × 10 _____
       (5) Tcom O_2 sat _____
       (6) BP _____/_____ Method _____
       (7) Race _____
           1 = Caucasian
           2 = Black
           3 = Hispanic
           4 = Other

Fig. 7-4 (continued)

(8) Head_____	(9) EENT_____
(10) Chest _____	(11) COR_____
(12) ABD_____	(13) GU _____
(14) MS _____	(15) Other _____

E. Neurologic exam:

DTRs_____	Head lag_____
Moro_____	Suck_____
Vert sling_____	Grasp_____
Clonus_____	Babinski_____
TNR_____	O-V nystagmus_____
Tone_____	Vision_____
Hearing_____	Socializing_____
Sym move_____	Speech/gait_____
Other _____	

F. Psychologic assessment
    (1) Name of tester_____
    (2) Test administered _____
        1 = Bayley mental scale
        2 = Stanford-Binet
        3 = Other
        4 = Observational data, not test administered
   *(3) Developmental age (to nearest half-month)_____

G. Physical therapy assessment
    (1) Name of tester_____
    (2) Movement postures/patterns_____
        1 = Normal
        2 = Abnormal
        3 = Suspect
    (3) Motor development range:
      *a. Fine motor_____
          Normal = 1
          Abnormal = 2
          Suspect = 3
          Reason _____

      *b. Gross motor _____ (use fine motor codes above)
          Reason _____

H. Referral and report information
   *(1) Date of next visit to IFUP (mo yr) _____/_____
    (2) At this visit, seen by: (1) _____ (2) _____ (3)_____
   *(3) Final impressions:
       a. _____
       b. _____
       c. _____
    (4) Lab results _____
    (5) Recommendations_____

    (6) Date IFUP report sent _____/_____/_____
       Copies sent to (include addresses):
       _____
       _____
       _____

    (7) At the next IFUP visit, the child needs to see:
       (1) _____ (2) _____ (3) _____
    (8) MD/RN signature _____

    IFUP code number _____ _____ _____ _____ (Office use only)

REFERENCES

Hack, M., and Faneroff, A. Changes in the delivery room care of the extremely small infant (<750 g): Effects on morbidity and outcome. *N. Engl. J. Med.* 314 : 660, 1986.

Sell, E. *Follow-up Programs for Intensive Care Nursery Survivors.* Privately printed with support from Ross Laboratories, Columbus, Ohio, and the Laidlaw Foundation, Tucson, Arizona, 1986.

8

Nursing Participation

Eunice Shishmanian and Patricia N. Rissmiller

I. Introduction

In many tertiary centers, an infant follow-up program (IFUP) collaborates with the pediatrician to offer assistance to parents in the management of their high-risk infant after discharge from the neonatal intensive care unit (NICU). In this chapter, we outline mechanisms for interaction between the NICU and IFUP, emphasizing the role played by nurses.

II. Parents' needs

Parents' prime concern when their infant is discharged from the NICU is to be able to care for their child, who for such a long time has been cared for by experts. Services available to parents after discharge fall into two categories, those involving immediate needs and those involving long-term needs. Immediate needs include medical care, community services, developmental services, and family support. Long-term needs include medical specialty visits and an IFUP. An IFUP should be well planned and include referral criteria, referral forms, a brochure, and a referral mechanism.

III. Coordination of care before discharge

A coordinated system between the NICU and IFUP ensures continuity of services for infant and family. Ideally, this role is facilitated by a health professional, often a nurse, who acts as a liaison between these two closely related areas.

A. Neonatal intensive care unit staff

Professional staff working within the NICU is responsible for giving information to parents about follow-up services and helping them develop a positive attitude toward these resources. They have managed the infant through multiple crises and are perceived as most knowledgeable about necessary and appropriate follow-up care. They have developed important relationships with families at a time when the families were feeling helpless and vulnerable. Therefore, effective referrals can only be accomplished when the NICU has a complete picture of the philosophy, services, management issues, and environment of the IFUP and other services available after discharge, such as early intervention programs (EIPs), community nursing services, and community social service networks.

B. Nurse-coordinator

The IFUP nurse-coordinator is, in many programs, the professional who facilitates referrals. Providers in the NICU and the IFUP must have knowledge of current treatments of the high-risk infant and family, available services, and treatment programs. Shared educational programs provide a forum for exchange of information, encourage development of positive attitudes, and enhance communication between IFUP and NICU staffs. Material might include (1) philosophy of the follow-up service, (2) criteria for referral, (3) mechanical aspects of scheduling clients, (4) information about services provided and assessments utilized, (5) management of infant and family on clinic visit, (6) community resources, and (7) sharing information and findings with family, NICU staff, pediatrician, and community services.

The nurse-coordinator can be helpful to the NICU primary care team in developing the discharge plan. He or she is a resource of information about community services and can identify the service or services that best meet individual infant's and family's needs. The NICU nurses can plan for the infant based on extended contact with the infant and family. Consideration can be given as to whether the infant meets criteria for IFUP; a verbal discussion is more meaningful than exchange of forms.

Time spent by the IFUP nurse-coordinator in meeting families in the NICU has several benefits. Parents are able to ask questions about the follow-up services of the person who participates in those services. In addition, the IFUP can be a contact that offers support to the family when the infant leaves the NICU.

C. Collaboration of neonatal intensive care staff and follow-up nurse-coordinator

Through a joint effort of the NICU staff and IFUP nurse-coordinator, a familiarity with each other's knowledge, shared concerns, and attitude toward patients is developed. Communication fosters the building of trust and credibility so that parents feel a sense of comfortable progression from one service area to another.

In summary, the nurse-coordinator, the NICU, and the IFUP staff can assist families in receiving appropriate services by (1) having clear criteria for the follow-up program, (2) sharing current knowledge about IFUP, (3) having a clear and easy system for referral of the patient to IFUP, (4) acting as liaison between IFUP and NICU to provide for communication about families, (5) identifying infants with special follow-up needs through chart review, and (6) being available to meet with selected families prior to discharge from NICU.

IV. Coordination of follow-up after infant is home

After the infant's discharge from the hospital, the nurse-coordinator can serve as a resource for families about follow-up services. High-risk infants are generally helped by a minimum of three service providers: the primary pediatrician, community nurse, and EIP. Parents retain a strong regard for and attachment to the tertiary medical center where restorative services were provided for their infant. They rely on and expect the continued expertise of professionals at the center as a resource. The IFUP can meet these expectations, and the nurse-coordinator assumes the role of contact person.

Contacting families approximately 2 to 4 weeks after discharge ensures continuity of services. A telephone call to the family at this time can demonstrate concern for child and family, determine progress, identify concerns, determine if referral visits have been accomplished, address problems, and schedule follow-up visits.

This contact indicates that the tertiary center continues to care about the family. The timing is important. The parents need time to be independent. Their questions 2 to 4 weeks after discharge are usually specific and address unanticipated problems. Information given during the stressful time of the hospitalization often needs to be repeated. The immediate needs of the infant may demand the total energy of the parents; scant energy remains for finding additional resources. Often the mother's attitude that she should be able to "do it all" for her infant can paralyze her and prevent her from seeking help when needed. Thus a skilled health professional can assess the situation and suggest strategies for alleviating problems. Recommendations may include referral to additional services, a visit to the IFUP, or merely a talking through of the problem. Frequency of contact is determined by individual need following general protocol for regular calls and visits.

V. Prototype infant follow-up program

Infant follow-up programs are usually based in tertiary care centers and are often called "high-risk follow-up clinics." They provide periodic assessment and longitudinal observations of the child's development by an interdisciplinary team. The team may include professionals from the fields of nursing, neurology, nutrition, developmental pediatrics, physical therapy, psychology, and social work. Services provided to the infant and family include (1) assessment of the child's growth and development, (2) identification of medical concerns, (3) provision of parent education and guidance, and (4) provision of a plan of recommendation with referral to services.

The goals of IFUP include those of patient care, teaching, and research. Concern over long-term consequences of aspects of intensive care has increased interest in IFUPs. It is hoped that the problems associated with use of diethylstilbestrol, thalidomide, sulfonamides, and oxygen for the developing fetus and newborn can be alleviated by consistent follow-up.

Although the goals of the program are clear, criteria for patient selection are commonly based on a combination of funding availability and the research activities. There continues to be a lack of consensus among health professionals on the need for and definition of such programs; therefore, minimal funding is available for follow-up. This view is not consistent with that of the parents of NICU graduates who are eager for quality developmental and medical information as well as other services for their infant. The responsibility of the IFUP is that of providing for the infant's and parents' needs.

A. Infant
   1. Comprehensive assessment of development
   2. Identification of concerns for early treatment
   3. Implementation of medical follow-up (e.g., audiologic, ophthalmologic)
   4. Coordination of information among caretakers

B. Parent
  1. Assessment of family capabilities geared to special needs of NICU graduates
  2. Reassurance and development of a sense of competency
  3. Information about caretaking
  4. Provision of environment for discussions about development

C. Common eligibility criteria are aimed at those infants at highest risk.

VI. Nursing perspectives within infant follow-up programs

Nursing uses a family-systems approach to its assessment of the premature infant and his or her family during the visit to the follow-up clinic. General systems theory is useful as an organizing framework for analyzing specific situations as well as for organizing assessment data collected during the family visit to the IFUP clinic.

General systems theory assigns families characteristics or properties, including wholeness, nonsummativity, and equifinality. Wholeness refers to the interdependence of family members. The needs and strengths of one family member cannot be assessed without seeing how they affect all family members. Nonsummativity refers to the interrelationship of all parts of the family system; thus the whole is more than the sum of its parts. A picture of family functioning cannot be obtained by a summation of individual scores. Equifinality describes the circular nature of interactions within families. One member's behavior affects the behavior of the other family members.

Using system concepts, families can be further described as having boundaries that define who can participate in the family system. Family boundaries also specify the degree to which members of that system allow input on information to flow in and out. The boundaries help families maintain equilibrium as well as allow the change and growth necessary to adaptation. Family members must continually modify their behavior and adjust to the demands and resources of both the outside environment and their own internal needs to function as an effective unit.

According to Sammons and Lewis (1985), visits to a follow-up clinic are a source of anxiety for the parents. This anxiety is present for parents who have been reassured that their infant is developing normally at the time of hospital discharge as well as for parents of infants for whom there is concern. When problems are suspected, parents worry if this is the visit that might document these problems. To help reduce parental anxiety about the follow-up visits, the family must be oriented to the clinic and its procedures to ensure that the visit will be comfortable and productive. The following must be carefully explained: mechanics of the evaluation, disciplines that will evaluate the infant, length of time involved in the clinic, procedure for sharing results of the evaluation, and procedure for implementing recommendations and referrals.

VII. Nursing goals

In addition to the responsibility for coordinating NICU and IFUP planning, nursing has the following overall goals:

Assessment of infant and family
Identification of family and infant needs
Communication of information to the family
Education and guidance of the family

The evaluation follows the usual nursing process of assessment, analysis of data, plan of intervention and further evaluation, and recommendations. Specific objectives of the nursing interview during the infant follow-up visit are to assess the family's management of the infant's day-to-day activities, the infant's health, the infant's developmental progress, and the relationships among family members vis-à-vis the infant.

VIII. Assessment

A. Nutrition, feeding, and growth
Information is collected about the infant's daily activities, including feeding, sleeping, elimination, and behavior patterns. Equally important is the impact on the family of the caretaking needs of the infant.
Feeding and weight gain cause great anxiety for the family of the premature infant. Parents know that medical complications are inversely related to an infant's weight, and great emphasis is therefore placed on feeding and weight gain from the first day. This pressure can continue after discharge, resulting in feedings becoming a battle between parent and infant rather than a relaxed time when infant and parent can enjoy each other.
It takes time for all parents to learn to understand the behavioral cues given by their infant. This is especially true for the premature infant who often does not give clear hunger or satiation signals. Parents may feel unsure about the adequacy of feedings. This doubt, coupled with the earlier emphasis on weight gain, often leads the parents to assume the infant is hungry each time he or she awakens. This miscommunication may result in fatigue of both parent and infant, poor intake during a feeding, mixed messages to the infant, and anxiety for the parents.
Parents benefit from information on judging the dietary intake of their infant, establishing feeding patterns, and reading behavioral cues to decrease the stress and worry associated with feeding. Frequency of voidings and patterns of sleeping between feedings are helpful as guides in assessing the adequacy of intake.
It is also important to elicit information from the parents about the feeding experience itself; this includes the time it takes, how it fits into the family schedule, the number of feeders, and the quality of the experience. The last issue is not easy to assess but is determined by listening to the caretakers' discussion of the infant's feeding experience as well as their perspective of his or her nutritional status. The following areas are important in the assessment process:
1. Nutrition
   a. Types of food eaten
   b. Amounts of food eaten

           c. Textures of foods
       2. Feeding behavior
           a. Development of feeding skills
           b. Feeding schedules and patterns
           c. Social interactions during mealtimes
       3. Growth
           a. Measurements of height, weight, and head circumference
           b. Plotting of growth measurements on growth charts

B. Elimination

Information is collected regarding the infant's elimination, including regularity, frequency, consistency, and use of medications. It is important to screen for indications of other problems, such as reflux, malabsorption, or food allergies.

C. Sleep patterns

Premature infants have difficulty establishing regular sleep-wake patterns during the first year of life owing to physiologic immaturity and the NICU experiences. Superimposed is the parents' concern and protectiveness. Often there is confusion as to whether to wake a child for feedings according to a schedule or to feed on demand. Waking the infant can cause distress and be costly in terms of energy. This situation should be evaluated and guidance based on the infant's nutritional state, medical problems, and tolerance for feedings. Promoting sleep also depends to a degree on the parents' knowledge and skill in reading the infant's behavioral cues (sleep states). Helping the parents recognize deep sleep (quiet state with regular breathing) and helping them feel comfortable about not waking the infant will result in a restful and relaxed infant who will with time achieve the skill of sleeping longer.

A composite of night sleep and naptime determines the amounts of sleep-wake times for the infant. Achieving a somewhat predictable sleep schedule for their infant also allows the parents a reasonable night's rest. Without sleep deprivation parents are usually able to deal with infant demands more effectively.

As the infant progresses, it is also important to assess bedtime behaviors. Comfortable routines aid the infant in finding ways to settle down with decreased dependence on parents.

D. Crying

Parents frequently need to be informed about crying. Considering the early days in the NICU when the infant's survival may have been questionable, it is not unusual for parents to feel uncomfortable about letting the infant cry. Recognizing the infant's capabilities to console him- or herself and finding ways to help this behavior can ease difficulties in managing fussing and crying.

E. Behavior

It is important to listen to parental reports of behavior because they can provide a more complete picture of their infant, including strengths and weaknesses. This contrasts to the assessments carried out during the follow-up visit, which is constrained by time and often seems more focused on the infant's problem areas than on his or her achievements. The relationship between infant and parents is characterized by reciprocity; each member is influenced by the other's personality and behavioral characteristics. Infants perceived as difficult, irritable, or fussy are at risk for maladaptive relationships with parents as it is difficult for some parents to be sensitive to the needs of such an infant. Frodi (1983) states that the mother's perception of her infant's temperament is one factor that influences both the attachment process and sociability.

As part of the nursing interview, parents are asked about the infant's general behavior, attention span, consolability, and activity levels. This information, in combination with observations of behavior during the visit and developmental assessments, provides a view of the infant's overall behavior and identifies infants who may benefit from intervention.

F. Adaptation between infant and family
The characteristics of the family as a social system discussed in sec. VI are especially useful for organizing data obtained in the nursing assessment. For example, because stress or problems in any family member affect all other parts of that system, it is important to collect information about the functioning of the family as a whole. Information should include employment of family members, changes imposed on the family, the loss of jobs of family members, persons living in the household, use of child care, and the health and educational concerns of the siblings.

Premature infants may be at risk for early disturbances in the parent-infant relationship for several reasons (Goldberg et al., 1980). The mother may not have been prepared psychologically for the birth owing to the infant's early arrival; the infant, because of his or her immature physiologic state, may not be as responsive or alert as a full-term infant; parents may have difficulty reading behavioral cues; and parents may have had the first months with their infant adversely affected by the NICU experiences. Parents' attachment to their infant may also be hindered owing to a phenomenon called the *vulnerable child concept* (Solnit and Green, 1977). After some children have recovered from a serious or life-threatening illness, parents may continue to believe and to treat the child as if at high risk. All of these factors may make parents reluctant to invest their emotional energies or can result in an overprotective attitude.

The nurse observes and listens carefully as the parents relate their perceptions and expectations of their infant. A comprehensive developmental profile of the infant is further summarized by the interdisciplinary team and shared with the parents.

G. Education
Although the emphasis is on assessment during the nursing interview, parent education and guidance are implicit throughout. Teaching is incorporated into each phase of the assessment with the following goals:
1. Promotion of infant development and health
2. Correction of parental misinformation or misconceptions

3. Facilitation of family management of the infant
4. Facilitation of family adaptation to the birth of a premature infant
5. Counseling of other family concerns
6. Prevention of recurrence of premature births

IV. Summary

In our experience, parents of former NICU infants value the opportunity to discuss problems with the nurse that they may be unable to discuss with the physician. In this way, nursing has a unique role in gaining important new information and in unraveling difficult management problems. Telephone contact and home visits can be invaluable in aiding the parents in caring for their "special" infant.

REFERENCES

Crnic, K., Ragozin, A., Greenberg, M., et al. Social interaction and developmental competence of preterm and full-term infants during the first year of life. *Child Dev.* 54 : 1199, 1983.

Frodi, A. Attachment behavior and sociability with strangers in premature and full-term infants. *Infant Ment. Health J.* No. 1, Spring 1983. P. 15.

Goldberg, S., Brachfield, S., and DeVitto, B. Feeding, Fussing and Play: Parent-Infant Interaction in the First Year as a Function of Prematurity and Perinatal Medical Problems. In T. Field (ed.), *High-Risk Infants and Children.* New York: Academic, 1980.

Johnson, S. M. *Parenting.* Philadelphia: Lippincott, 1979.

Miller, J., and Janosik, E. *Family Focused Care.* New York: McGraw-Hill, 1980.

Morris, P. G. Nutrition screening for the term and preterm infant. Long Beach, Calif.: Memorial Hospital Medical Center, 1983.

Sammons, W., and Lewis, J. *Premature Babies.* St. Louis: Mosby, 1985.

Solnit, A., and Green, M. Reactions to the Threatened Loss of a Child. In L. Schwarz (ed.), *Vulnerable Infants.* New York: McGraw-Hill, 1977.

VonBertalanffy, L. *General Systems Theory.* New York: Brazillen, 1968.

Wheelock College and The Children's Hospital. Access to developmental services for NICU graduates. A state-of-the-art paper at New England, Region I, 1985.

III

Assessment Procedures

Hearing Screening

Martin C. Schultz

I. Introduction

High-risk infants have a higher incidence (2.5–5.0%) of moderate to profound hearing loss than other infants (1%), suggesting that audiologic testing of high-risk infants is important. The 1982 Statement of the Joint Committee on Infant Hearing Screening* gives seven high-risk criteria for identifying children specifically at risk for hearing impairment (Table 9-1):

The hearing of infants who manifest any item on the list of risk criteria should be screened, preferably under the supervision of an audiologist, optimally by 3 months of age but not later than 6 months of age. The initial screening should include the observation of behavioral or electrophysiologic response to sound. (The Committee has no recommendations at this time regarding any specific device.) If consistent electrophysiologic or behavioral responses are detected at appropriate sound levels, then the screening process will be considered complete except in those cases in which there is a probability of a progressive hearing loss, e.g., family history of delayed onset or degenerative disease, or history of intrauterine infection. If results of initial screening of an infant manifesting any risk criteria are equivocal, then the infant should be referred for diagnostic testing.

II. Methods of screening

Within these general recommendations, a variety of procedures compete for adoption, with cost-benefit analyses only beginning to emerge.

A. Immitance audiometry (tympanometry, static compliance, and acoustic reflex thresholds) has been proposed as a screening procedure. However, acoustic reflexes can be obtained from only 12 percent of normal newborns between 3 and 132 hours of age (Stream et al., 1978). The poor results with newborns probably derive from an unlucky choice of probe-tone frequency by manufacturers of immitance equipment (Margolis et al., 1981) as well as the plasticity of the ear canal (i.e., tympanometry may appear normal but reflect movement of the canal wall only). The current procedure is inappropriate for use with infants less than 3 months of age.

B. One procedure uses the auropalpebral reflex or eyeblink to a loud transient sound (Wedenberg, 1956). The reflex is almost universal, although how the responsiveness of infants varies with postconceptional age (Men-

---

*The Joint Committee on Infant Hearing Screening comprised representatives from the American Academy of Pediatrics, Academy of Otolaryngology, Head and Neck Surgery, American Nurses Association, and the American Speech, Language and Hearing Association.

Table 9-1. Criteria for identification of infants at risk for hearing impairment

1. Family history of childhood hearing impairment
2. Congenital perinatal infection (e.g., cytomegalovirus, rubella, herpes, toxoplasmosis, syphilis)
3. Anatomic malformations involving the head or neck (e.g., dysmorphic appearance, including syndromal and nonsyndromal abnormalities; overt or submucous cleft palate; morphologic abnormalities of the pinna)
4. Birth weight less than 1,500 g
5. Hyperbilirubinemia level exceeding criterion level for exchange transfusion
6. Bacterial meningitis, especially *Haemophilus influenzae*
7. Severe asphyxia, which may include infants with Apgar scores from 0 to 3 or who fail to institute spontaneous respiration by 10 minutes

cher et al., 1985) and with signal parameters is only now being documented (Gerber, 1985). Currently, procedures and results vary widely, and routine application is not advisable (Jacobson and Morehouse, 1984).

C. The Crib-o-gram (Simmons, 1979) is a screening procedure involving delivery of a narrow band of intense noise (92 dB) at the ear canal and measuring the infant's gross body response with a sensitive motion detector under the mattress. A microprocessor analyzes motor response activity in 30 trials and indicates pass or fail. The procedure requires 1½ to 2 hours per child; a recent manufacturer's report states that testing time has been reduced to 30 minutes.

   In a recent report, 1,195 neonatal intensive care unit (NICU) infants (postconceptional age 6 to 13 months) were screened more than 1 hour after feeding and 1 to 3 days prior to discharge (1985 marketing publicity from Telesensory Systems, Inc., Palo Alto, Calif.). Infants with abnormal motor activity were not screened. This validation study found 5 percent hearing impairment with 60 percent of these children in the profound range and a 0 percent false-negative rate (no hearing-impaired infants were labeled as having normal hearing) from NICU graduates.

D. A screening procedure somewhat similar to the Crib-o-gram is the Auditory Response Cradle (Bennett and Wade, 1981; Shepard, 1983). The infant is placed in a specially designed cradle and is monitored for behavioral responses of total movement, head jerk or startle, head turn, and respiratory activity to an intense sound (85 dB from insert receivers in the external canals). A microprocessor analyzes and applies weights to the four classes of responses for a series of trials using equal numbers of sound and control periods. The infant is tested any time other than within the hour prior to or after feeding; testing time averages 5 to 10 minutes per child. Results for a well-baby nursery reveal an expected incidence of 0.32 percent (personal communication, Linco Ind., Calgary, Alberta, Canada).

E. A fifth procedure for screening is auditory brainstem response audiometry (ABR). Unlike the preceding four procedures, ABR is typically used for more than finding children with severe losses (>70 dB); rather it is used as a combination screening-diagnostic procedure to identify any loss. Equipment, procedures, and criteria differ. Results from one study for graduates from an NICU found 16 percent had hearing loss in one or both ears and 4 percent required hearing aids (Galambos et al., 1984). Cost of initial ABR screening in this study was estimated at $65 per patient. Used only as a double-criterion screening device (pass-fail response for each ear at both 60 and 30 dB [adult normal hearing level]), the procedure requires approximately 30 minutes.

III. Diagnosis of infants failing screening
Appropriate referral for children failing initial screening also was considered by the Joint Committee on Infant Hearing Screening (1982). Current ABR techniques typically yield definitive audiologic description of the magnitude of hearing loss before 6 months of age. Evaluation should begin as soon as hearing loss is suspected, and remediation should begin whenever the loss is documented. Overall recommendations include a general history and physical examination, with special attention to examination of the head and neck, followed by otoscopy and otomicroscopy. Special tests for perinatal infection or renal disease are indicated if hearing deficiencies are suspected. Comprehensive audiologic evaluation includes behavioral history, behavioral observation audiometry, and testing of auditory-evoked potentials (ABR), if indicated. After the age of 6 months, the following are also recommended: communication skills evaluation, impedance measurements, and selected tests of development.

IV. Managing the hearing-impaired infant
The diagnosis should be established and habilitation begun by 6 months of age. Services to the hearing-impaired infant include frequent evaluation, sound amplification, and genetic evaluation and counseling when indicated.

The psychologic support and education of parents who have a hearing-impaired infant are critical. Formulating an individualized education plan and sharing information about hearing impairment are key elements. A 1983 study considered data on 88 patients in a hospital-based program for hearing-impaired infants less than 3 years of age (Stein et al., 1983). The study examined the occurrence of risk factors and the ages when hearing loss was first suspected, when loss was diagnosed, and when habilitation was initiated. Results indicated that more than 25 percent of all hearing-impaired infants did not manifest high-risk factors. The median age for enrollment was approximately 20 months of age.

A partial explanation for the delay in entering children into intervention programs is that parents have difficulty dealing with the implications of having an "imperfect" child. Often they experience a grieving period preceding the stage when they can mobilize themselves for directed intervention.

V. Implications of hearing loss on speech and language development
Speech contains low-frequency, intense vowels, typically covering the range from 55 to 65 dB, and high-frequency, less intense consonants covering the range of 35 to 50 dB, delivered in background noise of about 30 dB. As back-

ground noise level increases, the talker reflexively increases speech loudness and becomes at the same time more precise. Speech tends to be no louder or more precise than it need be.

Table 9-2 presents a summary of the influences of hearing loss on speech and language (Madison, 1984).

The purpose of hearing aids is to make the consonants loud enough so that the child can hear and understand them in at least one ear over and above background noise. At the same time, the vowels cannot be so intense that their sound level damages or fatigues the ear, thereby masking the consonants. The child with a greater loss may use a personal FM system in the classroom to secure adequate speech levels from the teacher without the interfering classroom noise also being amplified.

Continuing audiologic management and monitoring are critical. The child requiring an aid should be fitted as early as the loss is documented, with ear choice aimed toward achieving balanced, aided binaural hearing, within normal range, if possible. A unilateral loss (binaural imbalance) presents problems of sound direction that are not trivial but need not influence language learning. Fluctuating hearing loss, because of recurring middle ear disease or variable hearing aid use, is associated with continued language problems. Early and consistent hearing aid use frequently results in normal language development.

New ear molds are required as the child grows, perhaps as frequently as 2 to 3 times per year. After initial adjustment, the aid(s) should be worn all waking hours. New aids need to be purchased every 3 to 5 years because of wear loss, damage, or technologic change.

Table 9-3 displays the options for habilitation typically associated with various magnitudes of hearing loss.

Table 9-2. Hearing loss effects on speech and language

| Type of loss | Voice | | | Articulation | | |
	Pitch	Loudness	Quality	Consonants	Vowels	Language
Unilateral	No	No	No	No	No	No
Fluctuating conductive	No	Perhaps low when present	No	Yes	No	Yes
Conductive	No	Low	No	Yes, dependent on onset and severity	No	Yes, dependent on onset and severity
Sensorineural, mild to moderate	Probably not	Possibly	Possibly	Yes, dependent on onset and severity	No	Yes, dependent on onset and severity
Sensorineural, moderate to severe (deaf)	Yes	Loud	Yes	Yes	Yes	Yes

Adapted from C. L. Madison. Speech and language difficulties of the hearing impaired. *Semin. Hear.* 5 : 204, 1984.

**Table 9-3. Habilitation considerations
associated with magnitude of hearing loss in children**

Degree of loss	Options*
0–15	Hearing within normal range; annual monitoring against increased loss
16–25 (borderline/mild)	Above plus special seating in classroom
26–40 (mild/moderate)	Above plus tutoring, speech/voice training, auditory skills training, language therapy, lip reading (speech reading)
41–55 (moderate)	Above plus tutoring, speech/voice training, auditory skills training, language therapy, lip reading (speech reading)
56–70 (moderate/severe)	Above plus special classroom (or school), sign language consideration
71–90 (severe)	Above plus special school
>90 (profound)	Above plus tactile aid(s)

*The child with a greater loss requires all the assistance given a child with a lesser loss plus additional help.

A general reference for orientation toward hearing, the development of auditory behavior, the testing of hearing of children, fitting of hearing aids and education of children with hearing losses is by Northern and Downs (1978). The work remains useful for parents and those who counsel them.

REFERENCES

Bennett, M. J., and Wade, H. K. Computerized hearing test for neonates. *Hear. Aid J.* 10 : 52, 1981.

deVries, L. S., Lary, S., and Dubowitz, L. M. S. Relationship of serum bilirubin levels to ototoxicity and deafness in high-risk low birth weight infants. *Pediatrics* 76 : 351, 1985.

Duara, S., Suter, C. M., Bessard, K. K., and Gutberlet, R. L. Neonatal screening with auditory brainstem responses: Results of follow-up audiometry and risk factor evaluation. *J. Pediatr.* 108 : 276, 1986.

Galambos, R., Hicks, G. E., and Wilson, M. J. The auditory brain stem response reliably predicts hearing loss in graduates of tertiary intensive care nursery. *Ear Hear.* 5 : 254, 1984.

Gerber, S. E. Stimulus, response and state variables in the testing of neonates. *Ear Hear.* 6 : 15, 1985.

Grimes, C. T. Audiologic evaluation in infancy and childhood. *Pediatr. Ann.* 14 : 211, 1985.

Jacobson, J. T., and Morehouse, C. R. A comparison of auditory brain stem response and behavioral screening in high risk and normal newborn infants. *Ear Hear.* 5 : 247, 1984.

Joint Committee on Infant Hearing position statement, 1982. *Ear Hear.* 4 : 3, 1983.

Madison, C. L. Speech and language difficulties of the hearing impaired. *Semin. Hear.* 5 : 204, 1984.

Margolis, R. H., Popelka, G. R., Handler, S. D., and Himmelfarb, M. Z. The Effects of Age on Acoustic Reflex Thresholds in Normal Hearing Subjects. In G. R. Popelka (ed.), *Hearing Assessment With the Acoustic Reflex.* New York: Grune & Stratton, 1981.

Mencher, G. T., Mencher, L. S., and Rohland, S. L. Maturation of behavioral response. *Ear Hear.* 6 : 10, 1985.

Northern, J. L., and Downs, M. P. *Hearing in Children.* Baltimore: Williams & Wilkins, 1978.

Rowe, L. Hearing loss: Profound benefits of early diagnosis. *Contemp. Pediatr.* 1985. Pp. 77–85.

Shepard, N. T. Newborn hearing screening using the Linco-Bennett auditory response cradle: A pilot study. *Ear Hear.* 4 : 5, 1983.

Simmons, F. B., McFarland, W. H., and Jones, F. R. An automated hearing screening technique for newborns. *Acta Otolaryngol.* 87 : 1, 1979.

Stein, L., Clark, S., and Kraus, N. The hearing-impaired infant: Patterns of identification and habilitation. *Ear Hear.* 4 : 232, 1983.

Stream, R. W., Stream, K. S., Walker, J. R., and Bremingstall, G. Emerging characteristics of the acoustic reflex in infants. *Otolaryngology* 86 : 628, 1978.

Wedenberg, E. Auditory tests on newborn infants. *Acta Otolaryngol.* 46 : 446, 1956.

Neuromotor Status

Claudine Amiel-Tison

I. Introduction

Awareness of the pattern and changes of motor function within the first year of life allows us to separate the normal from the abnormal and to assess whether motor abnormalities are transient or persistent. Assessment of neuromotor status is just one part of the neurologic evaluation. (Assessments of eyes, hearing, and social and behavioral development are discussed in other chapters.) Nonetheless, evaluation of neuromotor function is of paramount importance in establishing links between perinatal events and late outcome. Changes in neuromotor function observed during the first year of life seem closely linked with maturation of the central nervous system (CNS) and with the presence or absence of brain damage; moreover, these changes are relatively independent of familial and sociocultural background and the quality of parent-infant interaction. Therefore, it is useful to obtain information on the neuromotor function to document the perinatal origins of a later dysfunction or to demonstrate the effect of early intervention and recovery from injury (CNS plasticity).

II. Normal development of neuromotor function up to 1 year of age

A. Neurologic maturation from 28 to 40 weeks' gestation

Saint-Anne Dargassies (1955, 1974) first described the stages of development that characterize maturation between 28 and 40 weeks' gestational age. Her work is largely based on the methods developed by Thomas in the study of the full-term infant (1949, 1960). She has adapted Thomas's work to the study of the premature infant and relies to a large extent on the evaluation of reflexes and tone.

At 28 weeks' gestational age, the premature newborn is flaccid and lying in extension; legs and arms are almost lacking in tone. From 28 to 40 weeks' gestational age, tone increases in a caudocephalic direction, with increased tone in flexion observed first in the legs (around 34 weeks' gestational age) and later in the upper extremities (36–38 weeks' gestational age) (Fig. 10-1). This pattern is so precise and individual variations are so slight that incremental changes at 2-week intervals can be described. The full-term newborn when supine is in full flexion in all extremities with resistance to extension. During the same period, a caudocephalic increase of active tone is observed in the trunk (Fig. 10-2). When the infant is held upright, a righting reaction first appears in lower limbs (32 weeks' gestational age), later in the trunk (36 weeks' gestational age), and finally in the neck, allowing the infant to maintain the head in the axis for a few seconds (Amiel-Tison, 1968, 1974, 1985).

115

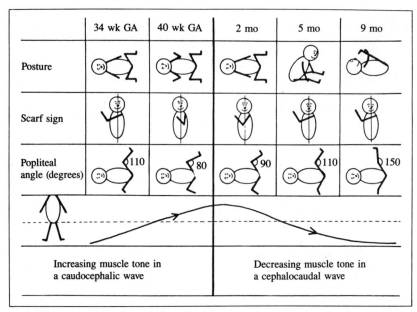

	34 wk GA	40 wk GA	2 mo	5 mo	9 mo
Posture					
Scarf sign					
Popliteal angle (degrees)	110	80	90	110	150

Increasing muscle tone in a caudocephalic wave	Decreasing muscle tone in a cephalocaudal wave

Fig. 10-1. Passive tone in upper and lower extremities. From 28 to 40 weeks' gestational age *(GA)*, muscle tone in flexor muscles increases in a caudocephalic progression, as indicated by posture, scarf sign (evaluating extensibility in upper limbs), and popliteal angle (evaluating extensibility in lower limbs). Within the first year of life, muscle tone in flexor muscles decreases in a cephalocaudal progression to reach a global hypotonia maximum at 8 to 10 months. (From C. Amiel-Tison, Pediatric Contribution to the Present Knowledge on the Neurobehavioral Status of Infants at Birth. In J. Mehler and R. Fox [eds.], *Neonate Cognition, Beyond the Blooming Buzzing Confusion.* Hillsdale, N.J.: Erlbaum, 1985. With permission.)

Besides the caudocephalic progression of tone, Saint-Anne Dargassies has shown that active tone develops earlier in the extensor muscles of the axis than in the flexor muscles, between 28 and 40 weeks' gestational age. A good example is the typical pattern at 34 weeks' gestational age: When the infant is pulled from supine to sitting, the head rolls on the shoulder, unable to pass forward in the axis of the trunk. When the infant is moved from sitting to supine, the head moves back with a consistent, sustained contraction of extensor muscles in the neck.

Evaluating neuromotor tone to determine gestational age relies on the dogma that maturation in the fetus progresses in an unvarying pattern regardless of environmental circumstances. Repeated observation has shown that there are exceptions to this rule (Amiel-Tison, 1980; Gould et al., 1972, 1977). Unfavorable intrauterine conditions (mainly hypertension during pregnancy and multiple pregnancies) may accelerate the development of the infant's CNS. However, the dogma remains valid for most infants. The very immature infant, upon reaching 40 weeks' post conceptional age, is similar in neuromotor tone to a 1-week old full-term newborn.

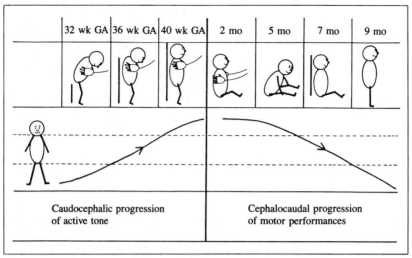

	32 wk GA	36 wk GA	40 wk GA	2 mo	5 mo	7 mo	9 mo

Caudocephalic progression of active tone

Cephalocaudal progression of motor performances

Fig. 10-2. Active tone in the axis. From 28 to 40 weeks' gestational age *(GA),* when the infant is held upright, a righting reaction first appears in the legs, later in the trunk, and finally in the neck and is maintained for a few seconds. Within the first year of life, head control is acquired first, later the sitting position; finally, at around 9 months, the infant can stand up and maintain the standing position for a while. From 4 to 7 months, at the time when the sitting position is being acquired, no righting reaction is observed when the infant is held in the upright position. (From C. Amiel-Tison, Pediatric Contribution to the Present Knowledge on the Neurobehavioral Status of Infants at Birth. In J. Mehler and R. Fox [eds.], *Neonate Cognition, Beyond the Blooming Buzzing Confusion.* Hillsdale, N.J.: Erlbaum, 1985. With permission.)

B. Neurologic maturation within the first year of life

Analysis of passive tone in the full-term infant during the first year of life allows us to recognize the general pattern of a decrease in flexor tone in the limbs (Amiel-Tison, 1978, 1985). In the first year of life, flexor tone first decreases in the upper extremities (beginning around 2 months after birth in the full-term infant), then in the lower limbs (from 4–8 months) (see Fig. 10-1). Later, tone slowly increases again, reaching during infancy norms already characteristic of the adult. Individual variations are greater in this postnatal change in the pattern of neuromotor tone than those occurring in late pregnancy, in terms of both timing and intensity. For example, maximum hypotonicity is attained any time between 3 and 15 months. The slower the overall development of the infant, the more the hypotonicity. In cases of extreme hypotonia, an infant will sit at a normal age but will not walk before 18 months, when hypotonicity begins to decrease.

At the same time, while this change in limb tone is observed, tone of the trunk also changes. An infant lifted and held with feet touching the examination table will straighten. This straightening reaction in the upright position follows fairly strict patterns (see Fig. 10-2). The straightening reaction prominent at 40 weeks' postconceptional age remains until 2 to 4 months postnatally. From 4 to 6 months, the straightening reaction disappears. At the same time, however, the ability to maintain a sitting position at 5 months demonstrates increasingly active tone in the axis. Around 7 months, the straightening reaction reappears. Awareness of these normal patterns of development and their individual variations is helpful for the diagnosis of abnormalities. As an example, the normal pattern at 5 months of age is a "tripod" sitting position with no straightening reaction in the standing position. An infant who has suffered perinatal asphyxia, however, often shows a persistence of strong straightening reactions in the upright position, where the delay in relaxation of the lower limbs makes sitting in the tripod position impossible.

The relationship between tone distribution and reflex activity is important for harmonious motor development. Since the straightening reaction is strong from birth to 4 months, automatic walking can easily be elicited. From 4 to 6 months, it is difficult to elicit automatic walking in a semiflexed child with no straightening reaction. This finding probably explains the discrepancies in the literature concerning the normal age of disappearance of automatic walking. It is only after 7 months that the postural changes allow for the beginning of voluntary steps. Furthermore, transitory hypotonicity in the lower limbs, pelvis, and spine may be considered a protective mechanism for the immature bones and articulations. Attempts to accelerate the acquisition of walking might be dangerous because of decreased muscle tone in the lower extremities during the period prior to 8 months or so.

C. Anatomic and physiologic correlates of neurologic development

Sarnat (1984) has proposed correlations between neuroanatomic processes and clinical development in early life, focusing mainly on synaptogenesis and myelinization. As the normal time course for the development of myelinization is well known, it is tempting to correlate this pattern with neurologic maturation, even though it is artificial to separate myelinization from other processes associated with maturation.

1. Between 28 and 40 weeks' gestational age, development as previously described can be explained by progressive myelinization of subcortical, and later cortical, motor pathways (Sarnat, 1984). Progressive caudocephalad development of muscle tone is probably linked with myelinization progressing in a caudocephalic direction for descending motor pathways. Differential development of tone in extensor and flexor muscles correlates with the successive myelinization of medial subcorticospinal, lateral subcorticospinal, and corticospinal pathways, according to the observations of Lawrence and Kuypers (1968a, b). These pathways affect different muscle groups: The medial subcortical pathway has a stimulating effect on extension and abduction of proximal joints, the lateral subcorticospinal pathway inhibits extension, and the corticospinal pathway has a stimulating effect on flexion and adduction of proximal joints. The pattern of differential development underlies the clinical pattern observed up to term when balance between flexor and extensor muscles in the trunk is achieved.

2. In the first year of life, the progressive cephalocaudal development of active tone in the trunk is probably linked with the progress in maturation of the corticospinal tract, which proceeds rostrocaudally from the

midbrain to the lumbosacral levels. The development of passive muscle tone waxes and wanes (Amiel-Tison, 1985), with tone increasing from foot to head between 28 and 40 weeks' gestational age. Passive muscle tone then decreases after term from head to foot throughout the first year. Active tone increases prior to term in a caudocephalic fashion.

After term, the acquisition of motor skills progresses from head to foot (e.g., head control precedes sitting, which precedes standing). These changes can be correlated first to the maturation of subcortical pathways and second to the maturation of corticospinal pathways.

III. Abnormal neuromotor development up to one year: Short-term outcome
Intraventricular hemorrhage (IVH) occurs in 50 percent of sick newborns weighing less than 1,500 g as documented by the systematic use of ultrasonographic examination. It is well known that late sequelae are more related to ventricular enlargement or loss of brain tissue than to the hemorrhage itself. Moreover, absence of IVH is not a guarantee of normal outcome in an immature infant. Prediction of risk after CNS insult in the sick newborn is difficult. Prediction of normal cerebral function in the first months of life is easier than prediction of abnormal outcome. The physician is most interested, however, in clues to late outcome, which means he or she is guessing the quality of cerebral functions that are not yet mature. Three periods have to be considered: the acute, initial stage; the term period and first 3 months; and the first year.

A. Acute initial stage
Methods are now available to make objective measurements of brain structure and function in the neonatal period and to provide predictive information, mainly by ultrasonographic brain imaging and by auditory brainstem response testing. These methods can be used in the smallest and sickest infants. Limitations of clinical evaluation of neuromotor status have long been recognized. For example, even in high-risk infants, neurologic evaluations performed every 2 weeks commonly demonstrate that neuromotor function is progressing smoothly in many infants up to term. We concluded 10 years ago (before ultrasonography) that this normal course is no guarantee of normal late outcome. Normal neuromotor development from 28 to 40 weeks' postconceptional age is not surprising in infants who later have abnormal cortical function, as the motor function at this stage is mainly related to the myelinization of subcortical pathways.

Stewart (1985a, b) described the association of major and minor neurodevelopmental disorders diagnosed by 18 months of age in very preterm infants (< 33 weeks' gestation) with neonatal ultrasonographic findings. In this study of 222 infants, including 96 with IVH, ultrasonographic studies were repeated once or twice a week for several weeks after birth. Abnormalities were defined as shown in Table 10-1. Serial neurologic evaluations were done within the first year; ophthalmologic examinations were done in the first 3 months of life; electrical and clinical audiologic function was tested at 6 to 9 months; and development was assessed with the Griffiths Baby Test by a psychologist at 12 months' corrected age.

Neurodevelopmental abnormalities identified by 12 to 18 months included cerebral palsy; sensorineural hearing loss; and visual disorders such

**Table 10-1. Definitions of lesions diagnosed
with ultrasonography in infants < 33 weeks' gestation**

PVH
  Hemorrhage originating in the region of the germinal layer with or without
    intraventricular hemorrhage

Uncomplicated PVH
  PVH without extension of hemorrhage into brain tissue or subsequent ventricular
    distention with CSF
Complex lesions
  Mild ventricular distention
    Distention of the ventricular system with CSF when the width of the lateral ventricle
      did not exceed 5 mm in excess of the mean + 2 SD for comparable normal infants
  Hydrocephalus
    Marked distention of the ventricular system with CSF so that the width of the lateral
      ventricle increased to more than 5 mm in excess of the mean + 2 SD for
      comparable normal infants
  Cerebral atrophy
    Either (a) persistent (usually irregular) enlargement of the ventricular system
      developing gradually in the absence of or several weeks after PVH, while cranial
      growth remained normal or delayed and there was no clinical evidence of raised
      intracranial pressure or (b) cysts developing at the site of a previous PVH or
      infarction

CSF = cerebrospinal fluid; PVH = periventricular hemorrhage; SD = standard deviation.
From A. Stewart. Early prediction of neurological outcome when the very preterm infant is discharged from
the intensive care unit. *Ann. Pediatr.* 32 : 27, 1985. With permission.

as delayed visual maturation, retinopathy of prematurity, and overall developmental delay of sufficient severity to predict mental retardation. All these
disorders, described as "major," were serious and disabling.

In addition to infants with major disabling neurodevelopmental disorders, other infants were identified with minor disorders causing little or no
functional disability, such as dystonia persisting to the end of the first year
of life. Ventriculoperitoneal shunts for the treatment of hydrocephalus in
infants who were otherwise developing normally were also included in
this category of minor neurodevelopmental disorders.

The predictive value of the lesions diagnosed by ultrasonography was investigated by calculation of the sensitivity (proportion of neurodevelop-
mentally abnormal children identified by a particular lesion), the specificity
(proportion of normal children recognized because the lesion was not present), and the accuracy (proportion of infants whose neurodevelopmental
status was correctly assigned on the basis of the ultrasonographic findings).
Probability estimates of an abnormal outcome (proportion of abnormal infants) were calculated for the ultrasonographic findings from logistical multiple regression analysis of the ultrasonographic and follow-up data. This
procedure also provided 95 percent confidence intervals of the lowest to
the highest probability estimates compatible with the data. The best overall
prediction of outcome was given by a diagnosis of complex lesions
thought to indicate hypoxic-ischemic damage (Table 10-2). As Tables 10-3
and 10-4 show, calculation of probability estimates from the ultrasono-

Table 10-2. Power of neonatal brain ultrasonographic findings to predict neurodevelopmental outcome at 12–18 mo*

Ultrasonographic findings	n	Accuracy (%)	Sensitivity (%)	Specificity (%)
Abnormal	103	65	77	62
IVH	96	63	64	62
Complex lesions	44	83	57	90

IVH = intraventricular hemorrhage.
*In 222 infants < 33 weeks' gestation at birth.
From A. Stewart. Assessment of Preterm Infant and Prognosis. In R. Beard and F. Sharp (eds.), *Preterm Labour and Its Consequences.* London: Royal College of Obstetricians and Surgeons, 1985. Pp. 25–36. With permission.

Table 10-3. Major and minor neurodevelopmental disorders according to neonatal brain ultrasonographic findings*

Ultrasonographic findings	n	Major and minor disorders		
		n	p	95% Confidence interval
Normal	119	11	11%	7–17%
Uncomplicated IVH	59	9	11%	7–17%
Mild ventricular distention	23	8	35%	18–56%
Hydrocephalus	5	4	80%	31–97%
Cerebral atrophy				
Cysts	8	8	94%	66–99%
General	8	7	94%	66–99%

IVH = intraventricular hemorrhage.
*In 222 infants <33 weeks' gestation at birth, age 12–18 mo.
From A. Stewart. Assessment of Preterm Infant and Prognosis. In R. Beard and F. Sharp (eds.), *Preterm Labour and Its Consequences.* London: Royal College of Obstetricians and Surgeons, 1985. Pp. 25–36. With permission.

graphic data classified in this way showed that uncomplicated IVH was a relatively innocuous lesion and had the same low probability of an adverse outcome as a normal scan. This finding is verified by clinical experience in terms of the excellent prognosis in those with grades I and II IVH without hydrocephalus. By contrast, the probability of an adverse outcome was great if there was evidence of hypoxic-ischemic damage, and the value depended on the type and extent of the damage (Tables 10-3 and 10-4).

The results of both neonatal ultrasonographic studies and neonatal neurologic examinations done at term were considered together in 110 very preterm (< 33 weeks) infants by Stewart (1985b). These findings were compared with neurodevelopmental outcome at 12 to 18 months. The neurologic abnormalities included imbalance of tone in extensor and flexor neck muscles and upper limbgirdle hypotonia (Table 10-5). Results indicate that neurologic abnormalities identified at term help in predicting outcome. In particular, when combined with the results of neonatal ultrasonographic studies, the clinical data help improve the recognition of normal infants.

**Table 10-4. Major neurodevelopmental disorders
according to neonatal brain ultrasonographic findings***

Ultrasonographic findings	n	Major disorders		95% Confidence interval
		n	p	
Normal	119	5	4%	2–8%
Uncomplicated IVH	59	2	4%	2–8%
Mild ventricular distention	23	7	30%	13–53%
Hydrocephalus	5	2	40%	5–85%
Cerebral atrophy				
Cysts	8	7	63%	35–85%
General	8	3	63%	35–85%

IVH = intraventricular hemorrhage.
*In 222 infants <33 weeks' gestation at birth, age 12–18 mo.
From A. Stewart. Assessment of Preterm Infant and Prognosis. In R. Beard and F. Sharp (eds.), *Preterm Labour and Its Consequences.* London: Royal College of Obstetricians and Surgeons, 1985. Pp. 25–36. With permission.

**Table 10-5. Neurologic and ultrasonographic prediction
of major and minor neurodevelopmental disability at 18 mo**

Findings	n	Sensitivity (%)	Specificity (%)
Abnormal neurologic signs	34	15/21 (71)	70/89 (79)
All abnormalities on ultrasonography	52	18/21 (86)	55/89 (62)
Complex lesions on ultrasonography	24	16/21 (76)	81/89 (91)
Abnormal neurologic signs + abnormal ultrasonographic findings	19	13/21 (62)	83/89 (93)
Abnormal neurologic signs + complex lesions on ultrasonography	12	11/21 (52)	88/89 (99)

From A. Stewart. Early prediction of neurological outcome when the very preterm infant is discharged from the intensive care unit. *Ann. Pediatr.* 32 : 27, 1985. With permission.

B. Term period and the first 3 months

This is a period of convalescence during which the examination is still impeded by continued difficulties in many infants (e.g., vasomotor instability, respiratory dysfunction, feeding problems, and metabolic adjustments). The infant's often poor tolerance of the examination is due to easy fatigability and cardiorespiratory instability. Neurologic abnormalities may be observed: The stages of maturation may be achieved with delay. For example, the progressive relaxation of passive tone may be slow (cephalocaudad), and poor progression of active tone (caudocephalic) may be observed in upper extremities, trunk, and neck. Primary reflexes may be present, but responses may remain slow and imperfect or exaggerated: The sucking reflex may remain weak and poorly synchronized with deglutition. Alertness and visual pursuit may not be achieved. Other neurologic signs, the most common of which are irritability and hypertonia in neck extensors, can appear at this time (oposthotonic posturing). When these abnormalities are prolonged, they correspond to the abnormal maturation of the corticospinal tract and therefore are more likely to persist.

C. First year of life

The most commonly observed transient neuromotor abnormalities in the first year of life are summarized in Figure 10-3. At the end of the first year, we are able to classify motor development as one of the following:

Fig. 10-3. Most commonly observed transient neuromotor anomalies in the first year of life. (From C. Amiel-Tison, *Neurologic Evaluation of the Newborn and the Infant*. New York: Masson, 1983.)

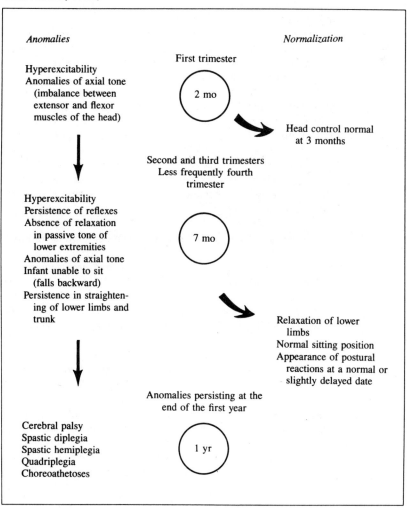

Normal throughout the first year
With transient abnormalities
With persisting abnormalities, mild or severe

After the first birthday, one motor event is particularly important, the age of independent walking. For a given child, it has no predictive value, as long as independent walking occurs before 18 months. Nonetheless, it is a very important milestone for group evaluation (Amiel-Tison et al., 1983; Chaplais et al., 1984).

The group of infants with so-called transient motor abnormalities may be a high-risk group for minimal brain dysfunction at school age (Amiel-Tison, 1978). These motor abnormalities are not really transient but appear so because of the wide range of normal. The rapidity and precision of motor development within the first year make it easy to use certain milestones to detect abnormalities. This is not so later on, and the ability to track mild motor disabilities after 18 months is lost until more sophisticated tests can be performed. Cerebral maturation and, more specifically, myelinization of motor pathways are still occurring within the first year. For example, continued maturation can compensate for mild lesions revealed by motor abnormalities identified by 7 months.

The high incidence of minimal brain dysfunction among infants who experience transient first-year motor difficulties suggests a possible causal relationship and points to the organic origin of abnormal signs at school age. Indeed, the transient motor signs may represent a minor form of cerebral palsy (i.e., a minor form of leukomalacia). Mild lesions of the white matter result in transient anomalies during the initial stages of development and a subtle deficit in fine motor control later in life. Concomitant cortical lesions only become evident later and determine the long-term prognosis on cognitive function.

IV. Prediction of long-term outcome in infants with neuromotor transient abnormalities

It has been my experience that children who had transitory neuromotor abnormalities during their first year, appeared normal at 1 year, and had a normal career in kindergarten from ages 3 to 6 would encounter scholastic difficulties between the ages of 8 and 10. We have tried to identify links between perinatal insults and later difficulties using a clinical neuromotor evaluation (Amiel-Tison et al., 1983).

In our work at the Port Royal Maternity Hospital in Paris, we selected a sample of 15 full-term newborns who had abnormal neurologic symptoms during their first week and neuromotor symptoms within the first year of life but not beyond. They all seemed normal at 1 year of age. At 5 to 6 years of age, these 15 children were reassessed and compared with 15 controls selected on the basis of a normal neurologic status in the first week of life (Table 10-6). Five of the 15 (33%) manifested no symptoms and succeeded in all the tests. These five should not encounter any scholastic difficulties. Four of 15 (27%) had abnormal test results. Also, they had problems in fine motor adjustments, manifested signs of dyspraxia, and scored less than 85 in the Terman-Merrill IQ test.

Table 10-6. Transitory neuromotor abnormalities within the first year of life

Number of cases	Categories at 5 to 6 yr		
	Abnormal	Intermediate	Normal
Target group (n = 15)	4	6	5
Control group (n = 15)	1	1	13

From C. Amiel-Tison, Pediatric Contribution to the Present Knowledge on the Neurobehavioral Status of Infants at Birth. In J. Mehler and R. Fox (eds.), *Neonate Cognition, Beyond the Blooming Buzzing Confusion.* Hillsdale, N.J.: Erlbaum, 1985. With permission.

The remaining six children had intermediate symptoms; no predictions could be made for their future. In the control group, 13 of 15 children were classified as normal, one was classified as abnormal, and one was in the intermediate group. Drillien and associates have shown the same link between the dystonic syndrome described in low-birth-weight infants (1972) and the late outcome at school (1980).

During successive evaluations of infants at risk for adverse CNS development, every cerebral function should be tested as soon as it appears. Language acquisition should be an excellent intermediate marker between ages 2 and 4. On the one hand, more systematic studies will be able to demonstrate better the continuum of CNS development. On the other hand, there is a tendency at each step in early infancy for the cerebral function to improve after a perinatal insult, and in the study of Drillien, as well as in my study, it appears that more than half of the cohort with transient motor abnormalities will be normal later in life.

To try to explain these observations, the theory of neurologic plasticity has been proposed, but it remains controversial. Some have been disillusioned by the failure to define specific risk criteria from prospective studies, despite the clear association of cerebral palsy and mental retardation with IVH or asphyxia. Others have discounted the importance of biologic risk and have emphasized the importance of social factors in the normal or abnormal CNS outcome of infants at risk. In practice, the processes concerned are so complex that it is not surprising that the relatively crude measures available in the past have failed to allow proper conclusions to be drawn. Perhaps now that objective measures of brain structure and function, including measures of cerebral energy metabolism, are being determined, it may be possible to learn more.

REFERENCES

Amiel-Tison, C. Neurological evaluation of the maturity of newborn infants. *Arch. Dis. Child.* 43 : 89, 1968.

Amiel-Tison, C. Neurological Evaluation of the Small Neonate: The Importance of Head Straightening Reactions. In L. Gluck (ed.), *Modern Perinatal Medicine.* Chicago: Year Book, 1974. Pp. 347–357.

Amiel-Tison, C. A Method for Neurological Evaluation Within the First Year of Life: Experience with Full-Term Newborn Infants with Birth Injury. *Ciba Found. Symp.* No. 59. 1978.

Amiel-Tison, C. Possible acceleration of neurological maturation following high risk pregnancy. *Am. J. Obstet. Gynecol.* 138 : 303, 1980.

Amiel-Tison, C. Pediatric Contribution to the Present Knowledge on the Neurobehavioral Status of Infants at Birth. In J. Mehler and R. Fox (eds.), *Neonate Cognition, Beyond the Blooming Buzzing Confusion.* Hillsdale, N.J.: Erlbaum, 1985. Pp. 365–380.

Amiel-Tison, C., Dube, R., Garel, M., and Jequier, J. C. Late outcome after transient neuromotor abnormalities within the first year of life. In L. Stern, H. Bard, and B. Friis-Hansen (eds.), *Intensive Care IV.* New York: Masson, 1983. Pp. 247–258.

Chaplais, J. D., and MacFarlane, J. N. A. A review of 404 "late walkers." *Arch. Dis. Child.* 59 : 512, 1984.

Drillien, C. M. Abnormal neurologic signs in the first year of life in low birth weight infants. Possible prognostic significance. *Dev. Med. Child Neurol.* 14 : 575, 1972.

Drillien, C. M., Thomson, A. J. M., and Burgoyne, K. Low birth weight children at early school age: A longitudinal study. *Dev. Med. Child Neurol.* 22 : 26, 1980.

Gould, J. B., Gluck, L., and Kulovich, M. V. The acceleration of neurological maturation in high stress pregnancy and its relation to fetal lung maturity. *Pediatr. Res.* 6 : 276, 1972.

Gould, J. B., Gluck, L., and Kulovich, M. V. The relationship between accelerated pulmonary maturity and accelerated neurological maturity in certain chronically stressed pregnancies. *Am. J. Obstet. Gynecol.* 127 : 181, 1977.

Hagberg, B., Hagberg, G., and Olow, I. The changing panorama of cerebral palsy in Sweden. *Acta Paediatr. Scand.* 73 : 433, 1984.

Lawrence, D. G., and Kuypers, H. G. J. M. The functional organization of the motor system in the monkey. I. The effects of bilateral pyramidal lesions. *Brain* 91 : 1, 1968a.

Lawrence, D. G., and Kuypers, H. G. J. M. The functional organization of the motor system in the monkey. II. The effects of lesions of the descending brainstem pathways. *Brain* 91 : 15, 1968b.

Saint-Anne Dargassies, S. La maturation neurologique du premature. Études neonatales. 4 : 71, 1955.

Saint-Anne Dargassies, S. *Le Développement Neurologique du Nouveau-né à Terme et Premature.* Paris: Masson, 1974.

Sarnat, H. B. Anatomic and Physiologic Correlates of Neurologic Development in Prematurity. In H. B. Sarnat (ed.), *Topics in Neonatal Neurology.* New York: Grune & Stratton, 1984. Pp. 1–25.

Stewart, A. Assessment of Preterm Infant and Prognosis. In R. Beard and F. Sharp (eds.), *Preterm Labour and its Consequences.* London: Royal College of Obstetricians and Surgeons, 1985a.

Stewart, A. Early prediction of neurological outcome when the very preterm infant is discharged from the intensive care unit. *Ann. Pediatr.* 32 : 27, 1985b.

Thomas, A., and Ajuriaguerra, J. de. *Étude Semeiologique du Tonus Musculaire.* Paris: Éditions Medicales Flammarion, 1949.

Thomas, A., and Autgaerden, S. Locomotion from pre to post-natal life. *Clin. Dev. Med. No. 24.* London: Spastics Society with Heinemann, 1966.

Thomas, A., Chesni, Y., and Saint-Anne Dargassies, S. The neurological examination of the infant. *Clin. Dev. Med. No. 1.* London: National Spastic Society, 1960.

11

Physical Therapy

Priscilla S. Osborne

I. Introduction

Physical therapists have been involved with the assessment and management of high-risk infants for many years. Parmelee and Huber (1973) defined the high-risk infant as "any newborn or young infant who has a high probability of manifesting in childhood a sensory or motor deficit and/or mental handicap." This chapter provides an overview of the physical therapy assessment and treatment approaches for infants at risk for motor disability. The physical therapist has several tasks: assessment and monitoring of motor function, direct treatment, and consultation to families and caretakers.

Hospitalized newborns may begin receiving physical therapy as inpatients. The physical therapist, at the time of the infant's discharge, provides for continuation of services, community referrals, and assessment and monitoring of the infant's motor behavior.

The underlying causes of motor problems vary. Alterations in movement pattern can result from neurologic abnormalities, musculoskeletal anomalies, sensory deficits, or a combination. The abnormality may be generalized, as in tone abnormalities, or it may be specific to an area of the body, as in the absence of a limb. Delay in motor development may be associated with an overall delay in development, with illness, or with environmental deprivation. Abnormal movement patterns and motor delay may occur in conjunction with one another and can have a variety of etiologies in the same infant.

II. Screening motor behavior in high-risk infants
Infants most commonly screened by physical therapists are

A. Infants who meet specific criteria known to be associated with a higher incidence of motor deficits:
1. Very low birth weight (Pape et al., 1978)
2. Intraventricular hemorrhage (Ment et al., 1982)
3. Bronchopulmonary dysplasia (Osborne, 1980)
4. Birth asphyxia (Mulligan et al., 1980)

B. Infants born with specific anomalies or syndromes known to be associated with motor deficits or problems, such as Down's syndrome and myelodysplasia

C. Infants with abnormal movement or abnormal postures

D. Infants with a possible delay in motor development

The results of the motor findings are integrated with other developmental and health findings so the physical therapist can help define the infant's strengths and weaknesses in relation to his or her overall functioning and suggest interventions if appropriate.

III. Physical therapy assessment of the infant

Physical therapy assessment of motor behavior evaluates movement patterns, postures, and motor development, emphasizing the area of concern in the referral. A history is essential for the assessment of motor function and, prior to the assessment, should be obtained by the examiner. Assessment of movement includes observation of the child free of intervention and handling as well as the child's response to various testing situations. These observations allow the examiner to evaluate spontaneous movement and to see the variation of movement without intervention.

A. Factors influencing motor testing
   1. Overall development status. If an infant has delays in other areas of development, motor function should be considered within the context of overall functioning so that relative strengths and weaknesses can be defined.
   2. Health status. Chronically ill infants or infants with recurrent illnesses may require special consideration during motor testing. The ill child may not have the strength, endurance, or motivation to perform motor skills. For these infants, assessment must be modified to accommodate health status, and results must be considered within the context of health findings. Repeat assessments as health improves assist in monitoring the progress of these infants.
   3. Behavioral state at the time of testing (Brazelton, 1973). Optimal motor function can only be achieved and observed when the infant is relaxed and comfortable. To be representative of the child's optimal performance, assessment should be planned, as much as possible, for a time when the infant is not acutely ill, tired, or hungry.

B. Assessment of movement patterns and postures
   Assessment of movement patterns and postures is qualitative in nature, focusing on the infant's patterns of movement. Abnormal movement patterns are energy consuming for the infant and may in some instances interfere with the development of more sophisticated movement (Bobath, 1965). The quality of the movement patterns is most influenced by the physical components that reflect the integrity and maturation of the musculoskeletal, neurologic, and sensory systems. These components include tone, muscle strength, joint range of motion, sensory perception, primitive reflexes, and postural reactions. Each component is assessed individually with particular attention to its influence on the development of normal movement.

   1. Tone. Muscle tone is assessed by feeling the resistance of muscles to passive movement and by observing the movement patterns and postures used by the infant (Amiel-Tison, 1976).

2. Muscle strength is evaluated through an adaptation of a procedure described by Daniels and Worthingham (1972) based on the ability of a muscle or group of muscles to move against gravity, with or without added resistance. In infants, muscle strength is formally assessed by a manual muscle-testing process and informally tested by observing the infant's ability to move against gravity.

3. Joint range of motion describes the ability of a body part to be moved passively through its anatomic arc. This function is assessed by passive manipulation of the infant's arms, legs, trunk, and neck. The arc is measured and compared to norms for infants (Zausmer, 1953).

4. Sensory perception is assessed by observing the infant's spontaneous movement and responses to specific sensory stimuli during testing. Touch, vision, hearing, and vestibular responses are the sensory areas of interest.

5. Primitive reflexes, when present normally, are thought to provide the framework for later volitional movement patterns (Milani-Comparetti and Gidoni, 1967). However, if these reflex patterns persist or are abnormally strong or weak, they may interfere with the development of normal movement (Bobath, 1965).

6. Postural reactions consist of righting reactions, protective reactions, and equilibrium reactions. Righting reactions allow the infant to maintain body alignment and adapt to upright positioning. Protective reactions are essential to prevent falling injuries when the center of gravity is displaced. Equilibrium reactions are necessary to maintain posture in space during stance and movement without losing balance. The emergence, maturation, and integration of these reflexes and responses influence the infant's ability to perform volitional movement (Milani-Comparetti and Gidoni, 1967).

In addition to these specific components, speed of movement, timing, ease of movement, and variability are observed in the assessment of motor function.

All of these components have a developmental aspect, changing as the infant matures, which must be considered when assessing an infant. Specific norms for infants and children in these areas are not fully defined, although some norms and general guidelines are available. Therefore, it is essential that the examiner have background knowledge and experience in growth and development to aid in the interpretation of these findings.

Because of the multiplicity of factors influencing the development of motor function in infants and children, prediction of motor outcome based on any one finding or even a group of factors is not possible. Serial assessments of movement address progression or resolution of the abnormal finding and its influence on the development of efficient patterns.

C. Assessment of the developmental aspects on motor behavior
Motor development proceeds in an established sequence most commonly noted by the attainment of motor milestones. This sequence represents a process of maturation and integration of many systems but particularly the nervous system, the musculoskeletal system, and the sensory system. Prin-

ciples associated with the maturation of these systems underlie the development of motor behavior in children. The usual sequence of development follows three general principles: (1) Development proceeds in a cephalocaudal direction (McGraw, 1963), (2) gross movement precedes fine movement (Milani-Comparetti and Gidoni, 1967), and (3) stability precedes mobility (Stockmeyer, 1967).

Motor development is measured through standardized tests that correlate an infant's motor achievements or milestones with a developmental age or the age at which most children achieve that task, according to the test. The results are expressed as an age level or developmental quotient, which compares the age level achieved on the test to the child's chronologic age.

The most commonly used standardized tests that measure motor development in infancy are the revised Gesell Developmental Schedules (Knobloch et al., 1980), Bayley Scales of Infant Development (Bayley, 1969), and the Peabody Developmental Motor Scales (Folio et al., 1983).

Each of these tests has strengths and weaknesses. The Peabody Developmental Motor Scales are unique in their attempt to provide a method of scoring that allows for partial completion of an item, thus noting the emergence of a skill.

As with other developmental tests, these tests are based primarily on cross-sectional data and not specifically on average rates of maturation of motor skills for groups of infants followed longitudinally. Therefore, there is a paucity of good data regarding progression of a particular skill from one age to another. Also, there is a lack of information about the normal rate of motor achievement. Knowledge in these two areas is essential when interpreting the results of motor tests in infants.

The Wolanski (Wolanski and Zdanska-Brincken, 1973), a test of gross motor development in the first year of life, attempts to address issues of variation in rates of development among children and attempts to correlate motor developmental milestones with the underlying maturational process. This test divides gross motor development into four areas and measures gains in "channels" of development. A child typically stays within his or her channel of development; a cross in channels indicates an unusual change in rate. Either end of the spectrum in rate of development is defined as unusual. This tool was standardized on Polish infants, however, and its applicability to U.S. infants is unknown.

Motor tests, standardized on normal children, do not address the quality of movement used to achieve the motor tasks. When an infant with abnormal movement patterns is only tested with a standardized motor development tool, the performance generally shows a scattering of motor abilities that would be scored as a delay. This conclusion could misrepresent the infant's motor development. To describe the infant's motor abilities further, quality of movement needs to be added to the assessment to qualify the results. Movement Assessment in Infants (Chandler et al., 1980), an assessment tool, combines the evaluation of movement patterns and motor development for infants less than 1 year of age. Although this test only has standardized norms for the 4-month age level and reliability studies are not complete, it can be used as a guide for the physical therapist in combining these two major aspects of motor assessment.

To determine the rate of a child's development in motor function and the direction of progress, serial testing is extremely important. One score is not predictive of later development.

To determine an infant's areas of strength and weakness within his or her motor abilities, it is necessary to look at more than the score from the motor testing. Items within the overall test need to be defined in terms of their association with motor principles, and the performance should be assessed in this manner.

When testing the motor development of premature infants, it is recommended that adjustment be made for their early gestational age at birth (Palisano, 1984). Corrected age is obtained by subtracting the amount of prematurity from the infant's chronologic age. Test results are compared with norms for the corrected age.

In summary, the results of motor developmental testing must be considered in conjunction with the assessment of the various components underlying the development of movement and the physical components that contribute to the establishment of normal movement patterns. Information about the infant's health and other developmental aspects is necessary when interpreting the results of the various motor tests.

IV. Physical therapy treatment

A. Goals

In general, the goal of physical therapy treatment is to optimize the motor function of an infant with emphasis on the establishment of functional movement that will allow the infant to explore the environment and manipulate objects in the most efficient manner. Physical therapists, using various treatment modalities, can help by (1) modifying abnormal movement patterns and postures into functional and effective patterns, (2) providing appropriate motor experiences, and (3) providing adaptations to enable compensation for motor deficits either temporarily or on a long-term basis.

Individual goals for a specific infant are based on the evaluation and are considered within the context of the infant's overall function and needs.

B. Principles of treatment

Multiple factors suggest that there is potential to change motor behavior in infants. At birth, the systems that influence motor development have undergone major growth and differentiation. This process continues postnatally, changing the motor behavior of the maturing infant and child. Animal studies have indicated that early experience influences the process of maturation of these systems (Buller et al., 1960; Hubel, 1979) and the process of recovery after injury (Bishop, 1982). The infant's ongoing awareness of his or her body will also enable the infant to adapt to movement and will provide motivation for movement (Gilfoyle et al., 1982).

To effect change in motor function, physical therapy uses neurophysiologic principles within a developmental model. The sensory modalities, including tactile, kinesthetic, proprioceptive, vestibular, auditory, and visual modalities, are used primarily to influence the motor system. Through the use of these sensory modalities, feedback is provided to enhance specific postures and motor patterns. The developmental framework pertains to the sequence of the progression of motor function as it relates to the maturation of the various systems that influence movement.

Compensatory adaptations for the infant may include positioning and mobility devices when postural abilities and movement do not allow these functions independently. The devices do not preclude the establishment of these basic motor activities but do allow the infants to participate in activities in a manner similar to their uninvolved peers.

These principles apply to the treatment of infants with isolated motor disability, such as a specific muscle tightness, as well as to infants with global involvement, such as those with cerebral palsy.

C. Treatment approaches for the infant
There are many treatment approaches for the infant with impaired motor skills. Two approaches are commonly used with infants who demonstrate abnormal movement patterns.

Bobath neurodevelopmental therapy (1965) emphasizes the use of the automatic postural responses within a developmental framework for the purpose of enhancing the development of volitional movement. Proprioceptive techniques, through the use of handling and positioning, are used to enhance normal movement and reduce the influence of abnormal movement patterns.

The Rood approach emphasizes a developmental framework that links posture and movement. Selected treatment techniques using various sensory inputs facilitate desired responses (Stockmeyer, 1967).

These descriptions are brief. Further research in each approach is recommended if a full comprehension of the treatment techniques is desired. The most effective approach is an integrated model drawing on components of each to obtain the best response from the infant (Farber, 1982).

In the infant and child, family participation is essential so that there is carryover and consistency of treatment goals throughout the day. The family should be frequently instructed in proper positioning and handling of the infant. The family should also help develop new activities for the infant.

D. Modes of treatment
It is not possible to specify clearly which type of motor disability requires which mode of therapeutic intervention. Direct treatment is most often required when abnormal movement patterns are present. Consultation as to what the next step in motor development is and how to encourage it may be the appropriate model for the child who requires only anticipatory guidance.

Direct treatment: Periodic, often frequent, treatment of the infant provided by the physical therapist with home instructions and consultation for the family and caretakers

Consultation: Guidance provided by the physical therapist periodically with suggestions to the family and caretakers or to other service providers

The mode of intervention may vary within the course of treatment. The therapist may at one time decide direct treatment is necessary and, at a different point, consultation only. The determination of the type of treatment needs to be considered within the context of other therapeutic, emotional, and social demands on the infant and family.

Although many of the same neurophysiologic principles apply, treatment of the infant varies greatly from that of the adult. Infants, particularly those with motor impairment, are carried, handled, and positioned by their families and caretakers throughout the day. The therapist advises families in handling, positioning techniques, and play activities that use the sensory modalities to enhance motor function. This approach varies from recommendation of specific exercises often used for adults. For infants, developmentally appropriate play activities incorporating therapeutic principles are provided to attain active participation of the infant in establishing movement patterns.

E. Frequency of treatment

The frequency of treatment varies with the developing and changing needs of the infant (Shea, 1983). At a time when a skill is emerging, frequent guidance or treatment is indicated; once a skill has emerged and is established, less frequent involvement is necessary. Frequency, duration, and mode of treatment delivery need to remain flexible. Periodic reassessment of effectiveness and appropriateness of a treatment mode is essential.

F. Treatment settings

Certain factors should be considered in choosing a treatment setting.

1. The need for an interdisciplinary setting. Because of the interrelationship of the various areas of development, an interdisciplinary approach may be optimal.
2. The need for home treatment. Because of health factors and the difficulty with which some infants adapt to new environments, home treatment may be the best choice.
3. Physical therapy expertise. Service should be provided by a physical therapist who has experience with both normal movement in infancy and with infants who have motor dysfunction.

Agencies that provide physical therapy services for infants vary from state to state. In many areas, public health (e.g., early intervention programs) and private agencies (e.g., United Cerebral Palsy Association) provide services for infants. The physical therapy departments of pediatric hospitals can also provide services for infants and make referrals to community agencies for physical therapy as appropriate. Available treatment settings should be evaluated individually as to their ability to meet the needs of a specific infant.

REFERENCES

Amiel-Tison, C. A method for neurological evaluation within the first years of life. *Curr. Probl. Pediatr.* 7 : 1, 1976.

Barnes, M., Critchfield, C., and Heriza, C. *The Neurophysiological Bases of Patient Treatment: Reflexes in Motor Development.* Morgantown, W. Va.: Stokesville, 1978. Vol. 2.

Bayley, N. *Manual for Bayley Scales of Infant Development.* Berkeley, Calif.: Psychological Corp., 1969.

Bishop, B. Neural plasticity. II. Postnatal maturation and function-induced plasticity. *Phys. Ther.* 62 : 1132, 1982.

Bobath, B. *Abnormal Postural Reflex Activity Caused by Brain Lesions.* London: Heinemann, 1965.

Brazelton, T. Neonatal behavioral assessment scale. *Clin. Dev. Med.* No. 50, 1973.

Buller, A., Eccles, J., and Eccles, R. Differentiation of fast and slow muscles in the cat hindlimb. *J. Physiol. (Lond.)* 150 : 399, 1960.

Chandler, L., Andrews, M., and Swanson, J. *Movement Assessment of Infants: A Manual.* Rolling Bay, Wash.: 1980.

Daniels, L., and Worthingham, C. *Muscle Testing Technique of Manual Examination* (3rd ed.). Philadelphia: Saunders, 1972.

Farber, S. D. (ed.). *Neurorehabilitation, A Multisensory Approach.* Philadelphia: Saunders, 1982.

Folio, R., and Fewell, R. *Peabody Developmental Motor Scales and Activity Cards, A Manual.* Allen, Tex.: D.L.M. Teaching Resources, 1983.

Gilfoyle, E., Grady, A., and Moore, J. *Children Adapt.* Thorofare, N.J.: Charles S. Slack, 1982.

Hubel, D. The visual cortex of the normal and deprived monkey. *Am. Sci.* 532, 1979.

Knobloch, H., Stevens, F., and Malone, A. *Manual of Developmental Diagnosis.* Hagerstown, Md.: Harper & Row, 1980.

McGraw, M. *The Neuromuscular Maturation of the Human Infant.* New York: Halfner, 1963.

Ment, L., Scott, D., Ehrenkranz, R., et al. Neonates of <1250 grams birth weight: Prospective neurodevelopmental evaluation during the first year post-term. *Pediatrics* 98 : 292, 1982.

Milani-Comparetti, A., and Gidoni, E. Pattern analysis of motor development and its disorders. *Dev. Med. Child Neurol.* 9 : 625, 1967.

Mulligan, J., Painter, M., O'Donnell, P., et al. Neonatal asphyxia. II. Neonatal mortality and long-term sequelae. *J. Pediatr.* 96 : 903, 1980.

Osborne, P. Effect of respiratory distress on motor ability in pre-terms (master's thesis). Boston University, Boston, Mass., 1980.

Palisano, R. Motor development in healthy premature and full-term infants (doctoral dissertation). Boston University, Boston, Mass., 1984.

Pape, K., Bunic, R., Ashby, S., and Fitzhardinge, P. The status at two years of low birth weight infants born in 1974 with birth weights of less than 1000 grams. *J. Pediatr.* 92 : 253, 1978.

Parmelee, A., and Huber, A. Who is the "risk infant"? *Clin. Obstet. Gynecol.* 16 : 376, 1973.

Shea, A. Physical Therapy. In M. Levine, W. Carey, A. Crocker, and R. Gross (eds.), *Developmental Behavioral Pediatrics.* Philadelphia: Saunders, 1983. Pp. 1121–1123.

Stockmeyer, S. An interpretation of the approach of Rood to the treatment of neuromuscular dysfunction. *Am. J. Phys. Med.* 46 : 900, 1967.

Wolanski, N., and Zdanska-Brincken, M. A new method for the evaluation of motor development of infants. *Pol. Psychol. Bull.* 4 : 43, 1973.

Zausmer, E. Evaluation of strength and motor development in infants. Part I. *Phys. Ther. Rev.* 33 : 575, 1953.

12

Cognitive Assessment

Janice Ware and Richard R. Schnell

I. Introduction

Controversy has always surrounded the theory and practice of infant intelligence testing. The appeal and the practical utility of early identification of intellectual disability are enormous. However, questions about the predictive validity of infant tests, coupled with concerns about the effects of detrimental labeling, continue to cloud the issue of the value of the tests.

Interest in developing a method of identifying children at risk for intellectual development problems grew in the United States in the early 1900s (Brooks and Weinraub, 1976). Binet's original intelligence test, conceived during the first decade of the twentieth century, was eventually standardized as the Stanford-Binet Intelligence Scale. Psychologists then began to promote the idea that infants inherited differing amounts of an entity called *intelligence* and that it could be empirically measured (Kagan et al., 1980). This premise, not present in Binet's original concept, was an alluring idea and stimulated psychologists to study intelligence during the early years of life. As a result, scales of infant intelligence were developed. Nancy Bayley and Arnold Gesell were leaders in this movement along with Psyche Cattell and Charlotte Buhler. Each of these researchers developed popular standardized infant assessment tools; which in turn stimulated research evaluating their predictive validity. Longitudinal follow-up studies on normal populations indicated little consistency in intelligence quotients (IQs) obtained during infancy or between infancy and later stages of development. Both Bayley (1955) and Cattell (1940) concluded that variability was marked and that their tests could not be relied on for long-range prediction. Even at 2 years of age the Bayley results yielded low correlations ($r \approx .30$) with IQ at 8 years. The closer together in time the tests were given and the older the child, the higher the correlation between an earlier and a later assessment (Bayley, 1955; Honzik, 1976). At 5 years of age IQ scores did not correlate with later IQ tests more than .70. These prediction study results stimulated Bayley to restate her view of intelligence as an emergent function, taking different forms at different times.

Factor-analytic studies of the Bayley Mental Scale (McCall et al., 1972) added further support to the position that standardized infant development tests do not have good predictive validity. McCall used early forms of the test administered monthly from 1 to 15 months of age and every 3 months from 16 to 30 months and other tests semiannually until 5 years of age. McCall's data revealed major discontinuities at 3, 8, 13, and 20 months. The correlations from 3 to 4, 5, 6, or 7 months were high, but the correlations from 3 to 8 months were low. Correlations were higher between adjacent ages that were within developmental eras, that is, between 3 and 7 months or 8 and 12 months.

McCall's data imply that major psychologic changes occur around 8 months of age and again after the first birthday. This low intraindividual stability is consistent with subsequent data reported by Kagan (1971). Both McCall and Kagan argue that their findings support the notion of invariance of developmental sequences, but that the lack of stability between stages implies that the emergence of new abilities may involve new structures and that earlier structures may vanish. For example, scores on measures of early sensorimotor development may not relate to later scores on language scales because a child's language development may not be directly related to his or her earlier sensorimotor development. Precursors of language development are not clear and therefore are not readily measurable.

Results from longitudinal studies with impaired and high-risk children show that infant development tests are effective predictors of continued patterns of impairment but are much less reliable for characterizing normality. Based on these findings, the value of the single IQ-like score generated by infant tests was questioned. Other studies of nonnormal populations showed greater predictive value for infant tests. These studies included large proportions of high-risk or handicapped children and yielded high correlations for prediction for the retarded portions of their samples (Broman and Nichols, 1975; Honzik, 1962; Illingworth, 1960; Knobloch and Pasamanick, 1974; MacRae, 1955). Drillien (1961), working solely with premature infants, demonstrated that standardized developmental tests adequately predicted subnormal intelligence. Of 16 children found unsuitable to enter ordinary school programs at 5 years (all had IQs < 70), 12 had performed at this low level at 6 months of age and at all ages tested up to 5 years. Similarly, Werner and colleagues (1968, 1971) have shown that Hawaiian infants with IQs on the Cattell Scale of Infant Intelligence of less than 80 at 20 months of age are very likely to have low IQs at 10 years of age. The continued interest in early detection of cognitive risk has been supported by findings from several longitudinal investigations (Field et al., 1983; Kopp and Vaughn, 1982; Siegel, 1983b). These studies indicated diminished predictive effects for global IQ scores but demonstrated the stability of a number of more subtle cognitive effects associated with learning disabilities. Consistent with these findings is the evidence of the association between specific risks such as respiratory distress syndrome (RDS) (Field et al., 1983), bronchopulmonary dysplasia (BPD) (Goldson, 1983), and intraventricular hemorrhage (IVH) (Gaiter, 1982) and subsequent intellectual impairments.

The reason that infant tests have such a high degree of predictive variability is complex and not thoroughly understood. Fagan and McGrath (1981) proposed that the abilities measured by infant tests are not the same as those measured by intelligence tests administered later in life, and therefore, little concurrence between tests measuring different abilities should be expected. This intuitively sensible argument lends support to theorists who question the idea of developmental continuity, the basic premise of infant development tests. Continuity theorists such as Bruner (1966) and Piaget (1960) emphasized the orderly, hierarchical organization of development and the relationship of one developmental stage to another. This idea supposes that success (or failure) at one stage is related to achievement at subsequent stages. Therefore, a strong relationship should exist between test performance at different stages of development.

Despite a substantial body of evidence questioning the ability of standardized assessment techniques to predict intelligence for normal populations, there continues to be a strong interest in the early evaluation of cognition. This appeal is partly based on the belief that developmental remediation is most effective when provided as early as possible, thus necessitating the identification of appropriate candidates for intervention. Although the value of infant development tests remains in question for long-term prediction of intelligence, infant tests do have concurrent validity: They provide an accurate measure of the child's present level of functioning that correlates well with other measures of intellectual behaviors in infancy as well as medical risk variables. Infant test results also provide an effective way to communicate with parents about their child's developmental strengths and weaknesses. The test score is generally not used in this situation. Test results can be reported to the parents by qualitatively describing the test performance, emphasizing the child's developmental strengths and weaknesses. Developmental age ranges can be used instead of single test scores to describe developmental functioning. Detailed and clear qualitative descriptions of test performance can provide the information necessary for parents to advocate appropriate remediation services.

II. Developmental abilities: What should be measured
One important outcome of intelligence prediction research is the dialogue on the nature of the child's characteristics defined as representing cognition in infancy. Data (Kagan, 1971; McCall, 1977) indicating that variation in developmental patterns can exist but is not necessarily indicative of impaired outcome led developmentalists to question the nature of the abilities measured by infant development tests. Generally speaking, there is agreement that a unitary concept called intelligence is not being measured. Perhaps Boring's (1923) definition of intelligence as "what intelligence tests measure" is most appropriate. Infant development tests measure the unfolding of developmental sequences and provide a current assessment of the child's competence and overall functioning. Many characteristics that play a major role in determining test outcome are assessed subjectively by the examiner and influence scoring of the test. Most notable among these characteristics are attention, persistence, responsiveness to the test situation, and motivation. Impairments in motor or sensory development (or both) also will directly affect test performance. Other important influences often implicated in cognitive status include a variety of maternal and family characteristics such as socioeconomic status, life stress, and amount and type of environmental stimulation available to the child. This combination of multiple factors with the child's actual pass-fail performance on individual test items is often defined as "cognition in infancy." Many would argue, however, that the multifactored judgments involved in the assessment process describe a general level of overall functioning or competence rather than a more unified concept of intelligence. Zigler and Trickett (1978) proposed the use of social competence measures as opposed to measures of intelligence. Included in their definition of social com-

petence are four categories of behavior: physical health, formal cognitive ability, achievement in school, and motivational-emotional variables. Their work is consistent with the growing interest in minimizing the use of a single developmental test score to characterize a child's level of functioning and maximizing the use of qualitative and descriptive assessments of the child's abilities. Scarr's thoughtful review (1981) discussed many of these ideas and advocated that the examiner have a clear understanding about what is being assessed, that the examiner carefully think through what he or she wants to know as a result of the cognitive evaluation, and further, that the examiner consider what decisions about the infant's life will be affected by the knowledge from the testing.

III. Infant assessments: Developmental tests of choice
The administration of tests to infants or their caretakers must follow standard procedures. Descriptive procedures for many tests are deceptively simple and are readily subject to misapplication. Extensive professional education, training, and supervision are necessary for appropriate use of the tests.

A. Assessments of development
Tests such as the Bayley Scales and the Denver Developmental Screening Test (DDST) enable examiners to make determinations about a child's abilities based on the number of developmental milestones achieved. Test performance is scored on a pass-fail basis. The developmental milestones assessed by infant development tests were empirically derived and not based on developmental theory. For example, during the first year of life, scores on infant tests are primarily determined by assessing a collection of the infant's neuromotor abilities. Because these scales assess behavior, they do include elements of sequential patterns of development, but they were not originally organized to measure these patterns. The score generated allows the examiner to compare the rate of sensorimotor development of the child taking the test with a normative sample consisting of other children of similar chronologic ages.

The tests most widely used for diagnostic purposes in the United States include the Gesell Developmental Schedules (Gesell and Amatruda, 1947; Knobloch and Pasamanick, 1974) and the Bayley Scales of Infant Development (1969). The Gesell Developmental Schedules present procedures for evaluating observed behavior of children from 1 month to 6 years of age. Gesell test items require either observation or direct assessment using tools from the test kit. Four scales compose the test: Motor Development, Adaptive Behavior, Language Development, and Personal-Social Behavior. The schedules do not have adequate norms, and little data are available on reliability and validity. The Gesell is employed as a screening tool as only age approximations can be obtained from each of the four scales. A rough developmental quotient, however, can be computed by dividing the developmental age by the chronologic age of the child.

Items from the Gesell Developmental Schedules have been widely used in other tests such as the Bayley Scales of Infant Development. The Bayley Scales comprise three separate scales: Mental, Motor, and Infant Behavior

Record. Of these three, the Mental Scale is most widely used. Norms for the Bayley Scales are considered to be the most representative for children from 2 to 30 months of age, and the scores have proved to be reliable. Overall standard scores, similar to IQs, are derived for the mental and motor scales. Developmental ages can also be obtained for these scales. Percentile ranks are available for each of the 24 ratings of the Infant Behavior Record. The Bayley is the test most often used to characterize infant developmental status.

Another test that uses Gesell items and is employed by many disciplines is the DDST (Frankenburg and Dodds, 1967; Frankenburg et al., 1971). The DDST is a series of developmental observations similar to those routinely made by a pediatrician. There are four scales assessing fine and gross motor abilities, language, and personal-social development. The scales are not numerically scored but are interpreted more impressionistically with a view to determining the maturity of the child. When examiners are well trained, the test reliability is relatively high. Although early reports indicated that it was an effective tool for identifying developmental problems, more recent evidence indicates that it may not be as useful as presumed, particularly with premature infants, because it is not a sensitive indicator of developmental delay (Elliman et al., 1985; Solomons and Solomons, 1975; Wacker, 1980).

One shortcoming of global function scores such as those generated by the DDST or the Bayley Scales is that they do not provide direct information about sequential patterns of development. Clinically useful data about the developmental stage aspects of a child's abilities must be gathered and recorded incidentally or by using a complementary test that characterizes the child's test performance descriptively. One example of a test designed to do this is the ordinal scales of infant development based on Piagetian tasks and developed by Uzgiris and Hunt (1975). Six scales are used to describe the child's sensorimotor stage placement. The scales assessing (1) the development of visual pursuit and the permanence of objects and (2) the development of means for obtaining desired environmental events are the most frequently used. No commercial test kit is available, but Uzgiris and Hunt (1975) describe the standard materials and test procedures for administration in their book. Other sensorimotor scales based on Piagetian theory such as the Casati-Lezine (1968) and the Decarie Scales (1965) are also widely used.

Another ordinal method of assessing development is the factor-analytic approach developed by Kohen-Raz (1967). This test uses 67 of the 163 items of the Bayley Mental Scale to assess developmental functioning within specific ability areas of the Bayley Scales. The Kohen-Raz method of scoring the Bayley divides Bayley items into five ordinal scales: eye-hand, manipulation, object relations, imitation-comprehension, and vocalization-social. Although promising, the factor-analytic approach has not received much clinical use.

Honzik (1976) believed that infant developmental test scores would be of greater value if specific abilities rather than global functions were measured. Recently more attention has been paid to using such measures with high-risk infants. Reports describing school performance (Rubin et al.,

1973), language development (Crawford, 1982; Siegel, 1983b), visual information processing (Rose, 1983; Ungerer and Sigman, 1983), and visual-motor abilities (Siegel, 1982) demonstrate differences between the performance of premature versus full-term children. Unfortunately, many of the specific ability measures (such as the Beery Developmental Test of Visual-Motor Integration and the McCarthy Scales of Children's Abilities) are not useful during the first 2 years of life.

B. Assessments of the environment

The younger the child, the more limited the range of abilities available for testing. Infant tests emphasize perceptual-motor exploration in the first 7 months of life, the understanding of means-end relationships at 8 to 13 months, the use of representation in the form of emerging communication skills at 14 to 18 months, and symbolic functioning and understanding of relationships beyond 18 months. Thus, early developmental testing primarily measures biologic functions and maturation of the neuromotor system.

As the child enters the second year, development becomes increasingly influenced by a broader range of factors, many of which have strong environmentally influenced determinants. Examples of environmentally influenced abilities include social adaptation, language development, and the ability to complete test tasks based on information and knowledge acquired through experience. The importance of the environment in relation to a child's development outcome is best described by Sameroff and Chandler's (1975) transactional model of child development. This model stresses the dynamic nature of both the child and environment, and the child's active role in shaping his or her environment over time. The child and environment interact and affect each other, and each adapts and changes over time as a result of these interactions. The chance that a negative developmental outcome will occur is enhanced when a high-risk infant is placed in an inadequate environment. In response to the recognition of the importance of environmental influences, test instruments have been developed to assess the quality of the home environment. Numerous studies show that availability of information about the home environment increases the accuracy of developmental prediction. Identification of positive and negative aspects of an infant's home environment combined with developmental test results may increase accuracy of prediction, particularly in borderline situations. For example, a mildly delayed infant in the first year of life who is raised in an extremely facilitative environment may be expected to function ultimately as a normal child. Likewise, an infant who develops normally in the first year of life growing up in an extremely deficient environment may not optimize his or her developmental potential (Escalona, 1982).

The instrument most commonly used for assessment of the home environment is the Home Observation for Measurement of the Environment (HOME) (Bradley and Caldwell, 1976). The infant HOME (birth to 36 months) comprises six subscales and is intended to measure the quality and quantity of social, emotional, and cognitive support available in the child's home. Scores on the HOME have been found to relate to later men-

tal development. Data are gathered from a combination of parental interviews and observation in the home. An obvious limitation of the HOME is
the requirement of a home visit. Unfortunately, staff time and resources
necessary for such visits are outside the reaches of most child evaluation
clinics. In an attempt to obtain information about the child's home environment within the confines of limited resources, several researchers have
developed adapted versions of the HOME for clinic use (see Chap. 13).

The HOME has also been used as one of the four techniques in the
Nursing Child Assessment Project (NCAST) (Barnard, 1978), which seeks
to serve as an early predictor of child health and development. A well-
organized program has been developed for training professionals to a high
level of interrater reliability in the use of the techniques so that they are
maximally effective. The NCAST system employs the Sleep/Activity Record,
which documents the newborn's and young infant's state-related behavior
patterns, and the Feeding and Teaching Scales, which assess the infant's and
parent's adaptive behaviors from observations of their interactions during
the first year of life.

Other scales that use information from parents or caretakers are called
"measures of adaptive behavior." They are measures of the behavior of
children that is effective in meeting the natural and social demands of the
environment (Grossman, 1973). These scales rely almost exclusively on
parental or caretaker reports. They provide information about the daily living skills of children who are thought to be developmentally delayed, and
these data can be compared to the same children's performance on measures of cognitive development. The newest and most extensively developed measure is the Vineland Adaptive Behavior Scales (Sparrow et al.,
1984), for use with children from birth through 18 years of age. The Vineland surveys four familiar domains of behavior: communication, socialization, daily living skills, and motor skills. Other adaptive behavior scales for
special groups are also available such as the Maxfield-Bucholz adaptation
of the old Vineland Social Maturity Scale for blind children (Maxfield and
Bucholz, 1957) and the Callier-Azusa Scale for deaf and blind children
(Stillman, 1975).

IV. Infant assessment test schedules: Who should be tested and when
The developmental testing of premature infants poses special challenges. As a
group, preterm infants are recognized as being at high risk for damage to the
central nervous system. Further, the more premature the infant, the higher the
risk for subsequent impairment (Drillien, 1972; Francis-Williams and Davies,
1974; Lubchenco et al., 1974). Because mental retardation in childhood resulting from damage to the central nervous system is frequently preceded by
developmental delays (Holden, 1972; Knobloch and Pasamanick, 1974; VanderVeer and Schweid, 1974), it is important to have an early and effective
means of monitoring the cognitive development of high-risk infants. An optimal developmental testing system maximizes contact with infants at highest
risk biologically and environmentally, while minimizing testing requirements
for healthy premature infants in stable environments. No clear-cut standard
exists to identify children in need of developmental testing. Environmental influences such as socioeconomic status must also be used to assess risk. Poor

and nonwhite women, for example, are at higher risk for delivering a premature child (Garn et al., 1977), and data from current studies report as much as a 30 percent IQ difference between the performance of economically advantaged and disadvantaged children, a result that may overshadow the influence of prematurity (Kopp, 1983). The most premature infants (< 28 weeks' gestational age) with complex medical and social risk histories clearly are candidates for continued monitoring of their developmental progress. The interactive effects of such risks are now well documented. Findings from longitudinal studies of premature infants conducted in the 1970s indicated that approximately 10 percent have severe handicapping conditions (Kopp, 1983). Because medical techniques for the care of premature infants continue to improve rapidly, this kind of figure is subject to change every few years. Many important perinatal problems and medical risks, however, have not been associated with problematic outcomes (Littman, 1979; Sigman and Parmelee, 1979), and these must be sorted out from the real contributors to risk. Longitudinal outcome research has reported major risk group differences, but many of these risks interact to effect risk for a particular infant, and the variability within risk groups has not been thoroughly explored. The present rule of thumb with respect to the use of infant scales such as the Bayley is to use scores greater than 1 standard deviation below the mean as indicators of developmental risk (Field, 1978).

V. Problems encountered in infant testing
    The developmental assessment of the premature infant poses special problems for the clinician and researcher. The question of how to deal with biologic immaturity, prematurity, and specific impairments (such as retrolental fibroplasia and cerebral palsy) remains unanswered. Standardized infant assessment tools do not provide guidelines for prorating scores based on degree of prematurity, nor do they provide guidelines for adapting test materials for specific impairments common to the premature infant.

    A. Testing the premature infant
        Calculation of scores for standardized infant development tests such as the Bayley are based on use of the child's chronologic age. Developmental delays as a function of prematurity were first described by Gesell and Amatruda (1945), who designated a newborn infant less than 40 weeks' gestation a fetal infant whose biologic timetable would proceed on its natural course despite the accident of premature birth. Full allowance for premature birth was suggested when evaluating development with the Gesell Developmental Schedules (Gesell and Amatruda, 1947). This practice has been widely adopted by persons working with premature infants, and for years it has been the custom to correct for the prematurity during the first 2 years of life (Hunt, 1981; Hunt and Rhodes, 1977). Kopp and Parmelee (1979) described two possible correction methods. In one system, age is calculated from time of expected date of birth (the term date rather than the actual birth date). For example, an infant with an expected birth date of June 1 is born April 1; June 1 is the date used to calculate subsequent age. An alternative strategy calculates the entire number of weeks from birth and subtracts the number of weeks of preterm birth. For exam-

ple, an infant with a total amount of extrauterine life equal to 38 weeks, born 6 weeks early, is considered to be 32 weeks, or approximately 8 months of age.

More recent data on the correction question suggest that full correction for the first 2 years of life results in overcorrection after the first 12 months of life. Siegel's (1983a) longitudinal study of the consequences of correcting developmental test scores for prematurity has strongly influenced this point of view. She found that in the first year of life corrected developmental test scores were more highly correlated with 3- and 5-year test scores. From 12 months of age on, uncorrected scores were more highly correlated. Based on these findings, Siegel suggested that use of corrected scores is probably most appropriate during the first months of life when development is strongly influenced by biologic factors. As the child matures and environmental factors become more important, it is appropriate then to use uncorrected scores. For clinical purposes, the child's score on the developmental test is less important than the pattern of the test, which should reflect increasing gains in developmental abilities.

B. Effects of impairment on test performance

Correcting for prematurity accounts for biologic immaturity but does not consider the effect of specific impairments on test performance. Current clinical practice is to adapt available tests and describe the child's performance qualitatively rather than quantitatively. The large number of test items evaluating perceptual-motor skills at the lower end of infant tests poses a problem for the young infant with clear indications of motor disability. Smoothly functioning motor coordination is needed to achieve a high score on the Bayley Scales at the lower end of the scale. For example, at 6 months of age, the child is expected to use his or her gross motor skills to reach out to grasp and manipulate objects and to transfer objects from hand to hand. Fine motor skill performance at this age level tests the infant's ability to use fingers to secure a string and to lift a cup by the handle. In addition to test items assessing motor proficiency, many Bayley and Gesell items testing other abilities rely heavily on motor skill development. For example, the Bayley tests the child's ability to produce secondary circular reactions such as relating two objects by banging them. To accomplish this task, the child must first be able to grasp and retain objects. A Bayley item assessing social responsivity is tested through observation of the child's playful patting response to his or her mirror image, again requiring arm and hand coordination abilities. Thus, the child with motor dysfunction will not be able to complete many early infant test items successfully, resulting in a lower test score. The nature and degree of motor impairment must be made clear in the description of the child's test results. Similar concerns are also raised if a child has a sensory impairment.

VI. Experimental infant testing strategies

Dissatisfaction with available infant development tests has led researchers to consider alternative methods of evaluating cognition in infancy (Fantz and Fagan, 1975; Kearsley, 1979; Rose, 1983; Zelazo, 1979). These researchers have concentrated on more direct assessments of cognitive processes such as habituation, visual discrimination and fixation, and recognition memory. In addition, an increasing number of researchers have begun to explore the predictive effectiveness of noncognitive indices of development such as heart-rate patterns (Fox and Porges, 1985; Porges, 1983) and temperamental inhibition (Garcia-Coll et al., 1984; Kagan et al., 1984). Researchers studying nontraditional approaches to behavioral assessment hope that such techniques will clarify the building blocks of more complex behaviors as well as function as a diagnostic window to the brain.

Studies of visual perception and memory have revealed interesting differences between full-term and preterm infants. Kopp and Vaughn (1982) found that sustained attention to presentation of test stimuli at 8 months of age was positively related to cognitive competence at 2 years of age as measured by both the Gesell and the Bayley. Ruddy and Bornstein (1982) found that attention at 4 months of age as measured by habituation rate or frequency was related to 12-month Bayley results. Sigman and associates (1973) found that full-term infants who were less attentive were more likely to have neurologic problems than those who were more attentive. Both Osofsky (1976) and Sigman and Beckwith (1980) related visual attentiveness to caretaking with their findings that full-term infants who were more attentive to visual and auditory stimuli during neonatal testing had mothers who were more attentive and sensitive to them. This finding is presumably based on the reasoning that more attentive infants elicit more positive caretaking responses from their mothers. When the same attention paradigm was administered to preterm infants, interesting, paradoxic findings were revealed. The preterm infants showed longer fixation times than full-term infants, but the maternal caretaking behaviors were inattentive and insensitive. Preterm infants with longer fixation times received less caretaking from their mothers. Also, high attentiveness in the preterm infant was negatively related to later Bayley scores in girls. Sigman and Beckwith (1980) concluded that in preterm infants high attentiveness reflects an inability to turn off stimulation rather than a state in which the ability to process information is maximal.

Recognition memory tasks administered early in infancy (Fagan and McGrath, 1981) were found to be statistically significant and moderately well correlated with later vocabulary-based tests of intelligence. The results were independent of differences on socioeconomic status, which adds further support to the view that assessments using information processing models may be less confounded by environmental influences.

VII. Recommendations

Despite the limitations and controversy surrounding available infant assessment techniques, they continue to have merit as effective means of identifying infants at risk for developmental disabilities. Identification of risk status can lead to provision of early intervention services aimed at prevention and amelioration of potential problems. The limitations of individual infant assessment techniques, however, must always be taken into account, and attempts to make long-term predictions about a child are not usually warranted. In this regard, infant assessors must be well-trained professionals who not only have a sound background in child development but have had training in the use of the measures and understand their strengths and limitations.

Three major issues must be addressed when assessing infants. The context in which the child exists must always be taken into account. Environmental and personal factors such as socioeconomic status of the parents, family stability, the child's health history, and sequelae of prematurity such as IVH or BPD need to be considered because they influence risk. Second, a combination of techniques should be used in evaluation. Taking a single score from a measure such as the Bayley Scales and using it alone to represent the child is not appropriate. Developmental levels in different areas such as adaptive skills, gross and fine motor development, language development, and cognitive development give a rounded picture of the child and might improve prediction. The use of developmental age scores, rather than standard scores, which often seem to parents like IQ scores, should be encouraged. Normative-based measures such as the Bayley Scale yield developmental levels and scores that may not lead parents to any better comprehension of their child's behavior. Piagetian measures such as the Uzgiris-Hunt Scales are not good predictors of future development, but may be employed to help parents understand how their children comprehend the world and respond to it. Parental insight can often lead to better parent-child interactions.

Third, prediction about an infant's development made to parents and others should initially be tentative and short-term. As an infant progresses in developing various skills over specific periods of time and under known conditions, better developmental predictions can be made. Infants at notable risk for developmental handicaps should be assessed at regular intervals. These assessments should be primarily for the parents to ask questions about the infant and to get to know their infant better. Only secondarily should the assessments be an exercise in discovering disability. With such an emphasis, assessment would be less likely to provoke anxiety, and more likely to contribute to parenting.

REFERENCES

Barnard, K. *Nursing Child Assessment Satellite Training: Instructor's Learning Resource Manual.* Seattle, Wash.: University of Washington School of Nursing, 1978.

Bayley, N. On the growth of intelligence. *Am. Psychol.* 10 : 805, 1955.

Bayley, N. *Bayley Scales of Infant Development: Birth to Two Years.* New York: Psychological Corp., 1969.

Boring, E. G. Intelligence as the test measures it. *New Republic* 35 : 35, 1923.

Bradley, R. H., and Caldwell, B. M. The relation of infants' home environment to mental test performance at fifty-four months: A follow-up study. *Child Dev.* 47 : 1172, 1976.

Broman, S., and Nichols, P. L. Early mental development, social class, and school-age IQ. Presented to the annual meeting of the American Psychological Association, Chicago, Sept. 1975.

Brooks, J., and Weinraub, M. A History of Infant Intelligence Testing. In M. Lewis (ed.), *Origins of Intelligence: Infancy and Early Childhood.* New York: Plenum, 1976.

Bruner, J. S. *Studies in Cognitive Growth.* New York: Wiley, 1966.

Caldwell, B. M., and Bradley, R. H. *Administration Manual: Home Observation for Measurement of the Environment* (rev. ed.). Little Rock, Ark.: University of Arkansas, 1984.

Casati, I., and Lezine, I. Les étapes de l'intelligence sensorimotrice. Les Éditions du Centre de Psychologie Appliquée. Paris, 1968.

Cattell, P. *The Measurement of Intelligence of Infants and Young Children.* New York: Psychological Corp., 1940.

Crawford, J. W. Mother-infant interaction in premature and full-term infants. *Child Dev.* 53 : 957, 1982.

Decarie, T. G. *Intelligence and Affectivity in Early Childhood.* New York: International Universities Press, 1965.

Drillien, C. M. A longitudinal study of the growth and development of prematurely and maturely born children. *Arch. Dis. Child.* 36 : 233, 1961.

Drillien, C. M. Abnormal neurological signs in the first year of life in low-birthweight infants: Possible prognostic significance. *Dev. Med. Child Neurol.* 14 : 575, 1972.

Elliman, A. M., Bryan, E. M., Elliman, A. D., et al. Denver Developmental Screening Test and preterm infants. *Arch. Dis. Child.* 60 : 20, 1985.

Escalona, S. K. Babies at double hazard: Early development of infants at biologic and social risk. *Pediatrics* 70 : 670, 1982.

Fagan, J. F., and McGrath, S. K. Infant recognition memory and later intelligence. *Intelligence* 5 : 121, 1981.

Fantz, R. L., and Fagan, J. F. Visual attention to size and number of pattern details by term and preterm infants during the first six months. *Child Dev.* 46 : 3, 1975.

Field, T., Dempsey, J., and Shuman, H. H. Five-year Follow-up of Preterm Respiratory Distress Syndrome and Post-term Postmaturity Syndrome Infants. In T. Field and A. Sostek (eds.), *Infants Born at Risk: Physiological, Perceptual, and Cognitive Processes.* New York: Grune & Stratton, 1983.

Field, T., Hallock, N., Ting, G., et al. A first year follow-up of high-risk infants: Formulating a cumulative risk index. *Child Dev.* 49 : 119, 1978.

Fox, N., and Porges, S. W. The relation between neonatal heart period patterns and developmental outcome. *Child Dev.* 56 : 28, 1985.

Francis-Williams, J., and Davies, P. A. Very low birthweight and later intelligence. *Dev. Med. Child Neurol.* 16 : 709, 1974.

Frankenburg, W. K., and Dodds, J. B. The Denver Developmental Screening Test. *J. Pediatr.* 71 : 181, 1967.

Frankenburg, W. K., Goldstein, A. D., and Camp, B. W. The revised Denver Developmental Screening Test: Its accuracy as a screening instrument. *Pediatrics* 20 : 988, 1971.

Gaiter, J. L. The effects of intraventricular hemorrhage on Bayley developmental performance in preterm infants. *Semin. Perinatol.* 6 : 305, 1982.

Garcia-Coll, C., Kagan, J., and Reznick, J. S. Behavioral inhibition in young children. *Child Dev.* 55 : 1005, 1984.

Garn, S. M., Shaw, H. A., and McCabe, K. D. Effects of Socioeconomic Status and Race on Weight-Defined and Gestational Prematurity in the United States. In D. W. Reed and F. J. Stanley (eds.), *The Epidemiology of Prematurity.* Baltimore and Munich: Urban & Schwarenberg, 1977.

Gesell, A., and Amatruda, C. S. *The Embryology of Behavior.* New York: Harper & Row, 1945.

Gesell, A., and Amatruda, C. S. *Developmental Diagnosis.* New York: Harper & Row, 1947.

Goldson, E. Bronchopulmonary Dysplasia: Its Relation to Two-year Developmental Functioning in the Very Low Birth Weight Infant. In T. Field and A. Sostek (eds.), *Infants Born at Risk: Physiological, Perceptual, and Cognitive Processes.* New York: Grune & Stratton, 1983.

Grossman, H. J. *Manual on Terminology and Classification in Mental Retardation* (rev. ed.). Baltimore: American Association on Mental Deficiency and Garamond/Pridemark, 1973.

Hirata, T., Epcar, J. T., Walsh, A., et al. Survival and outcome of infants 501 to 750 gm: A six-year experience. *J. Pediatr.* 102 : 741, 1983.

Holden, R. H. Prediction of mental retardation in infancy. *Ment. Retard.* 10 : 28, 1972.

Honzik, M. The mental and motor test performance of infants diagnosed or suspected of brain injury (unpublished manuscript). Berkeley, Calif., 1962.

Honzik, M. Value and Limitations of Infant Tests: An Overview. In M. Lewis (ed.), *Origins of Intelligence: Infancy and Early Childhood.* New York: Plenum, 1976.

Hunt, J. V. Predicting Intellectual Disorders in Childhood for Preterm Infants with Birthweights Below 1501 Grams. In S. L. Friedman and M. Sigman (eds.), *Preterm Birth and Psychological Development.* New York: Academic, 1981.

Hunt, J. V., and Rhodes, L. Mental development of infants during the first year. *Child Dev.* 49 : 204, 1977.

Illingworth, R. S. *The Development of the Infant and the Young Child: Normal and Abnormal.* London: Livingstone, 1960.

Kagan, J. *Change and Continuity in Infancy.* New York: Wiley, 1971.

Kagan, J., Kearsley, R. B., and Zelazo, P. R. *Infancy: Its Place in Human Development.* Cambridge, Mass.: Harvard University Press, 1980.

Kagan, J., Reznick, S., Clarke, C., et al. Behavioral inhibition to the unfamiliar. *Child Dev.* 55 : 2212, 1984.

Kearsley, R. B. Iatrogenic Retardation: A Syndrome of Learned Incompetence. In R. B. Kearsley and I. Sigel (eds.), *Infants at Risk: The Assessment of Cognitive Functioning.* Hillsdale, N.J.: Erlbaum, 1979.

Knobloch, H., and Pasamanick, B. (eds.). *Gesell and Amatruda's Developmental Diagnosis* (3rd ed.). New York: Harper & Row, 1974.

Kohen-Raz, R. Scalogram analysis of some developmental sequences of infant behavior as measured by the Bayley Infant Scale of Mental Development. *Genet. Psychol. Monogr.* 76 : 3, 1967.

Kopp, C. Risk Factors in Development. In M. Haith and J. Campos (eds.), *Infancy and the Biology of Development* (Manual of Child Development, P. Mussen, ed.). New York: Wiley, 1983. Vol. 2.

Kopp, C. B., and Parmelee, A. H. Prenatal and Perinatal Influences on Infant Behavior. In J. Osofsky (ed.), *Handbook of Infant Development.* New York: Wiley, 1979.

Kopp, C., and Vaughn, B. E. Sustained attention during exploratory manipulation as a predictor of cognitive competence in preterm infants. *Child Dev.* 53 : 174, 1982.

Littman, B. The Relationship of Medical Events to Infant Development. In T. Field, A. Sostek, S. Goldberg, and H. H. Shuman (eds.), *Infants Born at Risk.* New York: Spectrum, 1979.

Lubchenco, L. O., Bard, H., Goldman, A. L., et al. Newborn intensive care and long-term prognosis. *Dev. Med. Child Neurol.* 16 : 421, 1974.

MacRae, J. M. Retests of children given mental tests as infants. *J. Genet. Psychol.* 87 : 111, 1955.

Maxfield, K., and Bucholz, S. *The Maxfield-Bucholz Scale of Social Maturity.* New York: American Federation for the Blind, 1957.

McCall, R. B., Eichorn, D. H., and Hogarty, P. S. Transitions in early mental development. *Monogr. Soc. Res. Child Dev.* 42. Serial No. 171, 1977.

McCall, R. B., Hogarty, P. S., and Hurlburt, N. Transitions in infant sensorimotor development and the prediction of childhood IQ. *Am. Psychol.* 27 : 728, 1972.

Osofsky, J. D. Neonatal characteristics and mother-infant interaction in two observational situations. *Child Dev.* 47 : 1138, 1976.

Piaget, J. *Psychology of Intelligence.* Patterson, N.J.: Littlefield, Adams, 1960.

Porges, S. Heart Rate Patterns in Neonates: A Potential Diagnostic Window to the Brain. In T. Field and A. Sostek (eds.), *Infants Born at Risk: Physiological, Perceptual, and Cognitive Processes.* New York: Grune & Stratton, 1983.

Rose, S. A. Differential rates of visual information processing in full-term and preterm infants. *Child Dev.* 54 : 1189, 1983.

Ross, G., Lipper, E. G., and Auld, P. Consistency and change in the development of premature infants weighing less than 1,501 grams at birth. *Pediatrics* 76 : 885, 1985.

Rubin, R. A., Rosenblatt, C., and Balow, B. Psychological and educational sequelae of prematurity. *Pediatrics* 52 : 352, 1973.

Ruddy, M. G., and Bornstein, M. H. Cognitive correlates of infant attention and maternal stimulation over the first years of life. *Child Dev.* 53 : 183, 1982.

Sameroff, A. J., and Chandler, M. J. Reproductive Risk and the Continuum of Caretaking Casualty. In F. D. Horowitz (ed.), *Review of Child Development Research.* Chicago: University of Chicago Press, 1975. Vol. 4.

Scarr, S. Testing for children: Assessment and the many determinants of intellectual competence. *Am. Psychol.* 36 : 1159, 1981.

Siegel, L. S. Reproductive, perinatal, and environmental factors as predictors of the cognitive and language development of preterm and full-term infants. *Child Dev.* 54 : 963, 1982.

Siegel, L. S. Correction for prematurity and its consequences for the assessment of the very low birthweight infant. *Child Dev.* 54 : 1176, 1983a.

Siegel, L. S. The Prediction of Possible Learning Disabilities in Preterm and Full-term Children. In T. Field and A. Sostek (eds.), *Infants Born at Risk: Physiological, Perceptual, and Cognitive Processes.* New York: Grune & Stratton, 1983b.

Sigman, M., and Beckwith, L. Infant visual attentiveness in relation to caregiver-infant interaction and developmental outcome. *Infant Behav. Dev.* 3 : 141, 1980.

Sigman, M., Kopp, C. V., Parmelee, A. H., and Jeffrey, W. E. Visual attention and neurological organization in neonates. *Child Dev.* 44 : 461, 1973.

Sigman, M., and Parmelee, A. H. Longitudinal Evaluation of the High-Risk Infant. In T. M. Field, A. M. Sostek, S. Goldberg, and H. H. Shuman (eds.), *Infants Born at Risk.* New York: Spectrum, 1979.

Solomons, G., and Solomons, H. G. Motor development in Yucatan infants. *Dev. Med. Child Neurol.* 17 : 41, 1975.

Sparrow, S. S., Balla, D. A., and Cicchetti, D. A. *Vineland Adaptive Behavior Scales.* Circle Pines, Minn.: American Guidance Service, 1984.

Stillman, R. D. *Assessment of Deaf-Blind Children: The Callier-Azusa Scale.* Dallas: Callier Hearing and Speech Center, 1975.

Ungerer, J. A., and Sigman, M. Developmental lags in preterm infants from one to three years of age. *Child Dev.* 54 : 1217, 1983.

Uzgiris, I., and Hunt, J. M. *Assessment in Infancy: Ordinal Scales of Psychological Development.* Urbana, Ill.: University of Illinois Press, 1975.

VanderVeer, B., and Schweid, E. Infant assessment: Stability of mental functioning in young retarded children. *Am. J. Ment. Defic.* 78 : 1, 1974.

Wacker, D. Diagnostic efficiency of the Denver Developmental Screening Test. Presented to the annual meeting of the American Psychological Association, Montreal, Sept. 1980.

Werner, E. E., Bierman, J. M., and French, F. E. *The Children of Kauai: A Longitudinal Study from the Prenatal Period to Age 10.* Honolulu: University of Hawaii Press, 1971.

Werner, E. E., Honzik, M. P., and Smith, R. S. Prediction of intelligence and achievement at 10 years from 20 month pediatric and psychological examinations. *Child Dev.* 39 : 1063, 1968.

Zelazo, P. R. Infant Reactivity to Perceptual-Cognitive Events: Application for Infant Assessment. In R. B. Kearsley and I. Sigel (eds.), *Infants at Risk: The Assessment of Cognitive Functioning.* Hillsdale, N.J.: Erlbaum, 1979.

Zigler, E., and Trickett, P. K. IQ, social competence, and evaluation of early childhood intervention programs. *Am. Psychol.* 33 : 789, 1978.

13

The Home Environment

Patrick H. Casey and Robert H. Bradley

I. Introduction

Research and clinical experience have documented that the developmental and behavioral potential for most children is affected by the environment in which the child lives, to an extent at least comparable to the biologic constitution of the child. The most contemporary model of child development is the *transactional* model presented by Sameroff and Chandler (1975). This model stresses the dynamic nature of both the child and environment and the child's active role in shaping his or her environment over time. The child and environment interact and affect each other, and each adapts and changes over time as a result of these interactions. The child's health, physical appearance, gender, neurodevelopmental status, and temperament thus may affect the developmental-behavioral status directly at any point, but also indirectly by affecting the home environment. The more adaptable and competent the child and the more supportive and appropriately stimulating the home, the more likely that the child's development and behavior will be optimal. Problems with either the child or the environment create the potential for developmental and behavioral abnormalities. The probability of abnormalities increases when there are both a vulnerable child and an inadequate environment.

Premature and low-birth-weight infants are known to be at greater risk for developmental disabilities than full-term normal-sized newborns. Several studies have determined that the quality of the home environment of premature and low-birth-weight infants predicts developmental outcome better than any single biologic risk factor or aggregate of such risk factors (Sameroff and Chandler, 1975). For example, in Drillien's classic study of 595 premature infants, the developmental quotients (DQs) of the children at age 4 differed with each birth-weight group for each social class (Drillien, 1964). The greatest difference, 33 points, occurred between the smallest infants from the lowest social class and those from the highest social class (DQ of 64 versus 97).

Two recent prospective studies have shed light on the importance of the relation between biologic and environmental risk. Sigman and Parmelee (1979) followed 126 premature infants until the age of 25 months. A complex *cumulative risk* score quantitated medical, developmental, and social environmental factors. No correlations were found between the Obstetrical Complication Scale or the Postnatal Complication Scale and the infant's development at 24 months. When the infants were classified as high risk or low risk according to the original 14 criteria, there were no significant differences between the high-risk or low-risk infants in their 24-month developmental scores. However, when new risk classifications were made that included observation of mother-infant interaction, there were significant differences between high-risk and low-risk infants in their 24-month developmental scores. The best predictors of 24-month developmental status were the quality of the early infant-caretaker interaction and a 9-month developmental evaluation. In the second study, Siegel followed 53 premature and 51 term children in a longitudinal study until 3 years of age (Siegel, 1982). For the premature infants, socioeconomic status, birth order, and severity of perinatal illness were the best predictors of 3-year developmental status. Specific aspects of the home environment correlated with developmental outcome independent of socioeconomic status. Children considered at risk at 1 year but who were normal at 3 years came from families who provided better home environments. Children who were not thought to be at risk at 1 year but who were developmentally abnormal at 3 years came from families with less optimal home environments. In summary, the combination of perinatal and environmental variables allowed more accurate prediction of infants at risk for developmental problems.

Theorists and researchers have made major advances in conceptualizing the aspects of the environment that affect children's development and behavior. Infant development is most heavily influenced by those aspects of the environment most proximal to the child (parenting received, physical surroundings). These specific environmental factors are important to clinicians because they constantly change, are specific for individual families at various points in time, are measurable, and provide information that may be acted on clinically. The remainder of this chapter discusses clinical interpretations and recommendations based on the current status of an extremely active research field.

II. Vulnerability aspects of premature infants

Several characteristics of premature infants and the events surrounding their care make them vulnerable or liable to developmental and behavioral problems that go beyond the direct effects of the multiple medical problems that may affect their neurologic integrity. These factors increase the likelihood of problems by their effect on the parents and the home environment. For example, that premature infants are overrepresented in groups of abused children or children who fail to thrive suggests that these infants present problems to parents which may contribute to parenting failure.

A. Characteristics of premature infants
   1. Prolonged hospital stay and separation. Extended hospital stays in neonatal intensive care units (NICUs) structurally minimize the amount of physical and emotional contact between parent and child. Parents have less opportunity to interact with and to understand their infants as individuals. Bonding problems resulting from this separation have been well described by Klaus and Kennell (1976), among others.
   2. Health-related problems. Premature and low-birth-weight infants are clearly prone to serious illness after discharge from the NICU. For example, a recent study established that low-birth-weight infants were twice as likely as normal-birth-weight infants to be hospitalized in the first year of life, and that infants less than 1,500 g at birth are 4 times as likely to be rehospitalized (McCormick et al., 1980). Also, the concern with persisting apnea in premature infants and the trend to use home

apnea monitors (perhaps 50% of all premature infants currently discharged from NICUs) prolong the illness phase of these infants after discharge from the NICU.
3. Atypical behavioral characteristics. Premature infants, particularly sick
premature infants, present several problematic behavioral characteristics compared with healthy term infants, which make them difficult to
interact with as social partners (DiVitto and Goldberg, 1979). Some of
these characteristics are as follows:
a. More irritable, fussy, and restless
b. Less attentive and responsive to interaction
c. Less persistent in visual and auditory skills
d. Less coordinated in motor and feeding skills
4. Physical appearance. Premature infants seldom have the features that
attract parents and encourage positive interactions. Their elongated
heads, thin skins, and poorly integrated motor responses may create
fear and prevent formation of an emotional tie.

B. Characteristics of the home and parent-child interaction
1. Financial burden. The considerable financial burden that results from
neonatal medical care may negatively affect all aspects of the home environment. Financial problems may supersede all other difficulties.
2. Parent attitudes. Lack of preparation for premature birth, the NICU experience, the financial burden, and concern regarding the uncertain
health and developmental status of the infant all may affect parents' attitudes. These attitudes include guilt, grief, exhaustion, lack of self-
confidence, anxiety, and marked depression (Johnson, 1983). In addition,
the use of home apnea monitors may continue to contribute negatively to
these parent attitudes.
3. Parent-child interaction. The pattern of interaction between premature
infants and parents, as documented in multiple studies, differs from the
interaction of parents with term infants (Crawford, 1982; Field, 1980).
In the immediate neonatal period, parents of premature infants are less
actively involved with less body contact and less face-to-face contact
with less smiling and talking. However, during the first 6 months of life,
mothers of premature infants become more active, in control, and stimulating than mothers of term infants. This is seen as an adaptive approach because of the relative lack of activity and responsiveness from
the infants. This heightened level of stimulation is not necessarily positive as it is often not loving or sensitively attuned to the state of the infant. These interactional differences decrease over time and are not obviously different from term infants by the second year of life.

III. Clinically relevant aspects of the home environment
Most of the influences of the environment on infants' development are mediated through the social and nonsocial experiences directly encountered by the
child during the parenting process in the home. Because clinicians most often
influence the health and development of children through the parenting process, an understanding of some aspects of the home that influence the compe-

tency of parenting is important. This discussion does not deal with personal characteristics of the parent, such as mental and physical health, but rather with the aspects of the micro- and macro-environments that are germane to pediatric guidance (Belsky, 1983; Casey, 1982).

A. Microenvironment
   1. Socioemotional and cognitive home environment. The social home environment includes the degree of parental responsiveness, the amount of warmth and nurturance available, the level of encouragement provided for independence and maturity, the extent that parents restrict the child's behavior, and the type of discipline used. The cognitive home environment includes the quality and quantity of language used in the home, the variety of sensory and social experiences available, and the extent to which parents actually encourage achievement. The positive quality of parent-child relationships is clearly related to optimal development in premature infants (Beckwith and Cohen, 1980).
   2. Physical home. The physical environment is made up of attributes such as toys, learning materials, level of visual and auditory input, and the extent to which the environment is organized. Research has repeatedly shown that children benefit from a home that is well organized, rich in stimulating objects, and well structured (Bradley, 1982).

B. Macroenvironment
   1. Support. Werner and Smith (1982) found that if a family had strong social support networks, the family was more often able to provide the stimulating, nurturing, and predictable environment needed for good development. Social support includes emotional and instrumental-physical assistance, social expectations, and advice. Support is provided by significant others in the home, extended-family members, neighborhood and work contacts, and certain professionals. A major benefit of positive social support is that it provides a buffer against the negative consequences of stressful circumstances.
   2. Stress. Acute or chronic traumatic events and instabilities in economic, interpersonal, or situational areas may have a marked negative impact on parenting competency. Among traumatic events most frequently cited are divorce, interpersonal bickering, financial inadequacy, frequent moving, and hospitalizations.

IV. Assessment of home environment
   The method used to assess the clinically relevant aspects of the home environment is dependent on the resources available in the clinical situation in which the infant is being monitored. Some specialty clinics have access to social workers, visiting nurses, and others to gather information, whereas other primary care settings have only a general clinic nurse or aide to assist the pediatrician. While recognizing that there is no substitute for skilled, experienced clinicians who elicit information in a semistructured interview, what follows is a brief overview of standardized methods available to assess aspects of the home environment.

A. General approaches
   1. Home visit. A home visit to assess the quality of the child's physical environment and the interactional aspects of the social environment provides a vivid portrait of the condition in which a child is developing. The major advantage of using standard instruments during a home visit is the richness and naturalness of the information obtained. Moreover, the impressions gathered about the child's environment are not limited to those that are recorded on the standardized observation form. The obvious major limitation of the home visit is that it is time-consuming and often costly in terms of personnel.
   2. Questionnaires and office interviews. A more efficient means of assessing the child's environment is through questionnaires or structured interviews obtained during an office visit. Although questionnaires can provide valid and relatively comprehensive information about a child's environment, they lack the richness of direct observational measures because the interactions between parents and child are not measured. Also, parents may provide inaccurate information, either as a result of their ignorance or their wish to conceal events that are considered socially unacceptable.
   3. Clinical rating scales and direct observation. One means of measuring natural interactions between parent and child that does not involve a visit to the home is by systematically observing parent and child at a clinic. Medical office encounters provide excellent opportunities to observe the quality of parent-child interaction. For example, the health clinician usually notes whether the parent talks to the child during the examination, responds to the child's vocalization, comforts the child if upset, or expresses annoyance or strikes the child. Similarly, ratings of the parent-child interaction can be made in semistructured situations in an office or clinic. Although ratings based on observation of parent-child interaction during clinic visits can provide data about critical environmental transactions, such ratings have two limitations. First, their scope is limited as no information is obtained about the child's inanimate environment. Second, behavior observed in the clinic may not represent the typical behavior occurring in the house.

B. Specific assessments
   The following assessments have adequate psychometric characteristics and were developed for children and their families, and, as such, have potential for clinical usefulness.
   1. Microenvironment
      a. *Home Observation for Measurement of the Environment (HOME) Inventory* is the instrument most commonly used to assess the quality of the home environment during a home visit. There are three versions of the HOME Inventory: one for infants (birth to 3 years of age), one for preschoolers (3–6), and one for early elementary students (6–10). The inventory designed for assessing the home of infants contains 45 items grouped into six subscales: (1) maternal responsiveness, (2) acceptance of child, (3) organization of environment,

(4) provision of appropriate play material, (5) maternal involvement with child, and (6) variety of stimulation. Information to score the items is obtained through a combination of observation and interview in the context of a semistructured home interview with the child and primary caretaker. Items on the HOME Inventory are answered with either *yes* or *no*. Many studies have demonstrated that the HOME Inventory is reliable and valid and is an adequately sensitive screening instrument to assess the quality of children's home environments (Bradley, 1982).

b. Home Screening Questionnaire (HSQ) is a written questionnaire adapted from the HOME Inventory and is completed by the primary caretaker during a clinic visit. In a study of 73 low-income families, correlation of .71 was observed between the scores on the HSQ and scores on the HOME Inventory. The HSQ correctly identified 84 percent of those families with sufficiently low scores on the HOME to warrant some suspicion of the need for environmental intervention (Coons et al., 1982). The use of the HSQ has recently been advocated in the routine management of children from birth through 18 months of age in families in which at least one parent has less than a high-school education (Frankenburg, 1983). As previously noted, however, such questionnaires are unable to quantitate the interaction between parent and child.

c. *Pediatric Review of Children's Environmental Support and Stimulation (PROCESS)* is used by health clinicians during clinic visits to assess both social and inanimate aspects of the home environment of infants less than 18 months of age. It consists of two parts: (1) a written questionnaire with 24 items and a list of toys that assess the organization and developmental stimulation quality of the physical environment and (2) an observation rating scale with 20 items to measure the socioemotional support available in the parent-child interaction. The assessment is completed during a 15- to 20-minute semistructured health maintenance clinic visit. The PROCESS has acceptable interobservable reliability, internal consistency, and concurrent validity as demonstrated by extremely positive correlation of .84 with concurrently collected HOME Inventory, independent of income or education (Casey et al., 1985).

2. Macroenvironment

Theoretic and empirical understanding of the interacting relationship of environmental support and stress and their impact on children's development is an exceedingly active area of research. Perhaps as a reflection of this research, there is no consensus concerning the best way to measure social support and environmental stress. The following are suggested as potential instruments for clinical use, based on the criteria described at the beginning of B.

a. Support: Maternal Social Support Index (MSSI) consists of seven items gathered during an interview that assess the social and instrumental support available to the parent. (The MSSI does not measure financial support.) The items were selected to assess objective and subjective aspects of support. Used with 69 families 3 years after their infants' discharge from an NICU, the MSSI revealed a notable amount of variance of home stimulation, independent of socioeconomic status (Pascoe et al., 1981). In a different cohort of indigent multigravidas, mothers with high MSSI scores in the first trimester of pregnancy gave birth to larger neonates who had lower admission rates to the NICU than did mothers with low MSSI scores (6 versus 20%).

b. Stress. All measures of environmental stress are moderately long, as lists of potentially stressful events are presented. Some instruments inquire as to the relative severity and importance of these events to the family, whereas others ask only whether the events occurred.

(1) *Life Event Scale,* based on two earlier research instruments, rates the occurrence of 44 stressful events during the prior 9 months. Each item is rated on a four-point scale to assess the degree of disruption involved with that event. The instrument differentiated between a sample of 32 high-risk mothers who mistreated their children from a group of 33 mothers who provided adequate care (Egeland et al., 1980).

(2) *Life Experience Survey (LES)* rates a series of 46 life events as having occurred or not, whether the impact was "good" or "bad," and the relative degree of effect on the parent (Sarason et al., 1978). When used at 1 month of age with 52 mothers of premature infants and 53 mothers of term infants, the LES significantly predicted maternal attitudes at 1 month and mother-infant interaction behavior at 4 months of age (Crnic et al., 1983).

V. Clinical implications

Pediatricians should attempt to assess the premature and low-birth-weight infants' social and physical environments and screen for developmental problems to predict outcomes more adequately and to plan treatment effectively. As described earlier, methods of data gathering depend on the time and personnel resources available. The assessments previously described are different options that may be selected by these criteria. Extremely detailed information is not generally required to assist the basic pediatric guidance and counseling function. Thus, data gathering for clinical purposes often need not be lengthy or intrusive or threatening. Finally, few instruments available for measuring aspects of a child's environment are optimal for pediatric use in terms of psychometric properties, aspects of the environmental assessed, or reality features of time and personnel required. The instrument has to be carefully selected, keeping in mind the clinical action to be taken based on the information gathered.

How might information regarding the home environment be used by pediatricians? First, this information may increase accuracy of developmental prediction. Identification of positive and negative aspects of an infant's home environment combined with developmental test results may increase accuracy of prediction, particularly in borderline situations. For example, a mildly delayed infant in the first year of life who is raised in an extremely facilitative environment may be expected to function ultimately as a normal child. On the other hand, an infant who develops normally in the first year of life but who grows up in an extremely deficient environment may be expected to display less than optimal developmental skills eventually. Next, information regarding the home may help the pediatrician adopt appropriate treatment plans. For example, the pediatrician following a normal infant in a deficient environment may use an aggressive follow-up plan, including nurse home visitors, social workers, and early educational intervention programming. Finally, information regarding the home derived from office measures may serve as a basis for counseling parents about experiences that may be beneficial to children at risk for problems. This information may begin an effective dialogue with parents that may result in the transfer of information or values that may be favorable to the ultimate development of the child.

REFERENCES

Beckwith, L., and Cohen, S. E. Interaction of Preterm Infants and Their Caregivers and Test Performance at Age Two. In T. M. Field (ed.), *High-Risk Infants and Children: Adult and Peer Interactions.* New York: Academic, 1980.

Belsky, J. The determinants of parenting: A process model. *Child Dev.* 55 : 83, 1983.

Bradley, R. The HOME Inventory: A Review of the First 15 Years. In W. Frankenburg, N. Anastasiow, and A. Fandel (eds.), *Identifying the Developmentally Delayed Child.* Baltimore: University Park, 1982.

Casey, P. H., and Bradley, R. H. The impact of the home environment on children's development: Clinical relevance for the pediatrician. *Dev. Behav. Pediatr.* 3 : 146, 1982.

Casey, P. H., Bradley, R. H., Nelson, J., and Whaley, S. The clinical assessment of a child's social and physical environment during health visits. Presented to the Ambulatory Pediatrics Association, Washington, D.C., 1985.

Coons, C. E., Frankenburg, W. K., et al. Preliminary Results of a Combined Developmental/ Environmental Screening Project. In W. Frankenburg, N. Anastasiow, and A. Fandal (eds.), *Identifying the Developmentally Delayed Child.* Baltimore: University Park, 1982.

Crawford, J. W. Mother-infant interaction in premature and full-term infants. *Child Dev.* 53 : 957, 1982.

Crnic, K. A., Greenberg, M. T., Ragozin, A. S., et al. Effects of stress and social support on mothers and premature and full-term infants. *Child Dev.* 54 : 209, 1983.

DiVitto, B., and Goldberg, S. The Effects of Newborn Medical Status on Early Parent-Infant Interaction. In T. M. Field (ed.), *Infants Born at Risk: Behavior and Development.* Jamaica, N.Y.: Spectrum, 1979.

Drillien, C. M. *Growth and Development of the Prematurely Born Infant.* Edinburgh: Livingstone, 1964.

Egeland, B., Breitenbucher, M., and Rosenberg, D. Prospective study of the significance of life stress in the etiology of child abuse. *J. Consult. Clin. Psychol.* 48 : 195, 1980.

Field, T. M. Interactions of Preterm and Term Infants with Their Lower- and Middle-Class Teenage and Adult Mothers. In T. M. Field (ed.), *High-Risk Infants and Children: Adult and Peer Interactions.* New York: Academic, 1980.

Frankenburg, W. K. Infant and Preschool Developmental Screening. In M. D. Levine, W. B. Carey, A. C. Crocker, and R. T. Gross (eds.), *Developmental-Behavioral Pediatrics.* Philadelphia: Saunders, 1983.

Johnson, S. H. Parents of the Premature Infant. In R. A. Hoekelman and V. J. Sasserath (eds.), *Minimizing High-Risk Parenting.* Piscataway, N.J.: Johnson & Johnson, 1982.

Klaus, M. H., and Kennell, J. H. *Maternal Infant Bonding.* St. Louis: Mosby, 1976.

McCormick, M. C., Shapiro, S., and Starfield, B. H. Rehospitalization in the first year of life for high-risk survivors. *Pediatrics* 66 : 991, 1980.

Pascoe, J. M., Loda, F. A., Jeffries, V., and Earp, J. A. The association between mothers' social support and provision of stimulation to their children. *J. Dev. Behav. Pediatr.* 2 : 15, 1981.

Sameroff, A. J., and Chandler, M. J. Reproductive Risk and the Continuum of Care-taking Casualty. In F. D. Horowitz (ed.), *Review of Child Development Research*. Chicago: University of Chicago, 1975. Vol. 4.

Sarason, I. G., Johnson, J. H., and Siegel, J. M. Assessing the impact of life changes: Development of the Life Experiences Survey. *J. Consult. Clin. Psychol.* 46 : 932, 1978.

Siegel, L. S. Reproductive, perinatal, and environmental factors as predictors of the cognitive and language development of pre-term and full-term infants. *Child Dev.* 53 : 963, 1982.

Sigman, M., and Parmelee, A. H. Longitudinal Evaluation of the Pre-term Infant. In T. M. Field (ed.), *Infants Born at Risk: Behavior and Development*. Jamaica, N.Y.: Spectrum, 1979.

Werner, E., and Smith, R. *Vulnerable but Invincible: A Study of Resilient Children*. New York: McGraw-Hill, 1982.

14

The Preschool Period

Maureen Hack and Nancy K. Klein

I. Introduction

The spectrum of morbidity from perinatal insult continues well past the neonatal period. Adaptation or normalization does occur, however, during infancy and early childhood. Eventually most children, even those who initially had chronic diseases and some degree of neurologic abnormality, are healthy and functioning fairly well by their third year (Hack et al., 1983).

During the past 2 decades, important advances in perinatal care have improved survival and developmental outcome for very low birth weight (VLBW; < 1,500 g) infants. Before the 1960s, more than 50 percent of VLBW survivors exhibited neurodevelopmental impairment; most recent studies report a 10 to 18 percent incidence of severe neurologic or intellectual handicap among these infants (Douglas, 1956; Hack et al., 1979). However, these improved findings have not been reflected in the more complex arena of school performance (Bjerre and Hansen, 1976; Douglas, 1956; Drillien, 1969; Fitzhardinge and Ramsay, 1973; Francis-Williams and Davies, 1974; Hunt et al., 1982; Kitchen et al., 1980; Noble-Jamieson et al., 1982; Stewart, 1978).

School-age children who were the beneficiaries of modern medical technology as VLBW infants have been found to be at risk for learning problems in addition to neurodevelopmental delay (Fitzhardinge et al., 1973; Francis-Williams and Davies, 1974; Hunt et al., 1982; Kitchen et al., 1980; Noble-Jamieson et al., 1982). These school-related problems manifest as subtle motor, visual-motor, perceptual, language, and reading difficulties often accompanied by inappropriate classroom behavior. For example, Hunt and associates (1982) reported that 37 percent of VLBW children born after 1965 appear to have learning disabilities; Fitzhardinge and colleagues (1973) reported a 33 percent incidence of perceptual-motor difficulties; and Francis-Williams and Davies (1974) found a 20 percent incidence of learning problems at school age in VLBW infants. Similar findings were also noted prior to the introduction of modern neonatal intensive care (Douglas, 1956; Drillien, 1969). Klein and co-workers (1985) found that even among preschool-age children with normal intelligence there were significantly more visual-motor and visual-perceptual problems among VLBW children than among classmate controls matched for social class, race, and sex. Furthermore, teachers rated VLBW children as having significantly more problems attending to tasks and following directions. These children also tended to be shy and relatively withdrawn.

II. Preterm infants at 3 years of age: A summary of outcomes

A. Children with major neurologic sequelae (spastic diplegia and quadriple-

159

gia, hydrocephalus, blindness, and deafness) should be in appropriate intervention programs and may demonstrate functional improvement such as independent walking. Prior to this age, developmental assessment is heavily based on motor abilities. By 3 years of age language is well developed, and a valid assessment of cognitive function can be done, although performance is still affected by residual motor or behavioral problems.

B. Chronic pulmonary sequelae (bronchopulmonary dysplasia) should have resolved or considerably improved. There is, however, an increased incidence of asthma, bronchitis, or increased airway reactivity in children who had neonatal respiratory problems.

C. There is less need for rehospitalization.

D. Growth velocity should be normal; however, little catch-up growth occurs in children who had previous growth delay.

E. Subtle neurologic dysfunction such as clumsiness, poor coordination, and visual-motor function may become evident even in children with normal intelligence who were previously considered neurologically intact.

F. Behavioral problems may emerge as the child begins to interact with other children and to meet the demands of a preschool program.

G. Environmental or demographic factors, such as maternal education, marital status, and social class, demonstrate an increasingly dominant effect on the child's intellectual functioning (Drillien et al., 1982).

H. Hearing problems secondary to otitis media may occur. These are more common than sensorineural loss.

I. Subtle visual problems (myopia, astigmatism) may become evident.

J. High-risk children who are functioning within the normal range, with rare exceptions, will not be seen routinely in neonatal follow-up clinics. Thus the responsibility for the detection of any functional problems will lie with family caretakers, pediatricians, and educational personnel. In some cases parents may recontact neonatal follow-up programs when their children begin to experience school difficulties or behavior problems. The developmental specialist associated with the follow-up programs can provide consultation to parents through assessment of cognitive abilities and counseling. These services may assist parents in making decisions regarding their children's educational needs.

III. Preschool follow-up program

A. Goals
   The goals of a structured preschool follow-up program are to identify any

emerging medical, neurologic, behavioral, or functional problems and to refer children with these problems for appropriate diagnosis, intervention, or treatment.

B. Medical follow-up
   Medical assessment at this age includes
   1. Physical growth measures: weight, height, and head circumference
   2. A thorough physical examination, including specific attention to blood pressure, hearing, teeth, and any residual scars from neonatal procedures
   3. A standardized neurologic examination
   4. A behavioral hearing evaluation
   5. An ophthalmologic examination that includes vision and funduscopy

C. Developmental evaluation
   Developmental assessment should focus on general intellectual function, gross and fine motor skills, and language. It is not designed to substitute for the more comprehensive assessment provided by the schools for children with identified learning problems.
   The following is a list of instruments that are commonly employed in the longitudinal follow-up of children from 3 to 6 years of age.
   1. Intellectual development
      a. The Stanford-Binet Intelligence Scale (Terman, 1973) is highly reliable and widely used for assessing intellectual function during the preschool years. It yields a single global intelligence quotient (IQ) and includes items that assess language, concepts, and problem solving. Tasks are structured and call for a specific response. The Stanford-Binet is widely used for evaluating retarded children. The scale is highly predictive of school performance and is used extensively by researchers, schools, and clinicians who follow preterm children into early childhood.
      b. McCarthy Scales of Children's Abilities (McCarthy, 1972), a recently developed assessment tool, is being used increasingly by both researchers and clinicians because it subdivides cognitive abilities into Verbal, Perceptual/Performance (nonverbal/problem solving), and Quantitative (number knowledge and reasoning) Indexes, which make up the General Cognitive Index (GCI). Other function indexes reported are Memory and Motor Indexes. The scale is standardized for children from 2½ to 8 years of age. Objective scoring procedures for motor tasks are provided, and materials are attractive to children. It is not useful for children with IQs in the moderately and severely retarded range.
      c. Wechsler Preschool and Primary Scale of Intelligence (Wechsler, 1967) is standardized for children 4 to 6 years of age and includes verbal, visual-perceptual, motor, recall, and recognition skills. Norms are provided to convert scores to IQs.
      d. Peabody Picture Vocabulary Test, Revised (Dunn, 1981), is a measure of receptive language, standardized for use in persons from 2½ to 33 years of age. The tester provides a noun or verb, and the sub-

ject is required to select one of four pictures that describes the word. It is widely used in research as it is easy to administer and correlates well with measures of IQ. Mental age and IQ scores are derived from scores.

2. Visual-motor performance

   Developmental Test of Visual Motor Integration (Beery and Butenika, 1982), a form-copying test, requires that the child directly copy forms arranged from simple to complex. Norms are provided for children from preschool age through elementary years, and the test has been used extensively for identifying children with learning disabilities and by researchers following preterm children into the early school years.

3. Motor performance

   Bruiniks-Osterefsky Tests of Motor Proficiency (Bruiniks, 1978) can be used in combination with a neurologic examination. It provides objective assessment of gross motor skills (balance and coordination), fine motor skills (eye-hand coordination, tracking), speed of response, and lateralization. Norms are provided. The types of motor problems assessed have been documented to occur more frequently in preterm children.

4. Cognitive abilities

   a. The Woodcock-Johnson Psycho-Educational Battery Preschool Scale (Woodcock and Johnson, 1977) is a standardized test containing six subtests that assess visual and auditory aspects of cognitive function in children as young as 3 years. Subtests include spatial relations, picture vocabulary, memory for sentences, auditory-visual learning, blending, and quantitative concepts. At school age, the 11 subtests of the Cognitive Battery (part I) may be used separately or as verbal ability, reasoning, perceptual speed, and memory factors. Raw scores convert to grade- and age-equivalent scores.

   b. The Test of Language Development-Primary (Newcomer and Hammill, 1982) has been standardized for children 4 to 9 years of age. It assesses receptive and expressive language. Principal subtests include semantics and syntax; a supplemental phonology subtest is also included. Scores convert to language scores and standard scores. It is used extensively in schools and by researchers and clinicians.

5. Achievement tests

   For children 5 or more years of age, the following tests are suggested and have been used by researchers and clinicians studying preterm children.

   a. Wide Range Achievement Test (Jastak and Jastak, 1978). Level I is a standardized test that assesses reading word recognition, written spelling, and mathematic computation. Scores convert to grade-equivalent scores.

   b. Woodcock Reading Mastery Test Revised (Woodcock, in press) contains several subscales that assess many skills from word identification to reading comprehension. It is standardized for children from kindergarten through grade 12. The test is frequently used by researchers and schools. Norms are provided for individual subscales.

IV. Conclusion

The majority of premature children do well at school. However, the increased reported incidence of learning and behavioral problems in this population (Douglas, 1956; Klein et al., 1985) highlights the need for early identification of learning difficulties, both for the design and implementation of individual intervention programs and for the monitoring of children who were preterm infants into the early grades. Learning disabilities may be amenable to early intervention with carefully designed programs (Reynolds et al., 1983). It may thus be possible to prevent the compounding of these problems into more severe learning difficulties.

Most important, the continuity of high-risk follow-up until school age or even later is essential to measure the full impact of VLBW and perinatal care on function in society.

REFERENCES

Alberman, E., Benson, J., and McDonald, A. Cerebral palsy and severe educational subnormality in low birth weight children. *Lancet* 1 : 606, 1982.

Beery, K., and Butenika, H. A. *Developmental Test of Visual-Motor Integration.* Chicago: Follett, 1982.

Bjerre, I., and Hansen, E. Psychomotor development and school adjustment of 7-year-old children with low birth weight. *Acta Paediatr. Scand.* 65 : 88, 1976.

Bruiniks, R. H. *Bruiniks-Osterefsky Tests of Motor Proficiency. Examiners Manual 1978.* Circle Pines, Minn.: American Guidance Service, 1978.

Douglas, J. W. B. Mental ability and school achievement of premature children at 8 years of age. *Br. Med. J.* 1 : 1210, 1956.

Drillien, C. M. School disposal and performance for children of different birth weight born 1953–1960. *Arch. Dis. Child.* 44 : 562, 1969.

Drillien, C. M., Thomson, A. J. M., and Burgoyne, K. Low birth weight children at early school age: A longitudinal study. *Dev. Med. Child Neurol.* 22 : 26, 1982.

Dunn, L. M. *Peabody Picture Vocabulary Test, Revised.* Circle Pines, Minn.: American Guidance Service, 1981.

Fitzhardinge, P. M., and Ramsay, M. The improving outlook for the small prematurely born infant. *Dev. Med. Child Neurol.* 15 : 447, 1973.

Francis-Williams, J., and Davis, P. A. Very low birth weight and later intelligence. *Dev. Med. Child Neurol.* 16 : 709, 1974.

Hack, M., and Breslau, N. Very low birth weight infants: Effects of brain growth during infancy on intelligence quotient at 3 years of age. *Pediatrics* 77 : 196, 1986.

Hack, M., Fanaroff, A. A., and Merkatz, I. R. The low birth weight infant: Evolution of a changing outlook. *N. Engl. J. Med.* 301 : 1162, 1979.

Hack, M., Rivers, A., and Fanaroff, A. The very low birth weight infant: The broader spectrum of morbidity during infancy and early childhood. *J. Dev. Behav. Pediatr.* 4 : 343, 1983.

Hunt, J. V., Tooley, W. H., and Halvin, D. Learning disabilities in children with birth weight < 1500 grams. *Semin. Perinatol.* 6 : 280, 1982.

Jastak, J. F., and Jastak, S. *Wide Range Achievement Tests.* Los Angeles: Western Psychological Service, 1978.

Kitchen, W. H., Ryan, M. M., Richards, A., et al. A longitudinal study of very low birth weight infants: IV. An overview of performance at eight years of age. *Dev. Med. Child Neurol.* 22 : 172, 1980.

Klein, N., Hack, M., Gallagher, J., and Fanaroff, A. School performance of the normal intelligence very low birth weight infant. *Pediatrics* 75 : 531, 1985.

McCarthy, D. *Manual for the McCarthy Scales of Children's Abilities.* New York: Psychological Corp., 1972.

Newcomer, P., and Hammill, D. *Test of Language Development Primary (TOLD-P).* Austin, Tex.: PRO-ED, 1982.

Noble-Jamieson, C., Lukeman, D., Silverman, M., et al. Low birth weight children at school: Neurological, psychological and pulmonary function. *Semin. Perinatol.* 6 : 266, 1982.

Reynolds, L., Egan, R., and Lerner, J. Efficacy of early intervention on preacademic deficits: A review of the literature. *Top. Early Child. Spec. Ed.* 3 : 47, 1983.

Stewart, A. L. Outcome for infants at risk for major handicap. *Ciba Found. Symp.* 59 : 151, 1978.

Terman, L., and Merrill, M. *The Stanford-Binet Intelligence Scale, Third Revision.* Boston: Houghton Mifflin, 1973.

Wechsler, D. *Manual for the Wechsler Preschool and Primary Scale of Intelligence.* New York: Psychological Corp., 1967.

Woodcock, R. W. *Woodcock Reading Mastery Test.* Circle Pines, Minn.: American Guidance Service. In press.

Woodcock, R. W., and Johnson, M. B. *Woodcock-Johnson Psycho-Educational Battery.* Boston: Teaching Resources Corp., 1977.

Emotional Growth in Infants and Young Children with Unique Developmental Challenges

Stanley I. Greenspan

I. Introduction

Infants and young children with developmental delays, irregularities, or disorders present a unique challenge to their families. The 4-month-old infant with poor muscle tone may have a difficult time showing enjoyment of his or her parents' smiles and vocalizations, as the infant's ability to reveal joy with a bright smile or organized motor patterns may be limited. Similarly, the hypertonic infant may also have a difficult time providing focused joyful feedback to parents because the infant responds to stimulation by arching the back. This infant may look away from rather than toward his or her parents as they make facial gestures and vocalizations.

We have observed that parents and families may also manifest predictable emotional and social patterns when confronted with the unique challenge of their high-risk infant. Denial of their new infant, disinterest, depression, fear, overprotectiveness, and mechanical striving for perfection are not infrequently observed among parents of infants with developmental disorders.

Yet most infants with developmental problems or delays are capable of progressing through the adaptive stages of emotional and social development. To reach their potential, however, their caretakers may need to create and implement special patterns of care. For some parents, intuition and experience are sufficient; for many parents, professional guidance or peer support (or both) may be essential. For example, consider an infant who not only has a motor delay but also is sensitive to light touch and high-pitched sounds. The infant may require special approaches. Parents may be able to "woo" him or her into a pleasurable, even joyful, relationship if they use low-pitched sounds combined with clear facial gestures. Parents may need to learn to pay attention to even a subtle smile or motor gesture as a sign that their infant is joyful, since it may take a little longer for this infant to master the robust smile. The sense of trust and security attained may even be stronger for the extra effort. While parents may benefit from guidance in providing the special care needed, once an adaptive pattern gets started, it often takes on momentum of its own.

It is not only in the early months, however, that unique challenges are present. The 16-month-old infant learning to take initiative and organize behavior and emotions may find it difficult to strive toward independence if the infant's ability to communicate across space is compromised. If, because of motor or sensory processing problems, a toddler has difficulty gesturing or figuring out his or her parent's gestures or vocalizations, the toddler may become unsure of him- or herself when across the room. The parent's approving nod and "good boy!" may not be understood, and therefore, they may not provide the reassurance they potentially could. This toddler may need to return to the parent frequently for concrete reassurance. With extra patience and practice, special challenges such as these will also be mastered. But the potential is also present for a parent to overprotect, to resent a clinging toddler, or to become emotionally aloof, even while being physically available.

Knowledge of the adaptive and maladaptive emotional milestones will facilitate adaptive emotional development of the high-risk infant. It is often thought that only encouragement and love are needed, along with indicated physical or cognitive approaches. Love and encouragement are an essential foundation, but as is suggested in this chapter, each child requires attention to his or her changing emotional needs, in the context of a progression of emotional milestones and individual differences. For example, the 8-month-old wants his or her specific emotional signals read, and the 16-month-old wants his or her assertiveness and independence admired. Stage-specific emotional needs must be integrated with physical and intellectual needs. Knowledge of the stages of emotional organization will enable professionals and parents to provide experiences that will promote adaptive emotional patterns in the context of changing emotional needs and individual differences in infants and families. There are many ways for an infant to learn to be regulated, relate to others, communicate intentionally, form a complex self, and use emotional ideas to guide behavior and feelings. In this chapter, it is not possible to describe all the different pathways to adaptive emotional development. Describing the emotional milestones, however, provides a framework for working with each infant's and family's unique strengths and vulnerabilities.

Through clinical work and observational studies of infants and families with presumed normal functioning, developmental and emotional disorders, and risk patterns, we constructed a framework for the emotional milestones of both the infant and his or her caretakers. These milestones are also based on an impressive number of studies of presumed normal infant emotional functioning.

II. Emotional milestones

Although there are no large-scale studies of infants' and young children's affective patterns at different ages to partition the range of emotional patterns in the general population, there is extensive literature on the emotional development of presumed normal infants. Interestingly, during the past 15 years, there has been considerably greater documentation of normal emotional development in infants than probably any other age group.

It is now well documented that the infant is capable, even at birth or shortly thereafter, of organizing experiences in an adaptive fashion. He or she can respond to pleasure and displeasure (Lipsitt, 1966); change behavior as a function of its consequences (Gewirtz, 1965; 1969); form intimate bonds and make visual discriminations (Klaus and Kennell, 1976; Meltzoff and Moore, 1977); organize cycles and rhythms (e.g., sleep-wake cycles, alertness states) (Sander, 1962); evidence a variety of affects or affect-proclivities (Ekman, 1972; Izard, 1978; Tomkins, 1963); and demonstrate organized social responses in conjunction with increasing neurophysiologic organization (Emde et al., 1976). The infant from the early months demonstrates a unique capacity to enter into complex social and affective interactions (Brazelton et al., 1974; Stern, 1974a, 1974b, 1977). This empirically documented view of the infant is, in a general sense, consistent with Freud's early hypotheses (1911) and Hartmann's postulation (1939) of an early undifferentiated organizational matrix. That the organization of experience broadens during the early months of life to reflect increases in the capacity to experience and tolerate a range of stimuli, including responding in social interaction in stable and personal configurations, is also consistent with recent empirical data (Brazelton et al., 1974; Emde et al., 1976; Escalona, 1968; Murphy and Moriarty, 1976; Sander, 1962; Stern, 1974a, 1974b).

Increasingly complex patterns continue to emerge as the infant develops, as indicated by complex emotional responses such as surprise (Charlesworth, 1969) and affiliation, wariness, and fear (Ainsworth et al., 1974; Sroufe and Waters, 1977); exploration and "refueling" patterns (Mahler et al., 1975); behavior suggesting functional understanding of objects (Werner and Kaplan, 1963); and the eventual emergence of symbolic capacities (Bell, 1970; Gouin-Decarie, 1965; Piaget, 1962).

In these studies (and there are no dissenting studies), there is a consensus that, by 2 to 4 months of age at the latest and often much earlier, healthy infants are capable of responding to their caretakers' faces, smiles, and voices by brightening, alerting, and often smiling. Reciprocal responses such as vocalizations (suggesting positive affect) are often seen. Furthermore, the caretaker's interaction patterns become progressively characterized by more complex social interaction as development proceeds.

In addition to the studies on normal infant emotional development, important observations on disturbed development increase our knowledge of new integrated milestones. Interestingly, the study of psychopathology in infancy is a new area although the historic foundation for identifying disturbances in infancy dates to the early 1900s. Constitutional and maturational patterns that influence the formation of early relationship patterns were already noted in the early 1900s with descriptions of "babies of nervous inheritance" who exhaust their mothers (Cameron, 1919) and infants with "excessive nerve activity and a functionally immature" nervous system.

Winnicott, who as a pediatrician in the 1930s began describing the environment's role in early relationship problems (1931), was followed in the 1940s by the well-known studies describing the severe developmental disturbances of infants brought up in institutions or in other situations of emotional deprivation (Bakwin, 1942; Bowlby, 1951; Hunt, 1941; Lowrey, 1940; Spitz, 1945). Spitz's films resulted in the passing of laws in the United States prohibiting care of infants in institutions.

The role of individual differences in the infant based on constitutional maturational and early interactional patterns (i.e., "nervous" infants described by Cameron in 1919 and Rachford in 1905) again became a focus of inquiry, as evidenced by the observations of Burlingham and A. Freud (1942); Bergman and Escalona's descriptions of infants with "unusual sensitivities" (1949); Murphy and Moriarty's description of patterns of vulnerability (1976); Cravioto and DeLicardie's descriptions of the role of infant individual differences in malnutrition (1973); and the impressive emerging empirical literature on infants (Brazelton et al.,1974; Emde et al., 1976; Gewirtz, 1961; Lipsitt, 1966; Rheingold, 1966, 1969; Sander, 1962; Stern, 1974a, 1974b). More integrated approaches to understanding disturbances in infancy have been emphasized in descriptions of selected disorders and insightful clinical case studies (Greenspan et al., 1986; Provence, 1979).

To understand further both adaptive and disturbed infant functioning, an in-depth study was undertaken of normal and disturbed developmental patterns in infancy to develop a systematic comprehensive classification of adaptive and maladaptive infant and family patterns. Table 15-1 summarizes the observations made of the adaptive and maladaptive infant and family patterns and briefly describes these patterns. (See Greenspan, 1979, 1981; Greenspan et al., 1979; Greenspan and Lourie, 1981; and Greenspan and Porges, 1984, for detailed descriptions of these patterns.)

The capacities described by the stages are all present in some rudimentary form in very early infancy. The sequence presented suggests not when these capacities begin, but when they become relatively prominent in organizing behavior and furthering development.

The first milestone is the *achievement of homeostasis* (i.e., self-regulation and emerging interest in the world through the senses). Once the infant has achieved some capacity for regulation in the context of engaging the world, and the central nervous system (CNS) is maturing between 2 and 4 months of age, the infant becomes more attuned to social and interpersonal interaction. There is greater ability to respond to the external environment and to form a special relationship with important primary caretakers.

A second, closely related stage is *formation of a human attachment*. If an affective and relatively pleasurable attachment (an investment in the human, animate world) is formed, then as the infant matures, he or she develops complex patterns of communication in the context of this primary human relationship. Parallel with development of the infant's relationship to the inanimate world where basic schemes of causality (Piaget, 1972) are being developed, the infant becomes capable of complicated human communications (Brazelton et al., 1974; Charlesworth, 1969; Stern, 1974a; Tennes et al., 1972).

Causal relationships are established between the infant and the primary caretaker as evidenced in the infant's growing ability to discriminate primary caretakers from others. The infant also becomes able to differentiate his or her own actions from their consequences, affectively, somatically, behaviorally, and interpersonally. Usually by 8 months of age, the process of differentiation begins along a number of developmental lines (e.g., with sensorimotor integration, affects, relationships).

A third stage therefore may be formally termed *somatopsychologic differentiation* to indicate processes occurring at the somatic (e.g., sensorimotor) and emerging psychologic levels. (In this context, psychologic refers to higher level mental processes characterized by the capacity to form internal representations or symbols as a way to organize experience.) While schemes of causality are being established in the infant's relationship to the interpersonal world, it is not at all clear whether these schemes exist at an organized representational or symbolic level. Rather, they appear to exist mainly at a somatic level (Greenspan, 1979), even though the precursors of representational capacities are observed. Some are perhaps even prenatally determined (Lourie, 1971).

With appropriate reading of cues and systematic differential responses, the infant's or toddler's behavioral repertoire becomes complicated and communications take on more organized and meaningful configurations. By 12 months of age, the infant is connecting behavioral units into larger organizations as he or she exhibits complex emotional responses such as affiliation, wariness, and fear (Ainsworth et al., 1974; Sroufe and Waters, 1977). As the toddler moves further into the second year of life, in the context of the practicing subphase of the development of individuation (Mahler et al., 1975), there is an increased capacity for forming original behavioral schemes (Piaget, 1972) and imitative activity and intentionality.

A type of learning through imitation evidenced in earlier development now seems to assume a more dominant role. As imitations take on a more integrated personal form, it appears that the toddler is adopting or internalizing attributes of his or her caretakers.

To describe these new capacities it is useful to consider a fourth stage, that of *behavioral organization, initiative, and internalization.* As the toddler moves into the end of the second year, internal sensations and unstable images become organized in a mental representational form that can be evoked and is somewhat stable (Bell, 1970; Gouin-Decarie, 1965; Piaget, 1972). While this capacity is initially fragile (i.e., between 16 and 24 months), it soon appears to become a dominant mode in organizing the child's behavior.

A fifth stage can be documented: *forming mental representations or ideas.* Object permanence is relative and goes through a series of stages (Gouin-Decarie, 1965). It refers to the toddler's ability to search for hidden inanimate objects. *Representational capacity* refers to the ability to organize and evoke internal organized multisensory experiences of the animate object. The capacities to represent animate and inanimate experiences are related and depend on both CNS myelination and appropriate experiences. The process of internalization may be thought of as an intermediary process. Internalized experiences eventually become sufficiently organized to be considered representations.

At a representational level, the child again develops capacities for elaboration, integration, and differentiation. Just as causal schemes previously were developed at a somatic and behavioral level, in this stage they are developed at a representational level. The child begins to elaborate and eventually differentiate internal feelings, thoughts, and events that emanate from within and those that emanate from others. The child begins to differentiate his or her intentions from their impact on the world. This process gradually forms the basis for the differentiation of "self" representations from the external world, animate and inanimate, and also provides the basis for such crucial personality functions as knowing what is real from unreal, impulse and mood regulation, and the capacity to focus attention and concentrate to learn and interact.

The capacity for differentiating internal representations becomes consolidated as object constancy is established (Mahler et al., 1975). In middle childhood, representational capacity becomes reinforced by the child's ability to develop derivative representational systems tied to the original representation and transform them in accordance with adaptive and defensive goals. This process permits greater flexibility in dealing with perceptions, feelings, thoughts, and emerging ideals. Substages for these capacities include representational differentiation, consolidation of representational capacity, and the

Table 15-1. Developmental basis for psychopathology and adaptation in infancy and early childhood

Stage-specific tasks and capacities	Capacities		Environment (caretaker)	
	Adaptive	Maladaptive (pathologic)	Adaptive	Maladaptive
I. Homeostasis (0–3 mo); (self-regulation and interest in the world)	Internal regulation (harmony) and balanced interest in world	Unregulated (e.g., hyperexcitable, withdrawn, apathetic)	Invested, dedicated, protective, comforting, predictable, engaging, and interesting	Unavailable, chaotic, dangerous, abusive; hypostimulating or hyperstimulating; dull
II. Attachment (2–7 mo)	Rich, deep, multisensory emotional investment in animate world (especially with primary caretakers)	Total lack of, or nonaffective, shallow, impersonal, involvement (e.g., autistic patterns) in animate world	In love and woos infant to "fall in love"; affective multimodality pleasurable involvement	Emotionally distant, aloof, and/or impersonal (highly ambivalent)
III. Somatopsychologic differentiation (3–10 mo; purposeful cause and effect signaling or communication	Flexible, wide-ranging affective multisystem contingent (reciprocal) interactions (especially with primary caretakers)	Behavior and affects random and or chaotic, or narrow, rigid, and stereotyped	Reads and responds contingently to infant's communications across multiple sensory and affective systems	Ignores infant's communications (e.g., overly intrusive, preoccupied, or depressed) or misreads infant's communication (e.g., projection)
Behavioral organization, initiative, and internalization (9–24 mo)	Complex, organized, assertive, innovative, integrated behavioral and emotional patterns	Fragmented, stereotyped, and polarized behavior and emotions (e.g., withdrawn, compliant, hyperaggressive, or disorganized toddler)	Admiring of toddler's initiative and autonomy, yet available, tolerant, and firm; follows toddler's lead and helps organize diverse behavioral and affective elements	Overly intrusive, controlling; fragmented, fearful (especially of toddler's autonomy); abruptly and prematurely "separates"

IV. Representational capacity, differentiation, and consolidation (1½–4 yr; the use of ideas to guide play and behavior, and eventually thinking and planning)	Formation and elaboration of internal representations (imagery) Organization and differentiation of imagery pertaining to self and nonself; emergence of cognitive insight Stabilization of mood and gradual emergence of basic personality functions	No representational (symbolic) elaboration; behavior and affect concrete, shallow, and polarized; sense of self and other fragmented and indifferentiated or narrow and rigid; reality testing, impulse regulation, mood stabilization compromised or vulnerable (e.g., borderline psychotic and severe character problems)	Emotionally available to phase-appropriate regressions and dependency needs; reads, responds to, and encourages symbolic elaboration across emotional behavioral domains (e.g., love, pleasure, assertion) while fostering gradual reality orientation and internalization of limits	Fearful of or denies phase-appropriate needs; engages child only in concrete (nonsymbolic) modes generally or in certain realms (e.g., around pleasure) and/or misreads or responds noncontingently or nonrealistically to emerging communications (i.e., undermines reality orientation); overly permissive or punitive
V. Capacity for limited extended representational systems and multiple extended representational systems (middle childhood through adolescence)	Enhanced and eventually optimal flexibility to conserve and transform complex and organized representations of experience in the context of expanded relationship patterns and phase-expected developmental tasks	Derivative representational capacities limited or defective, as are latency and adolescent relationships and coping capacities	Supports complex, phase- and age-appropriate experiential and interpersonal development (i.e., into triangular and posttriangular patterns)	Conflicted over child's age-appropriate propensities (e.g., competitiveness, pleasure orientation, growing competence, assertiveness, and self-sufficiency); becomes aloof or maintains symbiotic tie; withdraws from or over-engages in competitive or pleasurable strivings

Adapted from S. I. Greenspan. Psychopathology and adaptation in infancy and early childhood; Principles of clinical diagnosis and preventive intervention. *Clin. Infant Rep.* No. 1, 1981; and S. I. Greenspan and N. T. Greenspan. *First Feelings; Milestones in the Emotional Development of Your Baby and Child.* New York: Viking, 1985.

capacity for forming limited derivative representational systems and multiple derivative representational systems (Greenspan, 1979).

III. Maldevelopment

At each of these stages in varying degrees, pathologic as well as adaptive development is possible (Table 15-1). These maldevelopments may be considered to be relative compromises in the range, depth, stability, or personal uniqueness of the experiential organization consolidated at each stage. The infant can form adaptive patterns of regulation in the earliest stages of development (stage I). Internal states are harmoniously regulated, and the infant is free to invest him- or herself in the animate and inanimate world, thereby setting the basis for rich emotional attachments to primary caretakers. On the other hand, if regulatory processes are not functioning properly and the infant is either hyposensitive or hypersensitive to sensations, he or she may evidence homeostatic difficulties. From relatively minor compromises, such as a tendency to withdraw or become hyperexcitable under stress, to a major deviation, such as overwhelming avoidance of the animate world, the degrees to which the infant, even in the first months of life, achieves a less-than-optimal adaptive structural organization can be observed.

Infants who, because of CNS immaturity, are especially sensitive to routine sensory stimulation (i.e., tactile, vestibular, auditory) provide a challenge to the caretaker to find experiences that are especially comforting. For example, firm holding and pressure may be helpful for the infant who is overly sensitive to touch, and use of large muscle groups may be helpful in facilitating an infant to attend more effectively. When motor coordination difficulties compromise expected control of body position or self-comforting behavior (e.g., hand to mouth), self-regulation is further challenged. Integrating special patterns of holding and movement with the aims of comfort, regulation, and interest in the world is therefore an important early goal.

When there have been distortions in the attachment process (stage II) (e.g., if a parent responds in a mechanical, remote manner or projects dependent feelings onto the infant), the infant may not learn to appreciate causal relationships between people at the level of compassionate and intimate feelings. This situation can occur even though causality seems to be developing in terms of the inanimate world and the impersonal human world.

The early attachments can be warm and engaging or shallow, insecure, and limited in their affective tone. The infant who is motor delayed has difficulty letting the caretaker know he or she is feeling joyful in the caretaker's presence. Poorly coordinated motor responses, lack of synchronous vocalizations, and even difficulty in organizing a smile challenge the caretaker to find a special look or gesture unique to the infant. The infant is likely to become doubly frustrated when unable to control his or her own body, and because of this, the infant cannot elicit emotionally satisfying responses.

There are differences between an infant who reads the signals of the caretakers and responds to multiple aspects of communication (with multiple affects and behavioral communications) in a rich, meaningful way and one who can respond only within a narrow range of affect (e.g., protest) or who cannot respond at all in a contingent or reciprocal manner (e.g., the seemingly apathetic, withdrawn, and depressed child who responds only to his or her own internal cues). During stage III, the ability to connect sensory experiences across the senses (e.g., auditory and visual), to connect sensory and motor experiences (e.g., look and reach), and to play and implement motor activities in accord with adaptive goals (e.g., exploring parent's mouth) are all important elements in learning to communicate purposefully (i.e., to take initiative and make things happen). It is also important at this stage to communicate purposefully across a range of emotions (e.g., dependency, by reaching out to be close; exploring, by examining parent's nose; or angrily protesting, by throwing down food), and to use all the sensory realms in support of affective interaction. Compromised motor planning, sensory discrimination, cross-sensory integration, and sensory motor coordination require special approaches to help an infant master this crucial emotional and cognitive stage.

As the toddler becomes behaviorally more organized (stage IV), and complex emotional patterns appear that reflect originality and initiative in the context of the separation and individuation subphase of development, we can observe those toddlers who manifest this full adaptive capacity. They may be compared with others who are stereotyped in their behavioral patterns (reflect no originality or intentionality); who remain fragmented (never connect pieces of behavior into more complicated patterns); or who evidence polarities of affect, showing no capacity to integrate emotions (the chronic negativistic aggressive toddler who cannot show interest, curiosity, or love).

The toddler who is motor delayed may have difficulty achieving a sense of self-control over space in relationship to balancing his or her needs for independence and dependence. Similarly, the motor-delayed toddler may understandably feel a lack of control over his or her own body. Large muscle activity associated with assertiveness and aggression may prove frightening, leading to avoidance of these important domains of emotional life. The toddler who, because of sensory processing lags, finds it difficult to discriminate auditory and visual cues across space (e.g., staying in emotional touch with the parent across the room by decoding vocalizations and gestures) may need to rely on proximal patterns (being held) or may become easily frightened. The task for stage V—to organize and integrate behavioral and emotional patterns—can therefore be especially challenging and require unique caretaking patterns.

In stage V, the child who can organize and create internal emotional imagery and integrate and differentiate a rich range of affective and ideational life can be distinguished from one who remains either without representational capacity or undifferentiated (i.e., deficits in reality testing, impulse control, focused concentration), or who may form and differentiate self and object representations only at the expense of extreme compromises in the range of tolerated experience (e.g., the schizoid child who withdraws from relationships). Similar adaptive or maladaptive structural organizations can be observed in later childhood (the triangular phase), latency, and adolescence.

To achieve these higher-level emotional and cognitive organizations, the child needs to be able to abstract his or her own motor-behavior patterns, sensory experiences, and somatically based affective experiences and form new higher-level symbolic (ideational) organizations, including an ideational sense of self and nonself. The ability to integrate across sensory, affective, and motor experience; to practice using ideas through "pretend play"; and to employ functional emotional language (e.g., "I am mad") is of obvious importance. Motor delays that compromise a child's ability to engage in make-believe play, to employ functional language, or to achieve sensory integration or sensory-motor coordination all create special challenges for the child and caretakers to find new ways to create and practice using "emotional ideas."

A more detailed discussion of this framework, including principles of prevention and intervention, is available (Greenspan, 1979, 1981; Greenspan and Greenspan, 1985). It should also be pointed out that, through videotaped analyses of infant-caretaker interactions (Greenspan and Lieberman, 1980), these patterns evidence temporal stability and can be reliably rated and new raters trained and kept at high levels of reliability (Hofheimer et al., 1981; Poisson et al., 1983). Most importantly, we have recently developed and are now piloting screening questionnaires based on these milestones for use in a variety of primary care settings.

IV. Clinical principles of integrating approaches and sensory, motor, and affective challenges

In the previous sections, it is suggested that, at each stage of emotional development, specific sensory or motor challenges create unique emotional challenges. How do we turn each challenge into a unique learning opportunity? For example, how do we help the infant with increased motor tone correct the motor difficulty and, at the same time, learn to use his or her motor system for "falling in love," cause-and-effect emotional signaling, emotional thinking, and so forth? In considering the objective of integrating the child's physical and emotional needs, a key guiding principle is immediately suggested.

Principle I   Each activity aimed at improving sensory, motor, or cognitive capacities should also have, as its goal, facilitation of the relevant, age-expected emotional pattern.

For example, the traditional approach to an 8-month-old with motor lags and increased motor tone involves lots of swaddling and flexion to decrease motor tone and specialized handling techniques to help the infant break up motor patterns (e.g., rotation patterns, gentle changes in position, and posture). In working with such an infant over a bolster, moving the elbow back and forth and rotating the shoulders slightly, how can an opportunity be created for the 8-month-old's emotional task of learning cause-and-effect emotional signaling? The infant might be taught to imitate the prescribed motor movements on his or her own: "I do it; now, you do it." The infant might be taught an emotional, relevant, intentional gesture indicating dependency such as reaching up to be held. To be sure, complex motor gestures are shaped through gradual approximations. However, if each approximation and eventually the complete pattern were emotionally age-appropriate and relevant and responded to with physical and emotional warmth, the infant would be learning in his or her own way to make things happen in the emotional world of closeness and dependency. The infant would learn "I can communicate my desire for closeness," rather than learn that closeness is random and the best he or she can do is remain passive or fragmented. As this example indicates, there are two parts to learning: (1) helping the child organize emotionally and socially relevant patterns, and (2) responding to each step in the sequence of the newly learned pattern in a pleasurable manner.

Principle II   Each emotionally or socially relevant pattern, either in its incipient stages or in its complete form, should receive a timely, "phase-specific," pleasurable, emotional response. This response includes the caretaker's position (e.g., when possible, in front of infant) and affective disposition (e.g., genuine pleasure at the infant's response).

The caretaker's response should be developmentally phase-appropriate. For example, a motor-delayed 15-month-old manages to crawl away from the caretaker and looks back with a smile of accomplishment. Clapping and admiring the infant's accomplishment from afar may at that moment be more phase-appropriate than a hugging and cuddling. The infant is learning to balance dependence and independence, and communicating across space with word and gesture. Distal communication modes, such as the use of words and gestures, support the infant's emerging ability to be close from across space. Because many motor exercises are carried out from behind the infant or child, innovative approaches to facilitate purposeful communication need to be developed to arrange for flexible enough positioning for appropriate, face-to-face, emotional interactions. A part of an infant's emerging communication capacities is his or her interest in self-control and initiative.

Principle III   Each emotionally relevant interaction should facilitate self-initiative (in generating similar emotional patterns) and the generalization (and abstraction) of these patterns to all areas and contexts of functioning.

For example, in facilitating phase-specific emotional patterns, one should always ask, "Am I doing it for the infant, or am I creating a learning opportunity where he or she is learning to take initiative?" The 9-month-old who hears "toot, toot" when pressing his or her hand near the parent's face is learning to take initiative and make things happen, but the 9-month-old who is only read to learns only to receive information passively. A new emotional skill should be applied to multiple contexts, such as touching Daddy's face to make Daddy say "toot, toot" and pulling Mommy's finger to get her to stick out her tongue. An older child's exploring the various ways G.I. Joe can destroy the "bad guys" facilitates the application of emotional-behavioral patterns and emotional-ideational patterns (through pretend play) to multiple contexts.

In addition to the challenge of learning to take initiative and generalize new coping capacities, the infant or child with developmental disabilities, as well as the infant or child with cognitive lags or difficulties, faces another important challenge. This challenge relates to the critical psychologic task of differentiating an emotional sense of self which is unique, encompasses the full range of human emotions, and is clearly separate from one's sense of others and non-self. Children with difficulties in sensory processing often have difficulty in discriminating subtle aspects of sensory-affective experience (e.g., "Is she happy or sad?" "Does he intend to hold me or hurt me?" "Am I angry or scared?" "Is my wish to bite a part of me?"). While such emotional interpretations relate to one's experiences, a basic difficulty in discriminating incoming information or information arising from one's own body (e.g., somatic affective cues) because of discrimination problems makes it extra difficult to interpret confusing experiences. Cognitive lags, in which abstracting abilities are limited, may contribute to an inability to abstract the difficult emotional aspects of one's self into an organized pattern. Similarly, motor planning or control difficulties create an extra challenge in developing a secure sense of self, in terms of body control, assertiveness, and handling aggression (e.g., "If I can't make my body do what I want it to, then what can I control, and where does my self-initiative and control end and someone else's begin?").

To facilitate a differentiated sense of self across the full range of human emotions in a child who has difficulties with sensory-affective discrimination, cognition, motor planning, or control requires that special experiences be made available.

Principle IV   Support and provide extra practice for self-differentiation. To accomplish this, provide extra opportunities for interpersonal interactions that have the elements of (1) the infant's or child's elaborating the full range of human emotions and inclinations, including closeness or dependency, pleasure, assertiveness and curiosity, anger, protest, self-limit-setting, and eventually empathy and consistent love, and (2) caretaker responses that are clear and accurate in regard to the child's elaborations, including feedback that provides a sense of being understood and at the same time supports further self-initiated elaboration.

For infants and children, special play time ("floor time") often provides the context for these types of interactions. Such play times, in which dolls or soldiers may carry forth the emotional theme, may demand a great deal from the caretakers, including understanding their own emotional reactions to the child's dependency or aggression, as well as extra patience and the realization that the child will need *extra* repetition at certain times and help with moving on at other times.

If emotional development is lagging, the goal should be to help the child catch up in emotion, as well as in motor development. For example, alertness, interest in the world, pleasure in others (a warm attachment), as well as intentional communication, are compromised in a 9-month-old infant with a severe motor lag and hypotonicity. While helping the child stabilize head, shoulders, and trunk, the caretaker should at the same time provide enough tactile, vestibular, and other sensory input to facilitate increased tone and alertness and interest in the world. Here, the first goal is to find ways to encourage and maintain alertness so that the child can eventually create those movement patterns and sensory experiences that support increased tone and alertness. At the same time, the caretaker is attempting to "woo" the infant so that he or she finds the human world especially lovable. A game of dance, nuzzle, and hugging, with gentle, light stroking, may combine the beneficial effects of movement and touch with the warm, pleasurable emotions of being close. The caretaker must be especially alert to even slight vocal or motor signals for interaction so that they can be quickly interpreted and responded to in a phase-appropriate manner. A seemingly disorganized slap on the nose during nuzzling may provide the opportunity for the caretaker to honk like a car, encouraging these touches to the nose with novel and entertaining "honks." Here, the caretaker is simultaneously providing movement; touch, head, shoulder, and trunk support; wooing (in a loving way); and cause-and-effect feedback for emerging motor patterns. A caretaker may encourage assertive exploration while an infant is secure in a bean bag chair, by making the caretaker's own body a multiresponsive human toy. The goal is to integrate the infant's need for increased motor tone and alertness, with sensory interest in the world, a loving attachment, and cause-and-effect emotional signaling.

The emotional milestones should also facilitate, for both professionals and parents, attention to predictable, but nonetheless potentially undermining, interaction patterns, including resentment and overexpectation early on, and overprotectiveness and inability to let the infant take initiative when capable later in development. The phase-specific emotional needs of the infant, therefore, also provide a context for the professional and parent to consider their own attitudes and expectations in relationship to the infant's emotional requirements.

This brief discussion highlights only a few examples and guiding principles. These provide a base from which innovative therapists and parents can develop their own way of working with the child's physical and emotional experiences. For example, a speech and language therapist may use pretend play to practice vocalizations and at the same time focus on the child's phase-specific interests and fantasies (e.g., a 3½-year-old interested in how the different parts of the doll's body work); a parent may help his or her 4-month-old who is disinterested in being in the prone position to roll over and tolerate the prone position by combining it with pleasurable, face-to-face interactions; or a health professional helping a parent of an irritable and crying 10-week-old may suggest that special postures, holding, and touching patterns be combined with extra practice in looking, listening, and gesturing to facilitate an "organizing" interest in the world. It is a valuable challenge for all those working with infants and children to provide opportunities for experiences that integrate emotional, intellectual, and physical goals.

V. The infant, the family, and the service system

Infants and children with unique capacities present special emotional challenges for their caretakers and families. These challenges can be understood in terms of the sequence of emotional milestones outlined in sec. II (Greenspan, 1981; 1985). With appropriate caretaker patterns, almost all infants and children are capable of negotiating these milestones in their own way. From learning to calm down and take an interest in sensory and affective information, to "falling in love" and learning to create ideas, to labeling and guiding feelings and behavior, infants can learn to use their special abilities to achieve these larger milestones.

For infants to master their emotional milestones, the special family challenges must also be understood. It is not unusual for the parent of an infant with a developmental disorder to go through a series of stages. Initially, they may have a hard time accepting their infant ("he is not a part of me"). This stage may be followed quickly by a feeling of guilt and overidentification ("she is me"), but if the parent has a negative self-concept and negative feelings about the infant, the predominate feeling may be that "it's a bad me." This stage also may last only a short time and a compensatory reaction may set in, and the parent will make him- or herself and the infant perfect ("it is going to be a perfect me"). These attitudes are often associated with characteristic interaction patterns. Withdrawal and apathy may be related to the feeling that the infant is not part of the family. Critical, intrusive, and even punitive behavior may be related to the feeling that the infant is part of a "bad me." Overprotectiveness, overcontrolling, and undermining (of autonomy) behavior may go along with the attitude that "it will be a perfect me." A "perfect me" attitude may also only marginally mask a feeling that the infant is inadequate "without me" and lead to difficulties when the child tries to become more independent. As the child becomes more self-sufficient and competent, either abrupt withdrawal or depression and excessive fears of injury or illness may ironically characterize the caretaker's behavior.

Each parent may have a different attitude, which may lead to marital conflict. The feelings about the challenging new infant may be so consuming that the parents have difficulty in being sensitive to each other's needs. In some instances, parents may feel so embarrassed about their "negative" private feelings that they may increasingly isolate themselves from their spouses. Siblings worry, "Will this happen to me?" "Did my anger and jealousy do this to him?" "Can I get love and attention this way?" Extended family members are often involved in these patterns, as well. Frequently, the infant becomes the focus of unresolved family issues centering on dependency, anger, damage, or loss. Lack of sleep, along with the expected physical and emotional stresses, may only further compromise caretaker coping capacities.

It may be useful to view caretakers as faced with a number of general challenges, that include (1) providing physical protection and care; (2) recognizing basic signals of pleasure and displeasure while providing an ongoing sense of acceptance and love; and (3) understanding and responding to the stage-specific, emotional, intellectual, and physical requirements of their infant, in the context of their infant's individual differences and unique abilities. For each stage of development, caretakers must understand their own reactions to provide special "experiential nutrients" that conform to the infant's special characteristics. For example, the infant at 2 to 4 months of age needs to be "wooed" to "fall in love." By 4 to 8 months, the infant requires cause-and-effect emotional interactions so that overtures for dependency (e.g., reaching out) are met and perceived differently than overtures indicating anger (e.g., banging or biting hard), which also require a response. But, the motor-delayed infant may find it difficult to return the caretaker's "wooing" and may communicate emotional inclinations in confusing rather than clear ways, leading to expected caretaker feelings of rejection, anger, or confusion. For example, the infant may communicate the need for closeness by flailing his or her arms. Special challenges for caretakers are therefore to provide physical protection and care; to recognize basic signals of pleasure and displeasure; and to facilitate their infant's physical, intellectual, and emotional progress in the context of changing developmental and emotional milestones and unique special characteristics.

Each infant, caretaker, and family may present a special challenge to the service providers. Just as a caretaker may become mechanical with and emotionally distant from his or her chaotic and disorganized infant, the clinician or team may become mechanical and avoid the intrusive, overanxious, disorganized caretaker or family. What is often seen clinically is a chain reaction in which the infant's special needs create a disequilibrium in the family (e.g., marital difficulties, alcoholic or psychosomatic problems), which in turn communicates stress to the service team. In this context, it is not unusual for the service team with the best intentions to wish to ignore the family's emotional patterns and in so doing themselves fall into a pattern of being covertly rejecting, critical and punitive, or overcontrolling or infantilizing.

It is critical for the service team not simply to react as one more link in the chain, but to (1) contain the reaction; (2) diagnose the infant's and family's emotional patterns; (3) introspectively figure out their own expected emotional reactions; and (4) NOT act on their immediate feelings, but use them to understand how the family feels and plan a corrective emotional strategy to be integrated with the specific treatment plan. For example, the service team may ask, "If they are getting us to feel disorganized and aversive or overcontrolling and bossy, perhaps that is how they are feeling. How can we be of assistance to them?" Team members can help each other. Sometimes the team member closest to the family is the one who most reacts or overidentifies, and others can help the involved team member see the larger pattern. Table 15-2 outlines common, clinically observed patterns in infants, caretakers, and service providers.

VI. Conclusion

Recent understanding of infant and family emotional functioning now makes it possible to pinpoint emotional milestones much like the neuromotor milestones. This "road map" will hopefully prove helpful in facilitating adaptive emotional growth in infants whose sensory, motor, or physical differences set into motion unique family challenges.

That there are "many roads to Rome" must always be remembered. Almost all infants and young children can learn—in different ways—to relate to others, interact intentionally, organize a sense of self, learn to use ideas to guide behavior and label feelings, test reality, modulate impulses and mood, experience positive self-esteem, and concentrate.

The challenge is to provide infants and children with the needed learning opportunities that are sensitive to their individual differences and unique potentials.

Table 15-2. Emotional milestones: Family and service system patterns

Stage-specific tasks and capacities	Maladaptive infant	Maladaptive family	Maladaptive service system	Adaptive service system
I. Homeostasis (0–3 mo; regulation and interest in the world)	Unregulated (e.g., hyperexcitable) or withdrawn (apathetic) behavior	Unavailable, chaotic, dangerous, abusive; hypo- or hyperstimulating; dull	Critical and punitive	Supply support structure and extra nurturing
II. Attachment (2–7 mo; falling in love)	Total lack of or nonaffective; shallow; impersonal involvement in animate world	Emotionally distant, aloof, and/or impersonal (highly ambivalent)	Angry and impatient covered by mask of impersonal professionalism	"Woo" caretaker into a relationship; point out pleasurable aspects of infant
III. Somatopsychologic differentiation (3–10 mo; purposeful communication)	Behavior and affects random and/or chaotic or narrow, rigid, and stereotyped	Ignores or misreads (e.g., projects) infant's communications (e.g., is overly intrusive, preoccupied, or depressed)	Vacillates between overcontrol and avoidance (of intrusive caretaker) or overprotectiveness (of depressed caretaker)	Combine empathy and limit setting with sensitivity to reading subtle emotional signals, help caretaker read infant's signals
IV. Behavioral organization, initiative, and internalization (9–24 mo; a complex sense of self)	Fragmented, stereotyped, and polarized behavior and emotions (e.g., withdrawn, compliant, hyperaggressive, or disorganized behavior)	Overly intrusive, controlling; fragmented, fearful (especially of toddler's autonomy); abruptly and prematurely "separates"	Premature separation from or rejection of family rationalized by notion: "They are okay now"	Support family self-sufficiency, but with admiration and more rather than less involvement
V. Representational capacity, differentiation and consolidation (1½–4 yr; creating ideas and emotional thinking)	No representational (symbolic) elaboration; behavior and affect concrete, shallow, and polarized; sense of self and "other" fragmented, undifferentiated or narrow and rigid; reality testing, impulse regulation, mood stabilization compromised or vulnerable (e.g., borderline psychotic and severe character problems)	Fears or denies phase-appropriate needs; engages child only in concrete (nonsymbolic) modes generally or in certain realms (e.g., around pleasure) and/or misreads or responds noncontingently or unrealistically to emerging communications (i.e., undermines reality orientation); overly permissive or punitive	Infantilizing and concrete with family providing instructions, but no explanations or real sense of partnership	Create atmosphere for working partnership; learn from caretakers and help them conceptualize their own approaches

REFERENCES

Ainsworth, M., Bell, S. M., and Stayton, D. Infant-Mother Attachment and Social Development: Socialization as a Product of Reciprocal Responsiveness to Signals. In M. Richards (ed.), *The Integration of the Child into a Social World.* Cambridge, Engl.: Cambridge University Press, 1974. Pp. 99–135.

Backwin, H. Loneliness in infants. *Am. J. Dis. Child.* 63 : 30, 1942.

Bell, S. The development of the concept of object as related to infant-mother attachment. *Child Dev.* 41 : 219, 1970.

Bergman, P., and Escalona, S. Unusual sensitivities in very young children. *Psychoanal. Study Child* 3 : 333, 1949.

Bowlby, J. Maternal care and mental health. *WHO Monogr.* No. 2, 1951.

Brazelton, T. B., Koslowski, B., and Main, M. The Origins of Reciprocity: The Early Mother-Infant Interaction. In M. Lewis and L. Rosenblum (eds.), *The Effect of the Infant on Its Care Giver.* New York: Wiley, 1974. Pp. 49–76.

Burlingham, D., and Freud, A. *Young Children in Wartime.* London: Allen & Unwin, 1942.

Cameron, H. C. *The Nervous Child.* London: Oxford Medical, 1919.

Charlesworth, W. R. The Role of Surprise in Cognitive Development. In E. Elkind and J. H. Flavell (eds.), *Studies in Cognitive Development: Essays in Honor of Jean Piaget.* London: Oxford University Press, 1969. Pp. 257–314.

Cravioto, J., and Delicardie, E. Environmental correlates of severe clinical malnutrition and language development in survivors from kwashiorkor or marasmus. In *Nutrition, the Nervous System and Behavior.* PAHO Scientific Publ. No. 251, Washington, D.C., 1973.

Ekman, P. Universals and cultural differences in facial expressions of emotion. *Nebraska Symposium on Motivation.* Lincoln: University of Nebraska Press, 1972.

Emde, R. N., Gaensbauer, T. J., and Harmon, R. J. Emotional expression in infancy: A bio-behavioral study. *Psychol. Issues* No. 37, 1976.

Escalona, S. K. *The Roots of Individuality.* Chicago: Aldine, 1968.

Freud, S. Formulation on the two principles of mental functioning (1911). In *The Standard Edition of the Complete Psychological Works of Sigmund Freud.* London: Hogarth, Vol. 12, pp. 218–226.

Gewirtz, J. L. The Course of Infant Smiling in Four Child-rearing Environments in Israel. In B. M. Foss (ed.), *Determinants of the Infant Behavior.* London: Methuen, 1965. Vol. 3, pp. 205–260.

Gewirtz, J. L. Levels of conceptual analysis in environment-infant interaction research. *Merrill-Palmer Q.* 15 : 9, 1969.

Gouin-Decarie, T. *Intelligence and Affectivity in Early Childhood: An Experimental Study of Jean Piaget's Object Concept and Object Relations.* New York: International Universities Press, 1965.

Greenspan, S. I. Intelligence and adaption: An integration of psychoanalytic and Piagetian developmental psychology. *Psychol. Issues* No. 47–48, 1979.

Greenspan, S. I. Psychopathology and adaption in infancy and early childhood: Principles of clinical diagnosis and preventive intervention. *Clin. Infant Rep.* No. 1, 1981.

Greenspan, S. I. A model for comprehensive preventive intervention services for infants, young children and their families. In S. I. Greenspan, S. Wieder, A. F. Lieberman, et al. (eds.), Infants in Multi-Risk Families; Case Studies of Preventive Intervention. *Clin. Infant Rep.* No. 3, 1984.

Greenspan, S. I., and Greenspan, N. T. *First Feelings: Milestones in the Emotional Development of Your Baby and Child.* New York: Viking, 1985.

Greenspan, S. I., and Lieberman, A. F. Infants, Mothers and Their Interactions: A Quantitative Clinical Approach to Developmental Assessment. In S. I. Greenspan and G. H. Pollock (eds.), *The Course of Life: Psychoanalytic Contributions Toward Understanding Personality Development. Vol. I: Infancy and Early Childhood.* Dept. of Health and Human Services publication (ADM) 80-786. Government Printing Office, 1980.

Greenspan, S. I., and Lourie, R. S. Developmental structuralist approach to the classification of adaptive and pathologic personality organization: Application to infancy and early childhood. *Am. J. Psychiatry* 138 : 6, 1981.

Greenspan, S. I., Lourie, R. S., and Nover, R. A. A Developmental Approach to the Classification of Psychopathology in Infancy and Early Childhood. In J. Noshpitz (ed.), *The Basic Handbook of Child Psychiatry.* New York: Basic Books, 1979. Vol. 2, pp. 157–164.

Greenspan, S. I., and Porges, S. W. Psychopathology in infancy and early childhood: Clinical perspectives on the organization of sensory and affective thematic experience. *Child. Dev.* 55 : 49, 1984.

Greenspan, S. I., and Weider, S. I. Dimensions and levels of the therapeutic process. *Psychotherapy* 1 : 21, 1984.

Hartmann, H. *Ego Psychology and the Problem of Adaptation.* New York: International Universities Press, 1939.

Hofheimer, J. A., Strauss, M. E., Poisson, S. S., and Greenspan, S. I. The reliability, validity and generalizability of assessments of transactions between infants and their caregivers: A multicenter design (working paper). Bethesda, Md.: Clinical Infant Development Program, National Institutes of Mental Health, 1981.

Hunt, J. M. Infants in an orphanage. *J. Abnorm. Soc. Psychol.* 36 : 338, 1941.

Izard, C. On the Development of Emotions and Emotion-Cognition Relationships in Infancy. In M. Lewis and L. Rosenblum (eds.), *The Development of Affect.* New York: Plenum, 1978.

Klaus, M., and Kennell, J. H. *Maternal-Infant Bonding: The Impact of Early Separation or Loss on Family Development.* St. Louis: Mosby, 1976.

Lipsitt, L. Learning processes of newborns. *Merrill-Palmer Q.* 12 : 45, 1966.

Lourie, R. S. The first three years of life: An overview of a new frontier for psychiatry. *Am. J. Psychiatry* 127 : 1457, 1971.

Lowrey, L. G. Personality distortion and early institutional care. *Am. J. Orthopsychiatry* 10 : 546, 1940.

Mahler, M. S., Pine, F., and Bergman, A. *The Psychological Birth of the Human Infant.* New York: Basic Books, 1975.

Meltzoff, A. N., and Moore, K. M. Imitation of facial and manual gestures by human neonates. *Science* 198 : 75, 1977.

Murphy, L. B., and Moriarty, A. E. *Vulnerability, Coping, and Growth.* New Haven, Conn.: Yale University Press, 1976.

Piaget, J. The Stages of the Intellectual Development of the Child. In S. I. Harrison and J. F. McDermott (eds.), *Childhood Psychopathology.* New York: International Universities Press, 1972. Pp. 157–166.

Poisson, S. S., Hofheimer, J. A., Strauss, M. E., and Greenspan, S. I. Inter-observer agreement and reliability assessments of the GLOS measures of caregiver infant interaction (unpublished manuscript). Bethesda, Md.: National Institutes of Mental Health, 1983.

Poisson, S. S., Lieberman, A. F., and Greenspan, S. I. Training manual for the Greenspan-Lieberman observation system (GLOS) (unpublished manuscript). Bethesda, Md.: National Institutes of Mental Health, 1981.

Rachford, B. K. *Neurotic Disorders of Childhood.* New York: E. B. Treat, 1905.

Rheingold, H. The development of social behavior in the human infant. *Monogr. Soc. Res. Child Dev.* 31 : 1, 1966.

Rheingold, H. Infancy. In D. Sills (ed.), *International Encyclopedia of the Social Sciences.* New York: Macmillan, 1969.

Sander, L. Issues in early mother-child interaction. *J. Am. Acad. Child Psychiatry* 1 : 141, 1962.

Spitz, R. A. Hospitalism. *Psychoanal. Study Child* 1 : 53, 1945.

Spitz, R. A. *The First Year of Life.* New York: International Universities Press, 1965.

Sroufe, L., and Waters, E. Attachment as an organizational construct. *Child. Dev.* 48 : 1184, 1977.

Stern, D. Mother and Infant at Play: The Dyadic Interaction Involving Facial, Vocal, and Gaze Behaviors. In M. Lewis and L. Rosenblum (eds.), *The Effect of the Infant on Its Caregiver.* New York: Wiley, 1974a. Pp. 187–213.

Stern, D. The goal and structure of mother-infant play. *J. Am. Acad. Child Psychiatry* 13 : 402, 1974b.

Stern, D. *The First Relationship: Infant and Mother.* Cambridge, Mass.: Harvard University Press, 1977.

Tennes, K., Emde, R., Kisley, A., and Metcalf, D. The Stimulus Barrier in Early Infancy: An Exploration of Some Formulations of John Benjamin. In R. Holt and E. Peterfreund (eds.), *Psychoanalysis and Contemporary Science.* New York: Macmillan, 1972. Vol. 1, pp. 206–234.

Tomkins, S. Affect, Imagery, Consciousness. New York: Springer, 1963. Vols. 1 and 2.

Werner, H. (1962). The Stages of the Intellectual Development of the Child. In S. Harrison and J. McDermott (eds.), *Childhood Psychopathology.* New York: International Universities Press, 1972.

Werner, H., and Kaplan, B. *Symbol Formation.* New York: Wiley, 1963.

Winnicott, D. W. *Clinical Notes on Disorders of Childhood,* London: Heinemann, 1931.

IV

Management of Specific Problems

16

Feeding and Growth of Premature and Small-for-Gestational-Age Infants

Karen E. Peterson and Deborah A. Frank

I. Introduction

Growth of premature and small-for-gestational-age (SGA) infants is assessed by comparison with the intrauterine and postnatal growth of full-term infants. Mean preterm growth velocities have been derived from several reference data sets (Table 16-1). Attained growth status of high-risk infants after term is assessed using the growth charts of the National Center for Health Statistics (NCHS) (Hamill et al., 1976). Incremental growth tables can be used to evaluate postterm growth velocities (Baumgartner et al., 1986) (Table 16-2).

Existing data on postnatal growth patterns of high-risk infants are descriptive and not necessarily normative. Patterns represent state-of-the-art medical care of high-risk neonates and may need to be revised as the techniques for sustaining growth in these infants are improved. Nutritional rehabilitation of premature and SGA infants should begin as soon as possible to approximate continued growth at intrauterine rates. In all infants, there is a brief period of physiologic weight loss postnatally, which may be exacerbated by illness or caloric deprivation. When the period of postnatal weight loss ends, catch-up growth should occur (Pereira and Barbosa, 1986). During catch-up growth, rates of gain for corrected age exceed intrauterine and postterm velocities of full-term infants.

II. Definitions

A. *Gestational age* refers to the period from the first day of the mother's last menstrual period to birth of the infant. Estimates of gestational age should be confirmed by clinical assessment of neurologic signs and external characteristics according to the Dubowitz method (Dubowitz et al., 1970).

B. *Postnatal age* is the time that has elapsed from birth of the infant to the present.

C. *Postmenstrual age* is the time that has elapsed from the first day of the mother's last menstrual period to the present and may be used in both the prenatal and postnatal periods to describe the age of the fetus or infant.

D. *Term* is 40 weeks of age, estimated from the first day of the last menstrual period, regardless of time of birth.

Table 16-1. Mean preterm growth velocities

Measurement	28–32 wk	32–36 wk	36–40 wk
Weight (g/day)	24.0	30.0	28.0
Length (cm/wk)	1.2	1.2	0.6
Head circumference (cm/wk)	0.9	0.8	0.4

Adapted from S. G. Babson. Growth of low birth weight infants. *Pediatrics* 77 : 11, 1970.

Table 16-2. Median (50th percentile) postterm growth velocities

	0–6 mo	6–12 mo	12–24 mo	24–36 mo
Weight (g/day)	23.0	14.4	6.8	5.5
Length (cm/mo)	2.8	1.6	1.0	0.7
Head circumference (cm/mo)	1.4	0.7	0.2	0.1

Note: Rates reflect mean of velocities for males and females combined. Values are rounded to the nearest tenth.
Adapted from R. N. Baumgartner, A. F. Roche, and J. H. Himes. Incremental growth tables: Supplementary to previously published charts. *Am. J. Clin. Nutr.* 43 : 711, 1986.

E. *Premature* or *preterm infants* are those born at 37 weeks or less of gestation. Moderately premature infants are born at 31 to 33 weeks of gestation; birth at 27 to 30 weeks' gestation indicates extreme prematurity (Babson, 1970).

F. *Corrected age* is postnatal age less the number of weeks the child was premature (the difference between 40 weeks and gestational age). Corrected age is used to assess growth and development of the infant after term. The difference between growth percentiles for corrected and uncorrected postnatal ages is statistically significant until 18 months to 3½ years, depending on whether head circumference, weight, or length is being assessed (see III.A) (Brandt, 1978). If uncorrected ages are used in growth data analysis, the severity of the growth deficits is overestimated.

G. *Relation of birth weight to gestational age.* Various intrauterine growth curves are used to classify the appropriateness of the birth weights of premature infants for gestational age. Infants weighing 2,500 g or less at birth are described as low birth weight (LBW). Very low birth weight (VLBW) infants weigh 1,500 g or less at birth. In contrast to assessments of postnatal growth, no universally accepted standard exists for determining intrauterine growth retardation. Growth curves vary according to the geographic and clinical population from which they were derived. For example, the 10th percentile on the Lubchenco charts lies close to the 3rd percentile on the other reference standards, because the Denver infants were smaller at given gestational ages than infants born at sea level, particularly after 38 postmenstrual weeks (Rosenberg and Jones, 1982).

Infants are classified as SGA if their weights are below the 10th percentile on Lubchenco charts (Lubchenco et al., 1963; 1966) or below the 3rd percentile (or − 2 SD) on charts of Babson (1970), Miller (1971), and Usher (1969). Recently the ratio of midarm circumference to head circumference has been proposed as a more useful measure than birth weight for identifying SGA infants at risk for perinatal metabolic complications. However, the implications of this classification scheme for later growth potential are as yet unknown (Georgieff et al., 1986; Sasanow et al., 1986).

H. *Classification of SGA infants.* Small-for-gestational-age infants constitute a heterogenous group that may be categorized into subgroups using the ponderal index (Rohrer, 1908).

$100 \times$ weight (g) ÷ length^3 (cm)

Symmetric SGA infants exhibit a ponderal index greater than the 10th percentile for gestational age on the Lubchenco charts or greater than the 3rd percentile on the Miller charts. These infants are also described as proportional and nonwasted and have an adequate ponderal index. Symmetric SGA infants have reduced linear skeletal growth, but normal soft tissue mass, suggesting a chronic growth-retarding process from early in gestation (Miller and Jekel, 1985; Woods et al., 1979). Head circumference in symmetric SGA infants is usually depressed (Villar et al., 1984).

Asymmetric SGA infants may exhibit normal or low birth weights but have a low ponderal index, less than the 10th percentile for gestational age on the Lubchenco charts or the 3rd percentile on the Miller charts. These infants are nonproportional or wasted, with reduced soft tissue mass but normal linear skeletal growth (Miller, 1985). Head circumference is similar to that of normal-birth-weight infants of the same gestational age (Villar et al., 1984). In these infants, the low ponderal index with adequate length suggests failure of adequate caloric transfer to the fetus in the third trimester (Woods et al., 1979).

III. Catch-up growth

A. Premature infants

Premature infants without a serious medical illness show maximal catch-up growth from 36 to 44 postmenstrual weeks, and growth measures are between the 10th and 90th percentiles of reference standards by 1 year corrected age (Brandt, 1978; Cruise, 1973; Fitzhardinge, 1975, 1976; Manser, 1984). Extremely premature infants or those with chronic medical problems exhibit slower catch-up growth occurring over a longer period. The distribution of attained growth is shifted so that median measures fall within the 3rd to 25th percentiles between 2 and 3 years (Manser, 1984).

1. Weight. From 32 postmenstrual weeks to 1 month postterm, mean attained weights of appropriate-for-gestational-age (AGA) infants follow the 10th percentile of intrauterine curves for normal full-term infants (Brandt, 1978). Mean weights of infants 2 to 18 months of age range from 0 to 1 SD below the mean. Weights follow the same weight curve as full-term controls from 2 to 5 years with nonsignificant but slightly lower values (Brandt, 1978). Weights should be corrected for gestation-

al age of the child at birth until 24 months, when differences between corrected and uncorrected ages are no longer statistically significant (Brandt, 1978).

From birth to term, rate of weight gain in premature infants is less than intrauterine curves of full-term infants if high-calorie feedings are not provided (Brandt, 1978). From term to between 1 and 2 months postterm, growth velocity of premature infants without a serious medical illness during the catch-up growth phase exceeds that of term infants of the same postmenstrual age. Velocities of both groups coincide after 2 months of age (Brandt, 1978).

2. Length. From 30 to 40 postmenstrual weeks, mean length of AGA infants falls below the 50th percentile of intrauterine curves (Brandt, 1978). After term, the mean length difference between AGA premature and full-term controls decreases from 2.5 cm at term to 1.2 cm at 18 months (Brandt, 1978). Length and height values should be corrected for gestational age to 3½ years, after which age a mean difference of 1 cm between corrected and uncorrected values will not show a significant difference in percentiles (Brandt, 1978).

   In the first month postterm, mean length velocities of AGA infants are similar to full-term controls. Catch-up growth rates in length of premature infants exceed velocities of full-term controls from 1.5 to 7.5 months postterm (Brandt, 1978). From 7.5 months to 5 years, AGA premature infants grow in length at the same rate or slightly faster (0.1–0.8 cm/year) than full-term infants.

3. Head circumference. The difference in mean head circumference of AGA premature infants at corrected and uncorrected ages decreases from 6.5 cm at birth to 0.5 cm at 17 months (Brandt, 1978). Head circumference is corrected for gestational age to 18 months postterm. Extrauterine head circumference velocities of premature infants are greater from 30 to 40 postmenstrual weeks than after term (Brandt, 1978). Maximal catch-up growth in head circumference is demonstrated during that period. Velocity decreases markedly from 6 months after term (Brandt, 1978).

B. Small-for-gestational-age infants

Small-for-gestational-age full-term infants who will demonstrate catch-up growth do so by 8 to 12 months' corrected age (Fitzhardinge and Steven, 1972; Hack et al., 1982; Villar et al., 1984). Prognoses for growth in individual children may vary by ponderal index classification (symmetric, asymmetric) (Davies et al., 1979; Villar et al., 1984). Symmetric SGA babies may not demonstrate catch-up growth in weight, height, or head circumference (Villar et al., 1984), or may have growth rates lower than those of asymmetric SGA infants (Davies et al., 1979). Growth for corrected age should, however, parallel norms for full-term infants.

Catch-up growth in asymmetric SGA infants is most rapid in the first 3 months of life (Davies, 1979; Villar et al., 1984). By 6 to 9 months, a new growth trajectory in a higher percentile is reached (Villar et al., 1984). Length velocity is similar among asymmetric, symmetric, and full-term infants to 36 months (Villar et al., 1984). Because of initial differences in length at birth, attained mean length of asymmetric infants is similar to that of normal infants but exceeds length of symmetric SGA babies from term to 36 months (Villar et al., 1984).

The SGA infants who exhibit catch-up head growth have smaller circumferences than AGA premature infants from 34 postmenstrual weeks to 12 months postterm (Brandt, 1978). However, by 2 months, these differences are negligible. At 12 months, the mean difference between the two groups is 0.2 cm. Compared with symmetric SGA infants, asymmetric SGA infants have significantly larger head circumferences up to 30 months of age (Villar et al., 1984).

Growth that is slower than expected requires the clinician not only to scrutinize dietary intake (see IV) but also to search for underlying medical problems such as urinary tract infections and cardiac, pulmonary, and neurologic difficulties. The clinician should be concerned about growth performance of premature and SGA infants when the child's anthropometric parameters show a progressive deviation from a previously established growth percentile for corrected age.

Also worrisome is the failure of premature and asymmetric SGA infants to show catch-up growth in the first 1 to 6 postnatal months. Abnormal rates of head growth may also indicate ongoing problems. For example, subnormal growth velocity in head circumference may indicate inadequate nutrition or impaired central nervous system (CNS) growth because of infection, cranial bleeding, or asphyxia. Excess growth velocity in head circumference may signal hydrocephalus.

IV. Feeding

The optimal diet for a preterm infant supports a rate of growth approximating the third trimester of intrauterine life (American Academy of Pediatrics, 1985). Promoting catch-up growth in premature and SGA infants should be strongly emphasized in the first 3 months of life, and efforts continued to 8 to 12 months' corrected age. During catch-up growth, nutrient requirements for premature and SGA infants per kg body weight or per 100 kcal exceed needs of normal full-term infants.

Premature and LBW infants should be fed their mothers' breast milk or formula designed for premature infants. Premature infant formulas provide an amino acid composition similar to breast milk and high concentrations of nutrients needed by the premature infant. Pooled mature breast milk, full-term infant formula, evaporated milk formula, soy-based formula, or formula supplemented with whey (Cooke and Nichoalds, 1986), should not be fed to preterm infants for reasons discussed in V.A. The LBW infant can be switched to full-term infant formula at 1,800 to 2,500 g or when discharged from the hospital.

During the first week of life, infants tolerate 50 to 100 kcal per kg (American Academy of Pediatrics, 1985). Daily weight gain of infants is monitored. If the rate of gain is inadequate, kcal per kg must be increased by increasing volume within limits tolerated by the infant or by increasing the caloric density of feedings from the standard 20 kcal per oz of breast milk or standard infant formula to 24 to 30 kcal per oz.

The premature or SGA infant who cannot tolerate sufficient volume of formula or breast milk to meet nutritional needs requires high-caloric-density feedings. Calories may be inadequate if the child has a disease that increases maintenance energy needs or requires volume restriction (bronchopulmonary dysplasia, congenital heart disease). Other problems necessitating increased caloric intake are neurologic and anatomic abnormalities that increase effort of feeding and limit volumes ingested (cleft palate, oral motor dysfunction).

Renal solute load of infants receiving high-calorie feedings needs close monitoring after each alteration in formula composition. Urine osmolality should be maintained between 300 and 400 mosm per liter (Gordon, 1984). Renal solute load of feedings can be estimated from 5.7 mosm urea per g dietary protein and 1 mosm urea per mEq sodium, potassium, and chloride (Gordon, 1984). Milligrams can be converted to milliequivalents by the formula

mg/atomic weight × valence = mEq

where

	ATOMIC WEIGHT	VALENCE
Chloride	35.5	1
Potassium	39	1
Sodium	23	1

Caloric density of feedings is increased gradually, from 20 kcal per oz in 2 kcal per oz increments. If caloric density is advanced too quickly, the child may get hyperosmotic diarrhea. Stool output should be monitored for reducing substances and blood since hyperosmolar feedings have been implicated as one of several factors possibly predisposing to necrotizing enterocolitis in asphyxiated VLBW infants less than 2 months of age (Reynolds, 1985). Vomiting or high postfeeding residue on nasogastric aspiration of the stomach may also indicate intolerance of high-caloric-density feedings.

Premature infant formulas provide 24 kcal per oz compared with 20 kcal per oz of full-term infant formulas and should be routinely used for preterm infants who are not breast-fed. Nutrient compositions of premature infant formulas are detailed in Table 16-3. Caloric density of premature infant formulas can be increased from 24 to 30 kcal per oz in 2 kcal per oz increments by using vegetable oil (corn or safflower), medium-chain triglycerides (MCT), and a glucose polymer (Polycose [Ross Laboratories], Moducal [Mead Johnson], Sumacal [Organon]). Increases in fat and carbohydrate should be proportional so that no one macronutrient is used in excess to increase caloric density. Proportions of macronutrients should be as follows: carbohydrate, 37 to 44 percent; protein, 10 to 12 percent; and fat, 40 to 50 percent.

Preterm breast-fed infants requiring caloric supplementation can be fed a mixture of their mother's milk and high-calorie premature infant formula (24–30 kcal/oz), alternately fed breast milk and high-calorie premature infant formula, or fed breast milk with added commercial fortifiers (Enfamil Human Milk Fortifier [Mead Johnson], Similac Natural Care [Ross]), MCT or vegetable oil, glucose polymer, human milk protein, or a combination (Ronnholm et al.,

Table 16-3. Composition of special formulas for premature infants[a]

Ingredient	Enfamil Premature	SMA "Preemie"	Similac Special Care
Protein (g/dl)	2.4	2.0	2.2
Fat (g/dl)	4.1	4.4	4.4
Medium-chain triglycerides	40%	12%	50%
Oleo oil	0	20%	0
Corn oil	40%	0	30%
Oleic oil	0	25%	0
Coconut oil	20%	25%	20%
Soy oil	0	18%	0
Carbohydrate (g/dl)	8.9	8.6	8.6
Lactose	40%	50%	50%
Glucose polymers	60%	50%	50%
Minerals (mg/dl)[b]			
Calcium	95 [48]	75 [37]	144 [72]
Phosphorus	48	40	72
Sodium	32 [14]	32 [14]	35 [15]
Potassium	90 [23]	75 [19]	100 [26]
Chloride	69 [19]	53 [15]	65 [18]
Magnesium	8	7	10
Zinc	0.8	0.5	1.2
Copper	0.073	0.07	0.2
Manganese	0.021	0.02	0.02
Iron	0.13	0.3	0.3
Iodine	0.006	0.008	0.015
Vitamins			
A (IU/L)	2,540	3,200	5,500
D (IU/L)	507	510	1,200
E (IU/L)	16	15	30
C (mg/L)	69	70	300
B_1 (mg/L)	0.63	0.8	2
B_2 (mg/L)	0.74	1.3	5
Niacin (mg/L)	10.1	6.3	40
B_6 (mg/L)	0.53	0.5	2
B_{12} (g/L)	2.5	2	4.5
Folic acid (g/L)	240	100	300
K_1 (mg/L)	0.08	0.07	0.1
Osmolality (mosm/kg H_2O)	300	270	300

[a]All formulas have a 60 : 40 whey protein-to-casein ratio; all contain 81 cal/dl.
[b]Values in brackets are mEq/L.
From American Academy of Pediatrics. Nutritional needs of low-birth-weight infants. *Pediatrics* 75 : 976, 1985. With permission.

1986). Powdered human milk fortifier (Enfamil) increases calorie density to 23 kcal per oz and increases protein and mineral concentrations and renal solute load. Unlike premature infant formula, human milk fortifier does not provide supplemental vitamins in amounts that meet the needs of premature infants. Liquid fortifier (Similac Natural Care) increases the caloric content and vitamin and mineral concentrations of breast milk to some extent, without increasing protein concentration. Use of liquid fortifier requires a reduction in the volume of breast milk in infant feedings.

No precise data are available for meeting caloric requirements after term. Clinical experience suggests that most infants may be fed standard infant formula when they weigh between 1,800 and 2,500 g. For children who do not exhibit expected catch-up growth for corrected age, caloric intake should be increased by increasing volume, if tolerated, or increasing caloric density of standard infant formula (or both). Caloric requirements per kg body weight for postterm infants with growth delay can be estimated with a formula used in nutritional rehabilitation of malnourished children (MacLean et al., 1980a):

$$\frac{120 \text{ kcal/kg} \times \text{kg ideal weight (50th percentile for corrected age)}}{\text{kg actual weight}}$$

Caloric density can be increased gradually in 2 kcal per oz increments until adequate rates of gain are demonstrated. Increasing calories can be achieved by changing from 20 kcal per oz in full-strength infant formula to 24 kcal per oz by concentration of the formula (less added water). Greater caloric densities are achieved by adding vegetable oil (corn, safflower), MCT oil, a glucose polymer, or a combination. Examples of recipes for increasing the caloric density of formula fed to infants after term are detailed in Table 16-4. Recipes for home use should include ingredients that can be easily and economically purchased in a supermarket or drugstore, unless special supplements are required for medical reasons. Corn syrup should not be routinely used to increase caloric density of formulas because it may cause diarrhea.

V. Composition of formulas

A. Protein
   A wide range of protein intakes (2.25–5.00 g/kg body weight) supports growth at the rate of the third trimester of intrauterine life (Cox and Filer,

Table 16-4. Recipes for increasing caloric density of infant formula

20 cal/oz
  Standard dilution
24 cal/oz by concentration
  13 oz can formula concentrate
  8 oz water
28 cal/oz by concentration (4 cal) and carbohydrate additive (4 cal)
  13 oz can formula concentrate
  8 oz water
  3 tbs + 2 tsp Polycose, Moducal, or Sumacal
30 cal/oz by concentration (4 cal), carbohydrate additive (4 cal), and MCT or corn oil (2 cal)
  13 oz can formula concentrate
  8 oz water
  3 tbs + 2 tsp Polycose, Moducal, or Sumacal
  1 tsp MCT or corn oil

MCT = medium-chain triglyceride.

1969). Low protein intakes are associated with low weight and height velocities and low serum protein and albumin levels (American Academy of Pediatrics, 1977). High intakes, between 6 and 9 g protein per kg, should be avoided because they may lead to high renal solute load, metabolic acidosis, elevated blood urea nitrogen (BUN) and ammonia levels, hyperpyrexia, lethargy, edema, and diarrhea (American Academy of Pediatrics, 1977). Recommended protein intakes are 4.0 g per kg for infants from 26 to 28 weeks' gestation, 3.5 g per kg from 29 to 31 weeks (Ziegler et al., 1981), and 3.0 g per kg from 32 weeks to term (Fomon, 1977).

Clinical practice indicates that protein intakes of 2.2 to 3.0 g per kg are usually adequate to promote catch-up growth in premature and SGA infants postterm. Adequacy of protein intake by children on restricted fluid volumes should be assessed. Breast milk of mothers of premature infants has a higher protein concentration (3.24 g/dl at 3 days postpartum to 1.81 g/dl at 28 days) than mature breast milk (2.29 g/dl at 3 days to 1.42 g/dl at 28 days), so preterm rather than pooled mature breast milk should be fed to preterm infants (Gross, 1983). Premature infant formulas provide 2.0 to 2.4 g protein per dl (American Academy of Pediatrics, 1985). Powdered human milk fortifier can be used to increase the protein concentration of breast milk.

The amino acid composition of breast milk and premature infant formulas is adapted to the physiologic requirements of the preterm infant. The 60 : 40 lactalbumin-to-casein ratio of breast milk and premature infant formula provides high concentrations of cystine (Raiha et al., 1976), which is required by the premature infant for protein synthesis, and taurine (American Academy of Pediatrics, 1985), which is needed for conjugation of bile salts and development of the retina and brain. High-protein, high-casein formulas (3 g protein/dl and 18 : 82 lactalbumin-to-casein ratio) have been associated with hypertyrosinemia, hyperphenylalaninemia, and metabolic acidosis in premature infants (Raiha et al., 1976). Full-term infant formulas with a 60 : 40 lactalbumin-to-casein ratio are inappropriate for preterm infants less than 1,800 g. Although the lactalbumin-to-casein ratio is favorable, caloric density and distribution of nutrients do not match the nutrient requirements of the premature infant.

After term, protein requirements for catch-up growth in infants taking low volumes can be met by concentrating formula to 24 kcal per oz. Soy protein–based infant formulas should not be routinely used for premature infants until further research is available. Reduced rates of weight and length gain, lower serum albumin and nitrogen retention values, and hypophosphatemia have been reported in premature infants fed soy-based formulas (Reynolds, 1985).

B. Fat

Fats are poorly absorbed by premature infants because of their low concentrations of intraluminal bile acids and pancreatic lipase (Maksimak, 1984). Vegetable oil, vegetable–animal fat blends, and breast milk fat are better absorbed than saturated animal fat (American Academy of Pediatrics, 1985). Medium-chain triglyceride oil enhances fat absorption, rate of weight gain, calcium absorption, and nitrogen retention (American Acade-

my of Pediatrics, 1985). However, excess MCT may cause intestinal disturbances such as abdominal distention, loose stools, and vomiting (Okamoto, 1982).

Premature infant formulas contain a mixture of MCT and unsaturated
vegetable oils. Fats should provide between 40 and 50 percent of calories
to avoid high protein concentrations, which increase renal solute load
(American Academy of Pediatrics, 1985). Essential fatty acids should constitute 3 percent of total calories (300 mg linoleic acid/100 kcal) (American
Academy of Pediatrics, 1985). Premature infants should not be fed evaporated milk formula, which contains butterfat, until at least 6 months' corrected age, if at all.

C. Carbohydrates
   Most intestinal disaccharidases: alpha-glucosidase (maltase), beta-fructo-
   furanosidase (sucrase), and isomaltase, reach full-term levels by 28 weeks'
   gestation (Lebenthal and Tucker, 1986; Winter, 1984). Beta-galactosidase
   (lactase) develops late in gestation, so premature infants less than 32
   weeks' gestational age may experience transient lactose intolerance (Winter, 1984). Lactose constitutes less than one-half of carbohydrates in premature infant formulas; the balance is supplied by sucrose or corn syrup
   solids (American Academy of Pediatrics, 1985). This formulation is associated with a lower incidence of diarrhea and metabolic acidosis. The inclu-
   sion of some lactose enhances calcium absorption in the small intestine;
   promotes fermentative, less putrefactive flora; and reduces constipation
   (American Academy of Pediatrics, 1977; MacLean and Fink, 1980). Clinical practice shows that infants less than 32 weeks' gestational age who do
   not tolerate the lactose concentration in premature infant formula fare better on their mother's breast milk, if available, or a lactose-free formula such
   as Nutramigen or Pregestimil (Winter, 1985).

D. Minerals and vitamins
   Premature infants are at risk of developing deficiencies of some micronutrients in the first 2 months of life for the following reasons (American Academy of Pediatrics, 1977):

   Two-thirds of minerals are deposited in the fetus in the last trimester of
     pregnancy. Small reserves in infants born too early to receive this trans-
     fer are rapidly depleted in postnatal growth.
   Gastrointestinal absorption of minerals and fat-soluble vitamins may be
     less effective in premature infants in contrast to intrauterine systemic
     transfer, so only 50 to 70 percent of ingested nutrients are retained.
   Precise requirements of premature infants for most vitamins and minerals
     are not known, but presumably are met at levels recommended for full-
     term infants. Vitamin and mineral concentrations in standard infant for-
     mulas are based on volumes taken by full-term infants.
   Premature infants may be unable to drink enough formula to meet daily
     requirements.

Preterm and postterm infants receiving breast milk should be given an infant multivitamin and mineral complex daily (e.g., Polyvisol with iron). Preterm infants fed premature infant formula do not need a multivitamin and mineral preparation. After term, infants taking inadequate volumes of full-term infant formula should receive a multivitamin and mineral complex daily.

Premature infants are prone to developing nutritional anemias, rickets, and possibly zinc deficiency. To prevent these deficiencies, supplements of certain micronutrients are required, in addition to standard formula or standard multivitamin and mineral complex designed for full-term infants.

A paradoxic interaction of several micronutrients requires staging supplementation to prevent nutritional anemias. Vitamin E, folate, and copper are required by the premature infant from birth. Iron supplementation is generally delayed either until the infant's birth weight doubles (Sabio, 1984) or 6 to 8 postnatal weeks to minimize the risk of hemolytic anemia.

1. Vitamin E. Requirements for vitamin E are elevated owing to poor absorption of fat-soluble substrates in premature infants and the interaction of dietary factors that favor the development of hemolytic anemia in VLBW infants between 4 and 6 weeks of age (Sabio, 1984). High intakes of polyunsaturated fatty acids, especially linoleic acid, provide a substrate for lipid peroxidation of the red cell membrane by iron and other oxidants. Vitamin E functions as an antioxidant to prevent hemolysis of the erythrocyte membrane. Iron supplementation is associated with decreased serum tocopherol and vitamin E lipid ratios (Gross, 1985).

   Vitamin E intake is maintained at a ratio of 1.0 IU per g of polyunsaturated fatty acids or 0.7 IU (0.5 mg alpha-tocopherol) per 100 kcal (American Academy of Pediatrics, 1985). A total supplement of 20 to 30 IU daily has been recommended for premature and VLBW infants (Kelts and Jones, 1984; Sabio, 1984). Recent research suggests that this level of supplementation may be required to prevent vitamin E deficiency only in infants fed premature infant formula (Gross, 1985). Breast-fed infants with and without iron supplementation showed no symptoms of vitamin E deficiency when provided with a standard multivitamin containing 4.1 IU alpha-tocopherol (Gross, 1985). Supplementation of vitamin E additional to the amount in multivitamin preparations can be discontinued after risk of hemolytic anemia is past (12 weeks' postnatal age or at term) unless the infant has underlying malabsorption. Vitamin E levels in serum should be monitored and maintained between 1.0 and 3.0 mg per dl (Pereira and Zucker, 1986).

2. Iron. Iron stores in premature, LBW infants may be depleted by 6 to 8 postnatal weeks to meet the demands of growth and the onset of normal active erythropoiesis (Sabio, 1984). Repeated blood sampling hastens depletion of iron stores. Small-for-gestational-age infants born at term have hemoglobin concentrations greater than AGA infants (Sabio, 1984), so reserves may be adequate to 3 to 4 months of age. Iron supplementation is begun when the risk of hemolytic anemia is past. If iron must be administered before 6 to 8 weeks, vitamin E supple-

ments should be given concurrently (American Academy of Pediatrics, 1985). Premature infants are provided with a total iron dose of 2 to 3 mg/kg/day from supplements and breast milk or formula, up to 6 months of age (American Academy of Pediatrics, 1985; Oski, 1985). Recommended intakes for infants with birth weights less than 1,000 g are increased to 4 mg/kg/day, continued to the age of 12 to 15 months (Siimes and Jarvenpaa, 1982). From 6 to 12 months of age, iron deficiency can usually be prevented in all but VLBW infants at levels recommended for full-term infants (1 mg/kg/day). These requirements can usually be met by diet alone. Dietary sources of iron include iron-fortified formulas (12 mg/liter) and infant cereals (3.6 mg/tbs).

3. Folate. The clinical importance of low plasma folate levels observed in premature infants between 1 and 3 months of age is not known (Sabio, 1984). Megaloblastic anemia is rarely observed. Folate is well absorbed and deficiency prevented with 50 μg per day (Sabio, 1984). Supplementation may be increased in infants who have recurrent infections or diarrhea, who receive phenytoin (Dilantin) therapy, or who drink goat's milk (Sabio, 1984). Folate supplements additional to the multivitamin preparation are necessary until the infant is 3 months of age, since folate is not present in routine multivitamin formulations (Pereira and Barbosa, 1986).

4. Copper. Copper stores of term infants are adequate to 6 months of age. Marginal stores of premature infants may be depleted by 2 to 3 months without supplementation (Sabio, 1984). Copper deficiency is manifest as a hypochromic, microcytic anemia, which is unresponsive to iron supplementation and may be associated with neutropenia (Sabio, 1984). The recommended intake of 60 μg per 100 kcal in full-term infants is increased to 90 μg per 100 kcal for preterm infants (American Academy of Pediatrics, 1985; Sabio, 1984). Deficiency is prevented in most high-risk infants by amounts present in breast milk and premature infant formulas. No routine recommendations for copper supplementation can be made on the basis of current literature. However, copper status of premature infants with protracted diarrhea and those receiving parenteral nutrition without supplementation should be monitored closely and treatment initiated as indicated (Sabio, 1984).

5. Calcium, phosphorus, and vitamin D. Breast milk and full-term infant formulas may provide insufficient calcium, phosphorus and vitamin D to prevent rickets in volumes ingested by the premature infant. Calcium and phosphorus intakes that exceed concentrations found in breast milk and unsupplemented formulas are required to maintain extrauterine bone mineralization at the same rate as intrauterine bone mineralization (American Academy of Pediatrics, 1985). Requirements for preterm infants have been estimated as calcium, 220 to 250 mg/kg/day, and phosphorus, 110 to 125 mg/kg/day (Venkataraman et al., 1985). The ratio of calcium to phosphorus should be maintained close to that of breast milk (2 : 1) in formulas fed to premature infants (American Academy of Pediatrics, 1977). Calcium and phosphorus supplementation is usually not required if infants are fed one of the recently introduced premature infant formulas. Infants fed breast milk and most other

formulas are supplemented with 3 ml/kg/day calcium gluconate suspension (100 mg/ml calcium gluconate powder = 9.4 mg calcium; e.g., Neo-Calglucon) (Kelts, 1984). Supplementation should be given at 1 mg per kg on day 1, then advanced by 1 mg per day to 3 mg per kg by day 3 (Kelts and Jones, 1984). Serum calcium and phosphorus are measured prior to supplementation and weekly thereafter. Supplements can be discontinued when the infant is discharged from the hospital if serum levels are within normal limits.

A total of 500 to 600 IU of vitamin D per day in addition to high oral intakes of calcium and phosphorus is recommended to prevent rickets in preterm infants (American Academy of Pediatrics, 1985). Very premature and VLBW infants may require higher levels of supplementation (800–1,000 IU) to prevent hypomineralization and low serum 25-OHD levels, but optimal doses are not presently known (Hillman et al., 1985). After hospital discharge, supplementation of 400 IU vitamin D contained in a standard multivitamin preparation is advised, in addition to vitamin D in formula and exposure to sunlight (American Academy of Pediatrics, 1985; Kelts, 1984).

6. Zinc. High fecal zinc losses and high requirements during rapid postnatal growth place the premature infant at risk of zinc deficiency. In the first 2 months of life, serum levels of zinc fall in premature infants and zinc balance remains negative (Reynolds, 1985). Zinc balance may be correlated with fat and nitrogen absorption, and positive zinc balance appears earlier when fat absorption is improved by providing 40 to 50 percent of fat as MCT (American Academy of Pediatrics, 1985).

Few infants manifest zinc deficiency, but generalized edema and hypoproteinemia have been reported between 5 and 9 weeks of age in VLBW infants fed their mothers' breast milk and supplemental full-term infant formula (Similac PM 60/40) (Kumar and Anday, 1984). Another group of infants who received total parenteral nutrition early in life and were later fed exclusively on their mothers' breast milk showed low serum concentrations and symptoms of zinc deficiency between 2 and 6 months: dermatitis, alopecia, diarrhea, irritability, anorexia, and growth delay (Ziegler, 1985). Current minimum zinc requirements for premature infants have been set at 500 μg per 100 kcal, the same recommendation as for full-term infants (American Academy of Pediatrics, 1985). Premature infant formulas provide concentrations up to 3 times this amount, although there is no evidence that this level of supplementation leads to positive balances (Reynolds, 1985).

VI. Feeding techniques

Premature infants may require medical and nutritional management in the intensive care unit where normal feeding interactions are limited and acquisition of developmental feeding skills delayed. Feeding experiences that foster attachment are denied the premature infant kept in an incubator or nourished by gavage feedings or hyperalimentation (Brazelton et al., 1984). Prolonged gavage feeding can produce an uncontrolled oral tactile hypersensitivity to nipples, spoons, or cups that results in choking, gagging, extensor thrusting of the tongue, or refusal of solids. Research suggests that preterm infants given pacifiers to suck during tube feedings require fewer total tube feedings, are able to start bottle feeding earlier than gavage-fed controls without pacifiers, exhibit greater weight gains, and can be discharged sooner from the hospital (Field et al., 1982).

Parents need education and support to tailor their expectations to the child's corrected rather than postnatal age for both feeding skills and introduction of new foods. The rate of progression to new feeding skills may vary with the degree of prematurity. Feeding capabilities appropriate for the child's corrected age can be predicted by observing oral motor skills (Table 16-5).

Referral to an occupational or physical therapist is indicated if the child fails to accomplish feeding skills as expected for corrected age or exhibits any of the following abnormal feeding behaviors (Morris, 1977):

Jaw thrust. Strong downward extension of jaw, which may appear stuck open. The child may have difficulty closing his or her mouth.

Tongue thrust. Strong movement of extension and protraction before or during feeding; tongue appears thick and bunched. It is difficult to insert nipple or spoon, and food may be ejected from mouth.

Tonic bite reflex. Strong closure of jaw when teeth or gums are stimulated. Child may have difficulty opening or closing jaw after reflex elicited.

Lip retraction. Tight drawing back of lips so that they form a tight line over mouth and cannot assist in sucking food from spoon or cup.

Tongue retraction. Pulling tongue back into pharyngeal space, which may interfere with breathing and make insertion of bottle difficult. Makes it difficult for child to handle food in mouth.

Nasal regurgitation. Loss of liquid or food through nose during sucking or swallowing.

Preterm infants may be hypersensitive to multimodal stimulation, especially in the early months. The feeding environment should be quiet and controlled, without noises from the television, radio, or telephone. The child may need to be fed alone with the caretaker and without other social stimulation.

Between 7 and 9 months' corrected age, many children begin to express independence in feeding behaviors. Although desire for autonomy indicates positive developmental progress, it may be frightening for parents who, perceiving the child as fragile and weak, wish to maintain control of feeding to ensure adequate intake. Paradoxically, once the child developmentally requires autonomy, self-feeding, although messy and time-consuming, results in greater

Table 16-5. Development of oral motor and feeding skills

Corrected age	Food types, textures	Oral skills	Adaptive skills
0–12 wk	Liquid: bottle- or breast-feeding	Rooting; sucking and swallowing; bite reflex; gag reflex; mouth usually closed; loses liquid from corners of mouth	Begins to get hand to mouth

Table 16-5 (continued)

Corrected age	Food types, textures	Oral skills	Adaptive skills
12–20 wk	May begin cereals or strained or pureed foods	Sucking and swallowing; bite reflex; gag reflex; decrease in loss of milk from corners of mouth; increased sucking strength	Begins opening mouth for nipple; begins mouthing objects; begins reaching purposefully
20–28 wk	Strained or junior foods mixed with mashed crackers; teething biscuits introduced	Possibly bite and sucking and swallowing reflexes; gag reflex; smacks lips; moves lips in eating	Begins positioning mouth for spoon insertion; transfers objects; drops objects
28–32 wk	Junior foods: mashed, cooked, canned	Clears spoon quickly and easily with lips; moves tongue laterally for early chewing	Begins finger feeding; holds 2 objects and bangs together
8–10 mo	Junior mashed foods minced fine; begin finger foods	Closes mouth on cup rim; bites on objects; "raspberries"; munches cracker	Finger feeds crackers; accepts 1 sip at a time from a cup; holds a bottle; extended reach and grasp
10–12 mo	Mashed and chopped fine foods	Licks food off lower lip; plays with tongue; moves tongue side to side in mouth; rotary chewing begins	Accepts 4–5 continuous sips from cup; finger feeds small pieces; begins to grasp spoon; picks up small objects—pincer; places objects on table
12–15 mo	Chopped fine foods; begin raw fruits and vegetables	Spits food; licks all of lower lip with tongue; decrease in drooling	Grasps spoon and attempts to take to mouth; assists in holding cup; decrease in mouthing objects; scribbles with crayon
18–24 mo	Regular table foods; some chopped fine meats	Mature rotary chewing	Feeds self messily with spoon; drinks from cup and places on table; off bottle; turns pages in book one at a time; unscrews lids

From J. A. Lewis, Oral Motor Assessment and Treatment of Feeding Difficulties. In P. J. Accardo (ed.), *Failure to Thrive in Infancy and Early Childhood*. Baltimore: University Park, 1982.

net intake. Conflicted force feeding may lead to secondary food refusal and even gagging and self-induced vomiting. Anticipatory guidance is important because caretakers may have difficulty tolerating the initial messiness of self-feeding. They may need support from health providers during this transient phase. Suggestions for feeding infants during this period include feeding the child in a high chair, not on the caretaker's lap; allowing the child to hold the spoon while the caretaker feeds the child; and encouraging finger feeding.

REFERENCES

American Academy of Pediatrics, Committee on Nutrition. Nutritional needs of low birth weight infants. *Pediatrics* 60 : 519, 1977.

American Academy of Pediatrics, Committee on Nutrition. Nutritional needs of low birth weight infants. *Pediatrics* 75 : 976, 1985.

Babson, S. G. Growth of low birth weight infants. *Pediatrics* 77 : 11, 1970.

Baumgartner, R. N., Roche, A. F., and Himes, J. H. Incremental growth tables: Supplementary to previously published charts. *Am. J. Clin. Nutr.* 43 : 711, 1986.

Brandt, I. Growth Dynamics of Low Birth Weight Infants with Emphasis on the Perinatal Period. In F. Falkner and J. M. Tanner (eds.), *Human Growth: Postnatal Growth*. New York: Plenum, 1978. Vol. 2.

Brazelton, T. B., Gatson, R. L., and Howard, R. D. Developmental Feeding Issues. In R. B. Howard and H. S. Winter (eds.), *Nutrition and Feeding of Infants and Toddlers*. Boston: Little, Brown, 1984.

Cooke, R. J., and Nichoalds, G. Nutrient retention in preterm infants fed standard infant formulas. *J. Pediatr.* 108 : 448, 1986.

Cox, W. M., Jr., and Filer, L. J., Jr. Protein intake for low birth weight infants. *J. Pediatr.* 74 : 1016, 1969.

Cruise, M. O. A longitudinal study of growth of low birth weight infants: I. Velocity and distance growth, birth to 3 years. *Pediatrics* 51 : 620, 1973.

Davies, D. P., Platts, P., Pritchard, J. M., and Wilkinson, P. W. Nutritional status of light for date infants at birth and its influence on early postnatal growth. *Arch. Dis. Child.* 54 : 703, 1979.

Dubowitz, L. M. S., Dubowitz, V., and Goldberg, C. Clinical assessment of gestational age in the newborn infant. *J. Pediatr.* 77 : 1, 1970.

Field, T., Ignatoff, E., Stringer, S., et al. Nonnutritive sucking during tube feedings: Effects on preterm neonates in an intensive care unit. *Pediatrics* 70 : 381, 1982.

Fitzhardinge, P. M. Early growth and development in low birth weight infants following treatment in an intensive care nursery. *Pediatrics* 56 : 162, 1975.

Fitzhardinge, P. M. Follow-up studies on the low birth weight infant. *Clin. Perinatol.* 3 : 503, 1976.

Fitzhardinge, P. M., and Steven, E. M. The small-for-date infant. I. Later growth patterns. *Pediatrics* 49 : 671, 1972.

Fomon, S., Ziegler, E., and Vazques, H. Human milk and the small premature infant. *Am. J. Dis. Child.* 131 : 463, 1977.

Georgieff, M. K., Sasanow, S. R., Mammel, M. C., and Pereira, G. R. Mid-arm circumference/head circumference ratios for identification of symptomatic LGA, AGA, and SGA newborn infants. *J. Pediatr.* 109 : 316, 1986.

Gordon, B. E. Nutritional Considerations for Infants with Congenital Heart Disease. In D. G. Kelts and E. G. Jones (eds.), *Manual of Pediatric Nutrition*. Boston: Little, Brown, 1984.

Gross, S. J. Growth and biochemical response of preterm infants fed human milk or modified infant formula. *N. Engl. J. Med.* 308 : 237, 1983.

Gross, S. J., and Gabriel, E. Vitamin E status in preterm infants fed human milk or infant formula. *J. Pediatr.* 106 : 635, 1985.

Hack, M., Merkatz, I. R., Gordon, D., et al. The prognostic significance of postnatal growth in very low-birth weight infants. *Am. J. Obstet. Gynecol.* 143 : 693, 1982.

Hamill, P. V. V., Drizd, T. A., Johnson, C. L., et al. NCHS growth charts. *Monthly Vital Statistics Report* 25, No. 3[suppl.]. U.S. Dept. of Health, Education and Welfare publication (HRA) 76. Government Printing Office, 1976.

Hillman, L. S., Hoff, N., Salmons, S. et al. Mineral homeostasis in very premature infants: Serial evaluation of serum 25-hydroxyvitamin D, serum minerals, and bone mineralization. *J. Pediatr.* 106 : 970, 1985.

Kelts, D. G., and Jones, E. G. Nutritional Supplements. In D. G. Kelts, and E. G. Jones (eds.), *Manual of Pediatric Nutrition*. Boston: Little, Brown, 1984.

Kumar, S. P., and Anday, E. K. Edema, hypoproteinemia, and zinc deficiency in low birth weight infants. *Pediatrics* 73 : 327, 1984.

Lebenthal, E., and Tucker, N. T. Carbohydrate digestion: Development in early infancy. *Clin. Perinatol.* 13 : 37, 1986.

Lubchenco, L. O., Hansman, C., and Boyd, E. Intrauterine growth in length and head circumference as estimated from live birth at gestational ages from 26 to 42 weeks. *Pediatrics* 37 : 403, 1966.

Lubchenco, L. O., Hansman, C., Dressler, M., and Boyd, E. Intrauterine growth as estimated from liveborn birth weight data at 24 to 42 weeks of gestation. *Pediatrics* 32 : 793, 1963.

MacLean, W. C., deRomaña, G. L., Masse, E., and Graham, G. G. Nutritional management of chronic diarrhea and malnutrition: Primary reliance on oral feeding. *J. Pediatr.* 97 : 316, 1980.

MacLean, W. C., and Fink, B. B. Lactose malabsorption by premature infants: Magnitude and clinical significance. *J. Pediatr.* 97 : 383, 1980.

Maksimak, J. The Premature Infant. In R. B. Howard and H. S. Winter (eds.), *Nutrition and Feeding of Infants and Toddlers*. Boston: Little, Brown, 1984.

Manser, J. I. Growth in the high-risk infant. *Clin. Perinatol.* 11 : 19, 1984.

Miller, H. C., and Hassanein, K. Diagnosis of impaired fetal growth in newborn infants. *Pediatrics* 48 : 511, 1971.

Miller, H. C., and Jekel, J. F. Diagnosing intrauterine growth retardation in newborn infants. *Perinatol. Neonatol.* Sept.–Oct. 1985, pp. 35–42.

Morris, S. E. Oral-Motor Development: Normal and Abnormal. In J. M. Wilson (ed.), *Oral-Motor Function and Dysfunction in Children*. Chapel Hill, N.C.: University of North Carolina, Division of Physical Therapy. 1977.

Okamoto, E., Muttart, C. R., Zucker, C. L., et al. Use of medium chain triglycerides in feeding the low birth weight infant. *Am. J. Dis. Child.* 136 : 428, 1982.

Oski, F. A. Nutritional Anemias. In W. A. Walker and J. B. Watkins (eds.), *Nutrition in Pediatrics*. Boston: Little, Brown, 1985.

Pereira, G. R., and Barbosa, N. M. Controversies in neonatal nutrition. *Pediatr. Clin. North Am.* 33 : 65, 1986.

Pereira, G. R., and Zucker, A. H. Nutritional deficiencies in the neonate. *Clin. Perinatol.* 13 : 175, 1986.

Raiha, N. C. Biochemical basis for nutritional management of preterm infants. *Pediatrics* 53 : 147, 1974.

Raiha, N. C., Heinonen, K., Rassin, D. K., and Gaull, G. E. Milk protein quantity and quality in low birth weight infants: I. Metabolic responses and effects on growth. *Pediatrics* 57 : 659, 1976.

Reynolds, J. W. Nutrition of the Low Birth Weight Infant. In W. A. Walker and J. B. Watkins (eds.), *Nutrition in Pediatrics*. Boston: Little, Brown, 1985.

Rohrer, F. Eine neue sormel zur bestimung der korperfulle, Korr.-B1. *Ges. Anthrophol.* 39 : 5, 1908.

Ronnholm, K. A., Perheentupa, and J., Siimes, M. A. Supplementation with human milk protein improves growth of small premature infants fed human milk. *Pediatrics* 77 : 649, 1986.

Rosenberg, A., and Jones, M. D. Growth Patterns of Small Infants. In P. J. Accardo (ed.), *Failure to Thrive in Infancy and Early Childhood.* Baltimore: University Park, 1982.

Sabio, H. Anemia in the high risk infant. *Clin. Perinatol.* 11 : 59, 1984.

Sasanow, S. R., Georgieff, M. K., and Pereira, G. R. Mid-arm circumference and mid-arm/ head circumference ratios: Standard curves for anthropometric assessment of neonatal nutritional status. *J. Pediatr.* 109 : 311, 1986.

Siimes, M. A., and Järvenpää, A. L. Prevention of anemia and iron-deficiency in very low birth weight infants. *J. Pediatr.* 101 : 277, 1982.

Usher, R., and McLean, F. Intrauterine growth of live-born Caucasian infants at sea level: Standards obtained from measurements in 7 dimensions of infants born between 25 and 44 weeks of gestation. *J. Pediatr.* 74 : 901, 1969.

Venkataraman, P., Koo, W., and Tsang, R. C. Calcium and Phosphorus in Infant Nutrition. W. A. Walker and J. B. Watkins (eds.), *Nutrition in Pediatrics.* Boston: Little, Brown, 1985.

Villar, J., Smeriglio, V., Martorell, R., et al. Heterogeneous growth and mental development of intrauterine growth-retarded infants during the first 3 years of life. *Pediatrics* 74 : 783, 1984.

Winter, H. S. Personal communication, 1985.

Winter, H. S. Development of the Gastrointestinal Tract. In R. B. Howard and H. S. Winter (eds.), *Nutrition and Feeding of Infants and Toddlers.* Boston: Little, Brown, 1984.

Woods, D. L., Malan, A. F., and Heese, H. de V. Patterns of retarded fetal growth. *Early Hum. Dev.* 3 : 257, 1979.

Ziegler, E. E. Infants of low birth weight: Special needs and problems. *Am. J. Clin. Nutr.* 41 : 440, 1985.

Ziegler, R., Biga, R., and Fomon, S. Nutritional Requirements of the Premature Infant. In R. M. Suskind (ed.), *Textbook of Pediatric Nutrition.* New York: Raven, 1981.

17

Apneic Spells After Discharge from Neonatal Intensive Care

H. William Taeusch and Frederick Mandell

I. Introduction

The main concern about apneic spells in an infant approaching neonatal intensive care unit (NICU) discharge is that the apneic spells may indicate increased risk for sudden infant death syndrome (SIDS). The causes and prevention of SIDS are largely unknown, and the relationship of SIDS to apneic spells is also unclear.

II. Incidence

Sudden infant death syndrome accounts for more than 20 percent of infant deaths in the United States. Infants discharged from NICUs are at higher risk than infants born at term. Estimates of risk for SIDS are as follows:

GROUP	SIDS/1,000 LIVE BIRTHS IN GROUP
NICU graduates	30
Twins	20
Maternal drug abuse	50
Birth weight <1,250 g	20
Bronchopulmonary dysplasia	100
All live births	2

III. Pathogenesis

Many believe that chronic or intermittent hypoxia, possibly associated with apneic spells, may precede death from SIDS. In this view, SIDS is seen as a manifestation of acute and chronic respiratory control immaturity, dysfunction, or both. However, work by Southall and colleagues (1982) on term infants did not indicate that apnea precedes SIDS. Nonetheless, with some apneic spells clearly associated with hypoxemia, these episodes in their most serious form are worth preventing in their own right.

IV. Management

A frequent management problem is that of a 2-month-old premature infant ready for discharge in terms of feeding, weight gain, and temperature control, but who nonetheless has between 2 and 10 apneic or bradycardic episodes per week. Our initial approach is to reassess diagnostic possibilities. Most often, we find no specific cause for the apnea or bradycardia, and we attribute it to immature respiratory control mechanisms. Nevertheless, a search for metabolic, central nervous system, or infectious causes is useful. Chronic metabolic acidosis, increasing cranial intraventricular dilatation, seizures, or cytomegalovirus-respiratory syncytial virus is reasonable to search for in this age group.

Our current management (if no specific remedial therapy is indicated) is to start oral theophylline in initial doses of 2 mg per kg of body weight every 6 to 8 hours. This dosage is adjusted to maintain blood levels of approximately 7 to 13 μg per ml. We keep the infant in the hospital for approximately 1 week on a monitor to observe cessation of spells. The monitor is relinquished a few days before discharge. The infant is discharged to home on theophylline without a monitor. Without complications, the infant is readmitted to the hospital at 3 months of age. With the infant on a monitor, theophylline is stopped, and the infant discharged if no spells occur in 3 days. If spells recur, theophylline is restarted for another 3 months before the hospital trial off therapy is repeated. Some experts prefer caffeine because of a less-frequent dosage schedule, and possibly because of less gastric irritability and tachycardia when compared with theophylline. Some infants have vomiting or irritability seemingly associated with acceptable blood levels of theophylline. If these symptoms are intolerable, the drug is stopped, and in some cases, home monitoring is started.

Some programs use cardiac-respiratory monitors in the home for infants with apnea. We have supported their use in the most severe cases or when parents clearly prefer what they perceive as the added protection of the home monitor. Most urban areas have home monitors for rent. Current rental prices in our area are approximately $200 per month. Medicaid usually covers the entire fee and most private insurers cover about 80 percent. If monitors are used, we strongly believe in measuring heart rate as well as the respiratory rate, because bradycardia of clinical importance may occur in the absence of apnea, and because obstructive apnea may be missed by some respiratory monitoring systems. There have been no clear indications for who should (or who should not) receive home monitoring, nor has home monitoring been shown to be more efficacious than other approaches to infants with apnea. Recently, this situation has been helped by the report of the Consensus Development Conference on Infantile Apnea and Home Monitoring (1986), which greatly restricts the indications for home monitoring.

Home monitoring is usually discontinued by 12 months of age. Indications for cessation of monitoring are unclear. The financial and emotional costs are great for families who have an infant on a home monitor (Wasserman, 1984). All experts agree that continuous professional help (technical, medical, and psychologic) should be available to parents who have an infant on a monitor at home. This recommendation is also valid for parents who have an infant with repetitive apneic spells who is not on a monitor.

Some programs use pneumograms (tape recordings of respirations and cardiograms that can be read by a computer for respiratory and cardiac pauses) to assess the need for respiratory stimulants or monitors. We believe that their use is justified only in unusual cases or as a research tool.

We are especially concerned about the possibility of sudden death in a special group of infants, those with bronchopulmonary dysplasia, because of the finding that 10 percent of this group may die suddenly in the first months of life. No doubt some of these deaths may not be classified as SIDS. Nonetheless, we suspect many are associated with delayed maturation of respiratory control mechanisms that are variably "loaded" with acute and chronic problems of compliance, resistance, repeated hypoxic episodes, and ventilation-perfusion abnormalities. While there is no known way of reducing this risk at present, we treat many of these infants with theophylline for 3 to 6 months after discharge. The mild diuretic and bronchodilator effects may be of added potential usefulness.

V. Summary

Approaches to the management of severe, repeated apneic spells and prevention of SIDS are inadequate despite years of intense study. In all probability, good management awaits better understanding of the mechanisms underlying these problems.

REFERENCES

American Academy of Pediatrics, Task Force on Prolonged Infantile Apnea. Prolonged infantile apnea: 1985. *Pediatrics* 76 : 129, 1985.

Black, L., David, R. J., Brouillette, R. T., and Hunt, C. E. Effects of birth weight and ethnicity on incidence of sudden infant death syndrome. *J. Pediatr.* 108 : 209, 1986.

Brady, J. P., and Gould, J. B. Sudden infant death syndrome: The physician's dilemma. *Adv. Pediatr.* 30 : 635, 1983.

Forster, J. The latest word on apnea monitoring: Summary of the Consensus Development Conference on Infantile Apnea and Home Monitoring, NIH. *Contemp. Pediatr.* Nov. 1986. P. 77.

Perlman, J. M., and Volpe, J. J. Episodes of apnea and bradycardia in the preterm newborn: Impact on cerebral circulation. *Pediatrics* 76 : 333, 1985.

Southall, D. P., Richards, J. M., Rhoden, K. J., et al. Prolonged apnea and cardiac arrhythmias in infants discharged from neonatal intensive care units: Failure to predict an increased risk for sudden infant death syndrome. *Pediatrics* 70 : 844, 1982.

Warburton, D., Stark, A., and Taeusch, W. Apnea monitor failure in infants with upper airway obstruction. *Pediatrics* 60 : 742, 1985.

Wasserman, A. L. A prospective study of the impact of home monitoring on the family. *Pediatrics* 74 : 323, 1984.

Werthammer, J., Brown, E., Neff, R., and Taeusch, W. Sudden infant death syndrome in infants with bronchopulmonary dysplasia. *Pediatrics* 69 : 301, 1982.

18

Rehospitalization of High-Risk Infants

Marie C. McCormick

I. Introduction

Although the mortality for infants born prematurely—especially those of very low birth weight—has dropped dramatically in the past 5 years, surviving infants now present a new morbidity of physical, neurologic, developmental, and behavioral problems. This chapter addresses one index of their health status, namely the incidence of rehospitalization after discharge from the neonatal intensive care unit (NICU).

II. Epidemiology of rehospitalization

A. Incidence of rehospitalization

High-risk infants are at increased risk of being readmitted to the hospital after their discharge. Among normal-birth-weight infants (NBW >2,500 g at birth), 8.4 percent are rehospitalized before their first birthday. The risk of rehospitalization increases with decreasing birth weight, and 17 percent of those born weighing between 1,501 and 2,500 g, and 33 to 38 percent of those weighing less than 1,500 g at birth, experience subsequent hospitalizations (Hack et al., 1981; McCormick et al., 1980).

Not only are very low birth weight (VLBW ≤ 1,500 g) infants admitted at higher rates than heavier infants, but they also average more days of hospitalization (all hospitalization combined) than heavier infants. The NBW infants who are rehospitalized average 7 to 8 days of hospitalization, whereas VLBW infants who are rehospitalized average 16 days.

After the first year, the rate of rehospitalization diminishes rapidly. Only 10 percent of VLBW infants in one series required hospitalization in the second year and 10 percent in the third year (Hack et al., 1983). However, of those hospitalized in the third year, about one-half (4 : 9) had a prior hospitalization, despite the fact that most of the hospitalizations after the first year were for conditions unrelated to prematurity. This finding suggests a continued vulnerability to ill health among a subgroup of VLBW infants that is serious enough to warrant admission.

B. Reasons for rehospitalization

Some of these rehospitalizations reflect sequelae of neonatal events such as bronchopulmonary dysplasia (BPD); others, however, appear due to higher rates of admission for routine problems of infancy, such as respiratory or gastrointestinal disorders. In one series, more than 80 percent of the 51 hospitalizations among 32 VLBW infants were attributed in about equal proportions to three sets of conditions: chronic conditions (BPD, patent

209

ductus arteriosus, and postnecrotizing enterocolitis treatment), respiratory and gastrointestinal infections, and hernia repair (McCormick et al., 1980).

The proportions were different in another series, probably due to differences in definitions (Hack et al., 1981). In this group, more than 60 percent of the admissions among 99 VLBW infants were due to infection and 21 percent were due to congenital anomalies and developmental delay.

Injury is not a major cause of hospitalization among VLBW infants in infancy with less than 15 percent of all children in this age range who have been injured requiring hospitalization (McCormick et al., 1981). This, in part, reflects a lag in developmental activities due to gestational age, in that VLBW infants begin walking and crawling at older chronologic ages than their NBW peers, and independent mobility is a risk factor for injury. There are few data that permit estimates for later childhood.

The presence of congenital anomalies and developmental delay is a major predictor of rehospitalization for all infants, including high-risk infants (Hack et al., 1981; McCormick, 1985; McCormick et al., 1980).

C. Other risk factors for rehospitalization
Socioeconomic disadvantages increase the risk of rehospitalization. Other risk factors for rehospitalization include nonwhite race, maternal age less than 17 at the time of birth, low family income, maternal education attainment less than high school, single-parent household, head of household unemployed, and Medicaid coverage. These factors increase the risk of hospitalization even when controlling for birth weight and the presence of congenital anomalies and developmental delay (McCormick et al., 1980).

These findings suggest that the socioeconomic disadvantage that increases the chance of a high-risk delivery confers an added risk of morbidity beyond a high-risk status in the newborn period (McCormick, 1985).

Many of the hospitalizations among disadvantaged children are considered potentially preventable because the conditions leading to hospitalization such as respiratory and gastrointestinal infections are preventable or readily treated at early stages on an ambulatory basis (Wadsworth and Morris, 1978). Preventing hospitalization assumes importance because of some of the acute and long-term sequelae noted in III.

III. Sequelae of rehospitalization

A. Acute distress due to separation
Hospitalization is a source of acute distress among preschool children, particularly at 6 months to 4 years (Rutter, 1979). During hospitalization, distress reflects separation from family members (not just the mother) and exposure to strange situations. Alteration of behavior may persist after the child comes home (Vernon et al., 1966). Regressive behavior was seen in 22 percent of normal children after one hospitalization, and in 38 percent after multiple hospitalizations (Douglas, 1975). The extent to which high-risk infants differ from low-risk infants in their acute reaction to hospitalization is unknown, but the proportion with adverse reaction is likely to be higher since the risk of adverse reaction is enhanced by socioeconomic disadvantage.

B. Long-term sequelae

Children with prolonged or multiple hospitalizations in the preschool period are at increased risk of behavioral and learning problems (Douglas, 1975; Quinton and Rutter, 1976). The risk of long-term behavioral problems is increased if the child comes from a disadvantaged family (Quinton and Rutter, 1976; Rutter, 1979). The mechanism by which such behavioral disturbances are related to rehospitalization is not known, but the data suggest that a single hospitalization may set up a situation in which subsequent separations cause substantial disruptions of parent-child interactions.

Again, few data address the long-term sequelae of hospitalization in high-risk infants. In the short term, hospitalization is associated with changes in the mother's assessment of the developmental progress of the child, independent of birth weight and measured developmental progress. Mothers of LBW infants who have been hospitalized are more likely to consider their children slow in development, even when developmental progress is appropriate for age (McCormick et al., 1982). Others have noted that prematurity is a risk factor for inappropriate medical care caused by parental anxiety when the older child is essentially healthy (Levy, 1979). Thus, some high-risk infants appear to have an increased chance of long-term sequelae as a result of socioeconomic disadvantage and of multiple or prolonged hospitalization.

IV. Prevention of rehospitalization and its sequelae

A. Prevention of rehospitalization

Some proportion of illness leading to hospitalization is preventable, although the proportion among high-risk infants remains to be established. Interventions designed to enhance parenting skills using home visitors with disadvantaged women have been shown to reduce morbidity, increase use of preventive services, and improve mother-infant interactions (Carpenter et al., 1983; Larson, 1980). Such findings suggest that the mothers of high-risk infants would benefit from continued, more intensive contact, possibly in the home, with specially trained workers to enhance their skills in caring for their children and recognizing early signs of illness. The conditions causing hospitalization would suggest that conscientious primary care focused on preventive strategies such as immunization, frequent monitoring, and prompt treatment of acute illness would be of benefit, but there is no empirical support for this recommendation.

B. Prevention of acute sequelae

The factors contributing to acute adverse reactions relating to hospitalization have been described (Rutter, 1979). These suggest that several interventions may reduce acute distress.

1. Encouraging the mother or another family member to accompany the child reduces the sense of separation.
2. When the admission can be anticipated, familiarizing the child with the surroundings and procedures helps reduce the distress from strange situations.

3. Continuity of other caretakers, such as nurses and physicians, during the admission or over repeated admissions, also reduces distress.

C. Prevention of long-term sequelae
The prevention of long-term sequelae remains more problematic. Clearly, however, the high-risk infant with multiple or prolonged hospitalization is doubly at risk for behavior problems. Such children should be targeted for especially close follow-up both for medical and behavioral problems. If disturbances of parent-child reaction or behavior problems are noted, then interventions aimed at enhancing child development and parental self-confidence should be initiated. These would include early education and stimulation programs, family counseling and psychotherapy, and education of parents to appropriate methods for altering child behavior.

REFERENCES

Carpenter, R. G., Gardner, A., Jepson, M., et al. Prevention of unexpected infant death. *Lancet* 1 : 723, 1983.

Douglas, J. W. B. Early hospital admissions and later disturbances of behavior and learning. *Dev. Med. Child Neurol.* 17 : 456, 1975.

Hack, M., DeMonterice, D., Merkatz, I. R., et al. Rehospitalization of the very-low-birth-weight infant. *Am. J. Dis. Child.* 135 : 263, 1981.

Hack, M., Rivers, A., and Fanaroff, A. A. The very low birthweight infant: The broader spectrum of morbidity during infancy and early childhood. *J. Behav. Dev. Pediatr.* 4 : 243, 1983.

Larson, C. P. Efficacy of prenatal and post-partum home visits on child health and development. *Pediatrics* 66 : 191, 1980.

Levy, J. C. Vulnerable children: Parents' perspectives and the use of medical care. *Pediatrics* 65 : 956, 1979.

McCormick, M. C. The contribution of low birthweight to infant mortality and childhood morbidity. *N. Engl. J. Med.* 312 : 82, 1985.

McCormick, M. C., Shapiro, S., and Starfield, B. H. Rehospitalization in the first year of life for high-risk survivors. *Pediatrics* 66 : 991, 1980.

McCormick, M. C., Shapiro, S., and Starfield, B. H. Injury and its correlates among one-year-old children. *Am. J. Dis. Child.* 135 : 159, 1981.

McCormick, M. C., Shapiro, S., and Starfield, B. H. Factors associated with maternal opinion development: Clues to the vulnerable child? *Pediatrics* 69 : 537, 1982.

Quinton, D., and Rutter, M. Early hospital admissions and late disturbances of behavior: An attempted replication of Douglas' findings. *Dev. Med. Child Neurol.* 18 : 417, 1976.

Rutter, M. Separation experiences: A new look at an old topic. *J. Pediatr.* 95 : 147, 1979.

Vernon, D., Schulman, J., and Foley, J. Changes in children's behavior after hospitalization. *Am. J. Dis. Child.* 111 : 581, 1966.

Wadsworth, M. E. J., and Morris, S. Assessing chances of hospital admission in preschool children. *Arch. Dis. Child.* 53 : 159, 1978.

19

Bronchopulmonary Dysplasia

Elizabeth R. Brown

I. Introduction

The term *bronchopulmonary dysplasia* (BPD) was first used by Northway et al., who described chronic lung changes in infants with respiratory distress syndrome (RDS) requiring prolonged ventilation with a high inspired oxygen concentration (Northway et al., 1967). The disease, according to these authors, develops through four stages:

1. Acute RDS (days 1–3)
2. Period of lung regeneration (days 4–10)
3. Period of transition to chronic disease (days 10–20)
4. Chronic disease (day 30+)

A well-accepted definition of BPD has been set forth in the recent excellent review by O'Brodovich and Mellins (1985). Essential elements of the diagnosis include

1. Initiating event: acute lung injury in first 2 weeks of life
2. Clinical findings: retractions, tachypnea
3. Radiographic findings: cystic and/or hyperinflated areas with fibrotic strands
4. Blood gas abnormalities if breathing room air
5. Age (diagnosis made after 1 month of age)

II. Incidence

The more immature the infant, the more likely the development of chronic lung changes. For ventilated infants less than 1,000 g birth weight, the incidence of BPD may reach 80 to 90 percent. For those over 1,500 g with RDS the incidence of BPD is about 10 percent. In recent years, the survival of very low birth weight infants has markedly increased. This increase in survival may be related to a variety of factors including fetal monitoring; maternal transport to a perinatal center; improved neonatal intensive care unit (NICU) care; and better methods of managing ventilator support, metabolic balance, and enteral and parenteral nutrition. With the increased survival of the very low birth weight infant, the prevalence of BPD has increased. In the last few years, the number of infants with this diagnosis has doubled, and the mean birth weight of infants with BPD has fallen.

III. Pathogenesis

Bronchopulmonary dysplasia occurs in some infants with immature lungs who are treated with exposure of increased FiO_2 delivered via an endotracheal tube under positive-pressure ventilation. Edwards and colleagues described a dose response relationship between oxygen exposure and risk of BPD (Edwards et al., 1977). They found that infants who were exposed to an FiO_2 of 0.8 to 1.0 for 6 days, 0.40 to 0.79 for 18 days, or 0.22 to 0.39 for 56 days had an increased risk of either death or development of BPD. Thus a high oxygen concentration for a short time and a lower oxygen concentration for a longer time are both associated with risk.

Reynolds and Taghizadeh (1974) reported that infants who died with chronic lung changes had been exposed to high peak inspiratory pressures (greater than 35 cm H_2O) and high respiratory frequencies (greater than 30 breaths/minute); moreover, they reported a decreased incidence of BPD when they adjusted respiratory settings to produce lower peak inspiratory pressures and lower respiratory rates by increasing the inspiratory-to-expiratory time ratio. They suggested that the major component of lung damage in BPD was barotrauma.

Pneumothorax, patent ductus arteriosus, and a high fluid intake in the first few days of life are additional factors implicated in the pathogenesis of BPD (Berg et al., 1975; Brown et al., 1978). More recently, lung effluent samples from ventilated infants showed that infants who developed BPD had increased neutrophils, macrophages, and elastase activity by the third day of life compared to samples from RDS infants who did not develop BPD (Merritt et al., 1983). Serum levels of alpha-1 antiprotease correlate with gestational age in the first 48 hours of life (McCarthy et al., 1984). Thus the least mature infants are the most susceptible to oxygen damage at a time when the protective mechanisms for free radicals are impaired (Frank, 1987).

IV. Pathology

The lung pathology in 21 infants who died from 7 to 217 days' postnatal age has been described by Bonikos and colleagues (1976). They found that these infants had no ciliary damage and accumulation of mucous secretions in terminal and respiratory bronchioles. These findings may result in impaired clearance of secretions from the airways and may be associated with respiratory infections seen in the infant with BPD. Also present were bronchial ulceration and necrosis with plugging of bronchial and bronchiolar lumina with mucus, epithelial debris, and inflammatory cells. The authors suggest that this type of bronchiolar injury may compromise further lung development. The proliferation of granular pneumocytes was most striking in those infants who survived longest. Widespread fibrosis involving both bronchiolar walls and alveolar septa was also commonly seen. The bronchiolar fibrosis resulted from widespread destruction of bronchiolar muscular and elastic tissue by a process of necrotizing bronchiolitis. Partial obliteration of bronchioles secondary to inflammatory changes may lead to air trapping. Inflammatory changes in the walls of terminal bronchioles may play an important role in the development of emphysema. Damage of peripheral airways probably results in increased airway resistance and wheezing with successive bouts of respiratory infection. These changes also result in a maldistribution of ventilation and perfusion that contributes to the hypoxemia seen in infants with BPD. Their final finding was right ventricular hypertrophy with cor pulmonale. Fibrotic areas of lung represent areas of high resistance to pulmonary blood flow. The combination of intermittent hypoxemia and lung fibrosis results in the development of cor pulmonale in infants most severely affected with BPD.

V. Mortality

The mortality for infants with BPD is about 20 percent in the first year of life. About 12 percent will die prior to NICU discharge and the remaining 8 percent after a period of time at home. The three major causes of death in this population are cor pulmonale, lower respiratory tract infections (particularly respiratory syncytial virus bronchiolitis), and sudden death (Werthammer et al., 1982).

VI. Management of infants with bronchopulmonary dysplasia

Increased oxygen must often be provided to prevent hypoxic vasoconstriction of the pulmonary vascular bed and to decrease the work of breathing. Decreased work of breathing allows the use of calories for growth. The oxygen source should be continuous. We have found that nasal-cannula oxygen best serves this purpose. Administration of oxygen by hood results in significant fluctuations of FiO_2 whenever the infant is handled (e.g., weighing, holding, bathing). Halliday studied the effect of lowering the PO_2 to less than 55 mm Hg in 4- to 18-week-old infants with BPD. Echocardiographic assessment of the ratio of right ventricular preejection times to right ventricular ejection times (RVPET/RVET) was made. This ratio correlates with pulmonary artery pressure. They found that the ratio of RVPET/RVET increased to a mean of 0.36 from 0.32 with lowering of PO_2 (Halliday et al., 1980). Fouron and colleagues (1980) found that BPD infants with RVPET/RVET ratios of greater than 0.30 for greater than 3 months had poor prognoses for survival. Hypoxic pulmonary vasoconstriction in some infants with BPD can be reversed by treatment with oxygen by nasal cannula (Abman et al., 1985). This finding reflects the dual nature of the etiology of cor pulmonale (i.e., hypoxic vasoconstriction plus increased resistance to blood flow across the fibrosed lung). A clue to the presence of intermittent hypoxemia in infants with BPD can be an increased reticulocyte count in conjunction with a high hematocrit.

Oxygen flow should be adjusted to keep the PO_2 greater than 55 mm Hg; therefore, the resting PO_2 should be at least 60 to 70 mm Hg. We have followed infants with BPD on home oxygen using both the transcutaneous oxygen monitor and digital oxygen saturation to evaluate adequacy of oxygenation. Infants should be studied at rest on oxygen and on room air, then under stress (feeding, for example). Weaning from oxygen should not be attempted until oxygenation on room air is greater than 55 mm Hg and until adequate growth has been established. Weaning too early from oxygen may result in diminished growth. Ultimately, improvement in lung function is dependent on increased lung size, so that maintenance of adequate growth is the most important consideration in the therapy for infants with BPD.

Infants who develop congestive heart failure secondary to cor pulmonale often require diuretics or fluid intake restriction. Diuretic therapy can be useful in the acute management of congestive heart failure, particularly early in the course of BPD. Kao and colleagues (1983) showed that administrating 1 mg per kg of furosemide to 10 infants with BPD at about 40 to 42 weeks' postconceptional age resulted in a decreased airway resistance and increased dynamic compliance. The mechanism of action of this response is not clear. Furosemide is a potent diuretic that inhibits the active reabsorption of chloride ion in the ascending loop of Henle. This action in the kidney is followed by a generalized reduction in plasma volume that allows for mobilization of water from extravascular fluid leaks, such as those seen with congestive heart failure. Isolated perfused lung studies in the lamb model, however, have shown a lung-specific effect on furosemide that results in increased net efflux of water from the lung. The propensity of the lungs to improve with diuretic therapy in some infants with BPD allows the diagnosis of "diuretic responsive interstitial pneumonopathy," according to William Tooley, M.D.

The chronic use of furosemide is more controversial. Numerous serious complications of such treatment have been described. These include secondary hyperparathyroidism (Venkataraman et al., 1983), hypercalcinuria (Taft and Roin, 1971), renal calcification (Hufnagle et al., 1982), and cholelithiasis with cholestasis (Callahan et al., 1982). One study has suggested that the use of a thiazide diuretic in conjunction with furosemide may decrease the hypercalcinuric effect and hence the long-term complications of chronic administration of furosemide (Callahan et al., 1982). An additional complication of furosemide administration may be the development of biochemical or overt rickets with pathologic fractures seen in a few infants.

Care should be taken to define the etiology of fluid retention when it occurs (i.e., fluid overload versus worsening of cor pulmonale). If the cause is hypoxic vasoconstriction of the pulmonary vascular bed, then the treatment is increased FiO_2, not increased diuretics. Acute administration of additional diuretic may be necessary, but this should be followed by increasing the inspired oxygen. Repeatedly increasing the diuretic dose for fluid retention can become a vicious circle of more diuretic for fluid retention but worsening of cor pulmonale secondary to chronic intermittent hypoxemia. This process leads to further fluid retention with increasing diuretic, and so on. With higher doses of diuretic, the complications of such therapy increase.

Monitoring of infants on diuretic therapy should include careful attention to sodium, potassium, and calcium balance. Serum electrolytes should be drawn frequently until stable and then should be monitored every 2 weeks.

Maintenance of an adequate growth rate is a requirement for improvement of lung function in infants with BPD. Adequate growth is difficult to achieve because of the need for many infants to maintain a restricted fluid intake to control congestive heart failure. Infants with BPD have an increased caloric expenditure because of both increased work of breathing and increased oxygen consumption. Therefore, nutritional counseling is an integral part of BPD management.

Methods for increasing caloric intake in the face of fluid restriction (often as little as 100–120 ml/kg/day) include concentration of the formula to 24 to 34 cal per oz by addition of caloric supplements using medium-chain triglycerides, polycose, or both (see Chap. 16). Since feeding is major exercise for BPD infants who are exercise intolerant, these infants often benefit from frequent small feedings. We rarely use feeding gastrostomies in infants with BPD.

Lower respiratory tract infections are a significant risk for infants with BPD in the first year of life. As many as 50 to 80 percent of infants with BPD will develop bronchiolitis or pneumonia (Pape et al., 1978; Vohr et al., 1982). The incidence is lower in the second year of life, but risk of infection still remains increased. The major cause of death with lower respiratory tract disease is respiratory failure secondary to respiratory syncytial virus bronchiolitis. Elective admission to a hospital, particularly a children's hospital, during winter months when this disease is epidemic should not be done. Exposure to the virus should be avoided whenever possible.

When an infant with BPD displays viral respiratory symptomatology, early aggressive management should be undertaken. Treatment may include increased FIO_2, increased diuretics, chest physical therapy, and sometimes admission to the hospital to fine-tune the management. Infants with BPD can develop respiratory insufficiency over a matter of hours, so they need to be carefully watched when lower respiratory tract disease is present.

Many wonder about the advisability of nursery school after the first year of age for infants who have had BPD because of potential vulnerability to respiratory tract infections. These risks are largely unknown. Special immunization protocols may afford some protection.

Other significant pulmonary complications seen in infants with BPD include tracheal stenosis (seen in about 8% of infants), upper airway obstruction secondary to subglottic cysts, and hoarseness secondary to partial or complete vocal cord paralysis. Whenever an infant with BPD has hoarseness or stridor, full evaluation by an ear, nose and throat specialist is indicated.

Pulmonary function studies in the first year of life have shown abnormalities consistent with an increased airway resistance. About 10 percent of infants with BPD will have persistent wheezing in the absence of respiratory infection, and most will wheeze with infections. In those who do wheeze, treatment with bronchodilators may be indicated.

There are few long-term follow-up studies of pulmonary function in this population. There is, however, growing evidence that infants who develop BPD do not recover completely. Smyth and coworkers (1981) reported that six of eight infants with severe BPD had bronchial hyperreactivity at a mean age of 8.4 years. Wheeler and coworkers (1984) recently reported that functional residual capacity and maximal expiratory flow rates were increased in a group of 7- to 9-year-old children with a history of BPD compared to other children who were preterm or term. Therefore, while the long-term pulmonary outcome for children who required respiratory assistance at birth is good, the subgroup of infants who develop BPD continues to show signs of pulmonary abnormalities associated with obstructive airway disease and ventilation-perfusion imbalance. Most of these children have no noticeable exercise limitation despite pulmonary function test abnormalities. Further studies are needed before the full impact of the disease process can be evaluated.

Some infants with BPD have developmental delay. Commonly, these infants have delayed development of gross motor skills related to hypotonia. Reasons for this severe, transient hypotonia are not always clear. In view of the delays in gross motor development often seen in the first and second years of life in BPD infants, care must be taken in the interpretation of tests of cognitive skills in this age group. Most early infant tests of central nervous system function rely heavily on motor skills to demonstrate cognitive functioning, and so reliable assessments of cognition can often be achieved only at an older age. Long-term studies of central nervous system outcome in infants with BPD are under-way. These infants are often those who have been ill for prolonged periods and have suffered intracranial hemorrhage and recurrent episodes of hypoxia and central nervous system ischemia. Formal retinoscopy and hearing testing should be carried out by 6 months of age. These infants are among those who frequently require the full panoply of follow-up services.

The stress placed on the family is considerable when an infant with severe BPD is cared for in the home (see Chap. 31). In addition to the physical effort of caring for the child, including administration and management of home oxygen therapy, administration of multiple medications and multiple small feedings, and physical therapy, there is the tension and anxiety generated by uncertainty about long-term outcome. The time commitment of the parents prevents them from spending time with other family members or attending to other activities in home or community. This limitation can result in disturbed family relationships between parents and among siblings. Many services are available to help families with chronically ill children. Visiting nurse associa-tions can provide home medical help, counseling, and parental and family support. Homemaking services should be provided where possible, as house-keeping may be neglected for the more important aspects of the child's medi-cal needs but can be a source of problems for other family members. Without such support systems, some parents cannot leave their infants for long periods of time. Early intervention programs play an important role in following the developmental progress of these infants as well as in providing physical thera-py, infant stimulation, social service support, respite care, parent groups, and eventually nursery schools. Such programs should be routinely utilized for the infant with BPD.

REFERENCES

Abman, S. H., Wolfe, R. R., Accurson, F. J., et al. Pulmonary vascular response to oxygen in infants with severe bronchopulmonary dysplasia. *Pediatrics* 75 : 80, 1985.

Berg, T. J., Pagtakhan, R. D., Reed, M. H., et al. Bronchopulmonary dysplasia and lung rup-ture in hyaline membrane disease: Influence of continuing distending pressure. *Pediatrics* 55 : 51, 1975.

Bland, R. D., McMillan, D. D., and Bressack, M. A. Decreased pulmonary transvascular fluid filtration in awake newborn lambs after intravenous furosemide. *J. Clin. Invest.* 60 : 601, 1978.

Bonikos, D. S., Bensch, K. G., Northway, W. H., and Edwards, D. K. Bronchopulmonary dysplasia: The pulmonary pathologic sequel of necrotizing bronchiolitis and pulmonary fi-brosis. *Hum. Pathol.* 7 : 643, 1976.

Brown, E. R., Stark, A., Sosenko, I., et al. Bronchopulmonary dysplasia: Possible relation-ship to pulmonary edema. *J. Pediatr.* 92 : 982, 1978.

Bryan, M. H., Hardie, M. J., Reilly, B. J., and Swyer, P. R. Pulmonary function studies dur-ing the first year of life in infants recovering from the respiratory distress syndrome. *Pediat-rics* 52 : 169, 1973.

Callahan, J., Haller, J. O., Cacciarelli, A. A., et al. Cholelithiasis in infants: Association with total parenteral nutrition and furosemide. *Radiology* 143 : 437, 1982.

Edwards, D. K., Dyer, W. M., and Northway, W. H. Twelve years' experience with bronchopulmonary dysplasia. *Pediatrics* 59 : 839, 1977.

Fouron, J. C., Le Guennec, J. C., Villemant, D., et al. Value of echocardiography in assessing the outcome of bronchopulmonary dysplasia of the newborn. *Pediatrics* 65 : 529, 1980.

Frank, L. Oxygen toxicity in neonatal rats: Effect of endotoxin on survival during and post O_2 exposure. *Pediatr. Res.* 21 : 109, 1987.

Hack, M., DeMonterice, D., Merkatz, I. R., et al. Rehospitalization of the very low birth weight infants. *Am. J. Dis. Child.* 135 : 263, 1981.

Halliday, H. L., Dumpit, F. M., and Brady, J. P. Effect of inspired oxygen on echocardiographic assessment of pulmonary vascular resistance and myocardial contractility in bronchopulmonary dysplasia. *Pediatrics* 65 : 536, 1980.

Hufnagle, K. G., Khan, S. N., Penn, D., et al. Renal calcifications. *Pediatrics* 70 : 360, 1982.

Kao, L. C., Warburton, D., Sargent, C. W., et al. Furosemide acutely decreases airway resistance in chronic bronchopulmonary dysplasia. *J. Pediatr.* 103 : 624, 1983.

Lamarre, A., Linsae, L., Reilly, B. J., et al. Residual pulmonary abnormalities in survivors of idiopathic respiratory distress syndrome. *Am. Rev. Resp. Dis.* 108 : 56, 1973.

Markestad, T., and Fitzhardinge, P. M. Growth and development in children recovering from bronchopulmonary dysplasia. *J. Pediatr.* 98 : 597, 1981.

McCarthy, K., Bhogal, M., Nardi, M., and Hart, D. Pathogenic factors in bronchopulmonary dysplasia. *Pediatr. Res.* 18 : 483, 1984.

Merritt, T. A., and Cochrane, C. C. Elastase and alpha-1 protease inhibitor activity in tracheal aspirates during respiratory distress syndrome. *J. Clin. Invest.* 72 : 656, 1983.

Mor, J., McLaughlin, J., Pintar, M., et al. Transcutaneous monitoring of oxygenation: What is normal? *J. Pediatr.* 108 : 365, 1986.

Northway, W. H., Rosan, R. C., and Porter, D. Y. Pulmonary disease following respirator therapy of hyaline membrane disease. *N. Engl. J. Med.* 276 : 357, 1967.

O'Brodovich, H., and Mellins, R. Bronchopulmonary dysplasia. *Am. Rev. Resp. Dis.* 132 : 694, 1985.

Pape, K. E., Buncic, R. J., Ashby, S., and Fitzhardinge, P. M. The status at two years of low-birth-weight infants born in 1974 with birth weights of less than 1001 gm. *J. Pediatr.* 92 : 253, 1978.

Perlman, J. M., Moore, V., Siegel, M. J., Dawson, J. Is chloride depletion an important contributing cause of death in infants with bronchopulmonary dysplasia? *Pediatrics* 77(2) : 212, 1986.

Reynolds, E. O. R., and Taghizadeh, A. Improved prognosis of infants mechanically ventilated for hyaline membrane disease. *Arch. Dis. Child.* 49 : 505, 1974.

Sauve, R., and Singhai, N. Long-term morbidity of infants with BPD. *Pediatrics* 76 : 725, 1985.

Smyth, J. A., Tabachnik, E., Duncan, W. J., et al. Pulmonary function and bronchial hyperactivity in long-term survivors of bronchopulmonary dysplasia. *Pediatrics* 682 : 336, 1981.

Stocks, J., and Godfrey, S. The role of artificial ventilation, oxygen, and CPAP in the pathogenesis of lung damage in neonates: Assessment by serial measurements of lung function. *Pediatrics* 57 : 352, 1976.

Taft, H., and Roin, J. Effect of furosemide administration on calcium excretion. *Br. Med. J.* 1 : 437, 1971.

Taghizadeh, A., and Reynolds, E. O. R. Pathogenesis of bronchopulmonary dysplasia following hyaline membrane disease. *Am. J. Pathol.* 82 : 241, 1976.

Tomashefski, J., Oppermann, H., Vawter, G., and Reid, L. Bronchopulmonary disease: A morphometric study with emphasis on pulmonary vascularity. *Pediatr. Pathol.* 2 : 469, 1984.

Unger, M., Atkins, M., Briscoe, W. A., and King, T. K. C. Potentiation of pulmonary vaso-constrictor response with repeated intermittent hypoxia. *J. Appl. Physiol.* 43 : 662, 1977.

Venkataraman, B. S., Han, B. K., Tsang, R. C., and Daugherty, C. C. Secondary hyperpara-thyroidism and bone disease in infants receiving long-term furosemide therapy. *Am. J. Dis. Child.* 137 : 1157, 1983.

Vohr, B. R., Bell, E. F., and Oh, W. Infants with bronchopulmonary dysplasia: Growth pat-tern and neurologic and developmental outcome. *Am. J. Dis. Child.* 136 : 443, 1982.

Weinstein, M. R., and Oh, W. Oxygen consumption in infants with bronchopulmonary dysplasia. *J. Pediatr.* 99 : 959, 1981.

Werthammer, J., Brown, E. R., Neff, R. K., and Taeusch, H. W. Sudden infant death syn-drome in infants with bronchopulmonary dysplasia. *Pediatrics* 69 : 301, 1982.

Wheeler, W. B., Castile, R. G., Brown, E. R., and Wohl, M. E. Pulmonary function in sur-vivors of prematurity. *Am. Rev. Resp. Dis.* 129 : 218, 1984.

20

Retinopathy of Prematurity

Robert A. Petersen

I. Introduction

Retinopathy of prematurity (ROP) is the current name for the vascular abnormalities that occur in some premature infants. The name ROP has superseded the term *retrolental fibroplasia* (RLF) as a general name for the process. Because fibrous tissue behind the lens never develops in the majority of infants who are afflicted, the old term is misleading and inaccurate.

II. Pathogenesis

The current understanding of the pathogenesis of ROP has been outlined by Flynn and coworkers (1979). The normal retinal vasculature begins growing out of the optic nerve from the central retinal artery and vein during the fourth month of gestation. By 40 weeks of gestation, the entire nasal retina is vascularized. Within the first 2 or 3 weeks after birth in a full-term infant, the temporal periphery of the retina has also been completely vascularized. Because the optic nerve is on the nasal side of the center of the retina, the vessels have a shorter distance to grow nasally than temporally. In some premature infants, for unknown reasons, the normal vascularization of the retina ceases sometime after birth, and abnormal vascular tissue develops. This typically takes the form of an elevated ridge of mesenchymal tissue containing budding capillaries and forming a syncytium of primitive vascular channels. Depending on the postconceptional age of the infant, this so-called mesenchymal shelf may be circumferential or limited to the temporal periphery. The more premature the infant, the more likely the abnormality is to be further posterior in the retina and the more extensive it is likely to be. The larger and more extensive the mesenchymal shelf, the more it behaves as a large arteriovenous shunt. Fundus examination reveals the mesenchymal shelf with retinal blood vessels ending suddenly in it, which appears as an elevated ridge of tissue with the avascular retina peripheral to it. Because of the shunting, the retinal blood vessels may be more or less dilated and tortuous posterior to the mesenchymal shelf.

The process may resolve if normal intraretinal vascularization of the retina peripheral to the shunt resumes with gradual flattening of the mesenchymal shelf. When resolution is complete, the peripheral retina may contain retinal blood vessels, which are excessively numerous or relatively sparse, and they may be too straight in their orientation. There may be arteriovenous loops remaining in the peripheral retina. Sometimes a white line can be seen in the retina where the mesenchymal shelf had been. The posterior retinal blood vessels may remain somewhat tortuous. In most infants, however, ROP resolves without leaving any trace of abnormality.

221

In patients who do not resolve spontaneously, extraretinal neovascularization occurs either on the surface of the retina, usually coming off the posterior edge of the mesenchymal shelf or vertically into the vitreous. Neovascularization occurring vertically into the vitreous may be accompanied by a large amount of fibrous tissue. Retinal detachment may also occur, which may be due to exudation of fluid beneath the retina. In some infants, retinal detachment occurs later, in the cicatricial phase of the disease with the fibrovascular proliferation causing a traction detachment. At any stage in this process, spontaneous remission may occur with resolution of the abnormalities and resumption of normal vascularization of the peripheral retina, regression of abnormal blood vessels and fibrous tissue, and spontaneous reattachment of the retina.

III. Classification

A new classification of ROP has recently been proposed by the Committee for the Classification of Retinopathy of Prematurity (1984a, b), which makes it possible to conduct organized follow-up on ROP patients and to describe the findings precisely to other physicians. The classification divides the retina into zones to localize the abnormalities (Fig. 20-1) and stages the disease to describe the level of vascular abnormalities observed. Stage 1 is the presence of a demarcation line, which is a thin, flat structure separating the peripheral avascular retina from vascularized posterior retina. The retinal blood vessels branch abnormally and stop suddenly at this demarcation line. Stage 2 involves the formation of a ridge, the aforementioned mesenchymal shelf, which is elevated and has width. Stage 3 includes extraretinal fibrovascular

Fig. 20-1. Scheme of retina of right eye *(RE)* and left eye *(LE)* showing zone borders and clock hours to describe location and extent of retinopathy of prematurity. (From Committee for the Classification of Retinopathy of Prematurity. An international classification of retinopathy of prematurity. Published simultaneously in *Arch. Ophthalmol.* 102 : 1130, 1984, and *Pediatrics* 74 : 127, 1984. With permission.)

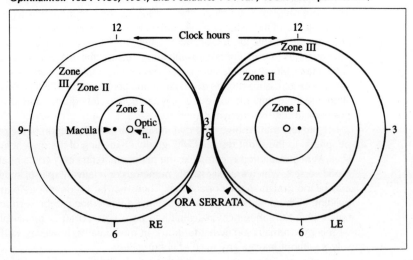

proliferative tissue coming off the posterior edge of the ridge or growing vertically into the vitreous off the ridge. Stage 4 includes the preceding abnormalities plus retinal detachment, either serous or exudative, or a traction detachment. A traction detachment is a transition between ROP and the cicatricial phase of the disease, which may still be called RLF.

If stages 1 through 4 are accompanied by dilation and tortuosity of the posterior veins and arterioles, the new classification adds the designation "plus" to the stage described (i.e., 2+). A copy of the examination record for the organized recording of these findings is shown in Fig. 20-2.

The classification of cicatricial RLF by Reese and colleagues (1953) is still in use. It describes the final outcome of ROP when the pathologic process has run its course and ended in a stable situation. The classification was established when the retina could be examined only with the direct ophthalmoscope, so it mainly describes relatively posterior abnormalities. Grade I includes vitreoretinal membranes and myopia, to which many ophthalmologists now add peripheral retinal scarring not severe enough to cause posterior retinal distortion. Grade II includes distortion of the posterior retina with displacement of the macula, usually in a temporal direction. Grades I and II are compatible with relatively normal corrected vision. Grade III includes a retinal fold that usually extends temporally from the disc through the macular area leading to an opaque temporal vitreoretinal mass. Grade IV has an incomplete retrolental membrane, usually temporally, and grade V exhibits a complete retrolental membrane.

IV. Causative factors

In our group of patients at the Joint Program in Neonatology* (JPN), the major factors correlating with the development of ROP have been short gestational age and low birth weight. Duration of treatment with oxygen and duration of mechanical ventilation also correlate with the development of ROP, but no correlation with elevated PaO_2 even with continuous transcutaneous monitoring, has been found. This finding agrees with the large cooperative study of Kinsey and associates (1977). The failure to correlate PaO_2 with the development of ROP makes it seem unlikely that oxygen has a direct etiologic role. It seems more likely that other factors are involved in the smallest, sickest infants who require prolonged oxygen and mechanical ventilation and also tend to develop ROP. We have seen very small premature infants who developed ROP but who received neither oxygen nor mechanical ventilation.

V. Criteria for examination

Retinopathy of prematurity almost always begins when the patient is still in the neonatal intensive care unit (NICU), generally before 32 weeks postconception. Patients who meet one of the following generally accepted criteria should be examined while still in the NICU: birth weight of 1,500 g or less, a gestational age of 32 weeks or less, an oxygen requirement of 30 percent or more for 4 hours or longer, or mechanical ventilation. An ophthalmologist skilled in the examination of newborn infants, usually a pediatric ophthal-

*The JPN is affiliated with Harvard Medical School, Beth Israel Hospital, Brigham and Women's Hospital, and The Children's Hospital, Boston.

International Classification of ROP

Retinopathy of Prematurity (ROP) Ophthalmic Examination Record

Biographic data

Name ______________________ Hospital # __ __ __ __ __ __ __

Birth date
(Mo/D/Yr) __ __ / __ __ / __ __ Sex (M = 1, F = 2) __

Birth weight (grams) __ __ __ __ Gestational age (weeks) __ __

Multiple births (single = 1, twin = 2, triplet = 3) __

Examination

Date of exam __ __ / __ __ / __ __ Examiner's initials or # __ __ __

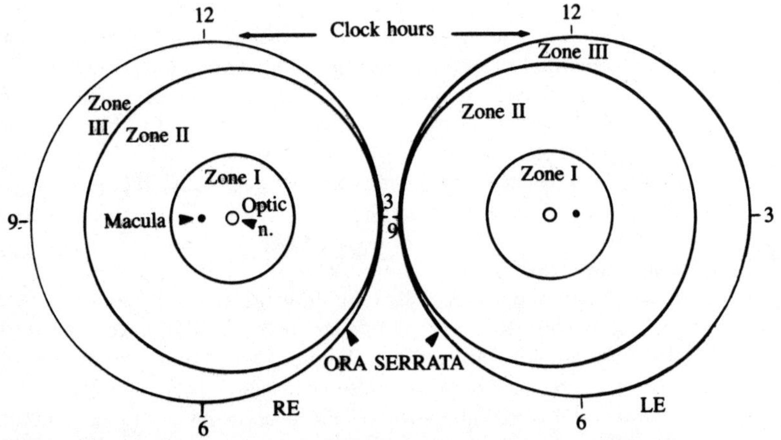

Fig. 20-2. Examination record for recording detailed examination results. *LE* = left eye; *OD* = oculus dexter (right eye); *OS* = oculus sinister (left eye); *RE* = right eye; *RLF* = retrolental fibroplasia; *Z* = zone. (From Committee for the Classification of Retinopathy of Prematurity. An international classification of retinopathy of prematurity. Published simultaneously in *Arch. Ophthalmol.* 102 : 1130, 1984, and *Pediatrics* 74 : 127, 1984. With permission.)

mologist or retina surgeon, should examine all infants meeting these criteria before discharge from the nursery. The most expeditious time for the examination of most infants is 32 to 34 weeks postconception, but infants with birth weights less than 1,000 g should be examined earlier. It cannot be predicted whether ROP will occur before 32 to 34 weeks postconception.

A problem arises in many tertiary level NICUs because infants frequently return to their community hospitals before 32 weeks postconception. The ophthalmologist experienced with ROP cannot rule it out prior to transfer, and there may not be an ophthalmologist knowledgeable about ROP available

Zone

Mark with 'X'

Z I   Z II   Z III   Z I   Z II   Z III
☐   ☐   ☐   ☐   ☐   ☐

Stage at clock hours

Blank = normal
1 = Demarcation line
2 = Ridge
3 = 2 + Extraret prolif
4 = 3 + Retinal detach
9 = No information

Mark highest stage at every clock hour

☐   If stage 3: 1 = mild, 2 = moderate, 3 = severe   ☐

☐   If stage 4: 1 = exudative, 2 = tractional, 3 = combined   ☐

Other findings

OD   Mark with 'X'   OS

☐   A   Dilatation/tortuosity posterior vessels   ☐

☐   B   Iris vessel dilatation   ☐

☐   C   Pupil rigidity   ☐

☐   D   Vitreous haze   ☐

☐   E   Hemorrhages   ☐

Cicatricial RLF (Reese, 1953)

OD   Mark with 'X'   OS

☐   I.   Small mass opaque tissue in periphery without detachment   ☐

☐   II.   Larger mass opaque tissue in periphery with localized detachment ☐

☐   III. Larger mass in periphery with traction fold to disc   ☐

☐   IV.   Retrolental tissue covering part of pupil   ☐

☐   V.   Retrolental tissue covering entire pupillary area   ☐

Comments:

_____
Signature

Fig. 20-2 (continued)

to the community hospital nursery. These patients should be reexamined by the experienced ophthalmologist after discharge from the community hospital nursery. Reassurances about the normality of the retina in an infant less than 32 weeks postconception should not be given, as ROP might still develop. All infants meeting the aforementioned criteria should be examined with the indirect ophthalmoscope after the pupils have been fully dilated with 1% cyclopentolate (Cyclogyl), one drop in each eye, repeated in 5 minutes with the examination a half-hour later.

VI. Diagnosis

Visual acuity can be tested early in infancy by a behavioral method, the Preferential Looking Test (Fulton et al., 1978). Attempts to test premature infants with this technique before 40 weeks postconception have not been successful (Manning et al., 1982). In our group of patients, this test has been most effectively used approximately 48 weeks postconception in high-risk premature infants.

Special modifications of the visual evoked potential recording can also be used to measure visual acuity in infancy (Sokol, 1978). A pediatrician or ophthalmologist without special equipment can estimate the visual behavior of a child by assessing the patient's ability to fix and follow. The age at which infants are capable of this kind of visual behavior varies, especially in high-risk premature infants. The most effective targets for estimating a child's visual behavior are the examiner's face and a penlight.

VII. Treatment

Cryotherapy and photocoagulation of the abnormal blood vessels or of the peripheral avascular retina anterior to the ridge in the more severe stages of ROP have possibly benefited some patients (Nagata et al., 1982; Sasaki et al., 1976). In a disease that is subject to spontaneous remission at all stages of its development, it is difficult to evaluate treatments that have been reported so far. A large, collaborative, randomized, carefully controlled clinical trial is currently underway in the United States. Cryotherapy is given anterior to the ridge of tissue in patients who are selected for treatment. Until the results of the collaborative study are known, this treatment should be considered investigational.

In patients who have progressed to severe cicatricial RLF, vitreoretinal surgery has been performed to remove the scar tissue and reattach the retina (Charles, 1983; Hirose, 1985). The anatomic success rate is approximately 50 percent, but only about 10 percent of the patients have achieved useful vision. At this end stage of the disease, there is no other hope for vision, so that even the modest success with vitrectomy seems justified in suitable patients.

Patients with lesser degrees of RLF need to be followed indefinitely because of the possibility of late rhegmatogenous retinal detachments (Faris et al., 1969). If retinal holes and localized detachments are discovered and treated early, extensive detachment may be prevented, preserving vision.

VIII. Prognosis

The prognosis for untreated infants with ROP is good. Of 2,500 high-risk infants meeting the criteria in V who were examined between 1975 and 1985 at the JPN nurseries, 11 percent of them had ROP. Of these, only 12 infants (0.48% of the high-risk group) progressed to grade IV or V cicatricial RLF in one or both eyes. Of the 11 percent who had ROP, about 62 percent experienced complete resolution. Twenty-eight percent had mild cicatricial RLF (grade I or mild grade II), without visual impairment. Most of these patients had mild vascular changes visible only in the extreme periphery, a few were myopic, and a few had mild distortion of the retinal vessels in the posterior pole without macular ectopia. Seven percent had grade II or III RLF, some with decreased visual acuity because of retinal folds running through the macula but with good peripheral vision. Of the infants with ROP, 4.4 percent (i.e., 0.48% of the overall high-risk group) had grade IV or V RLF with blindness, or only light perception vision, in one or both eyes.

IX. Follow-up

Depending on the severity, activity, and extent of the abnormalities, infants who are identified as having ROP should be seen every few days to once every 2 weeks. Generally there is a relatively prolonged period of uncertainty in the course of ROP, which may be difficult for the nurses, pediatricians, and parents to tolerate. In most individual patients there is no way of predicting the final outcome, and prognosis mostly involves describing the statistical probabilities. During this time it is helpful for the primary nurse, the neonatologist, and the ophthalmologist to maintain contact with the parents. The period of uncertainty may last as long as 4 to 5 months with little or no change taking place and then progression or ultimate resolution.

X. Prevention

Because the etiology of ROP is obscure, it is not clear what preventive measures might be added to the care that patients already receive. A suggestion that large doses of vitamin E administered prophylactically from birth might ameliorate the severity of ROP (Hittner et al., 1981) has not been confirmed by recent studies (Phelps et al., in press; Schaffer et al., 1985).

XI. Support for families

Aside from the support that can be offered to parents and children with visual impairment from RLF by their physicians, social agencies and volunteer groups should be contacted. If a child is legally blind, he or she should be reported to the state's commission for the blind and division of special education. More and more preschool programs are becoming available for visually handicapped children. An example is the preschool program at the Perkins School for the Blind in Watertown, Massachusetts. Information about programs and parent support groups can be obtained from the International Institute for the Visually Impaired, Age Birth to Seven.* This organization has also published books that are helpful to parents of visually impaired children. *Move It* (1977) and *Get a Wiggle On* (1975), both by Sherry Raynor and Richard Drouillard, are two such books, available directly from the Institute.

XII. Summary

It is fortunate that the vast majority of high-risk infants who are discharged from NICUs have no major eye or visual problems. It is important to identify children who do have difficulties and ensure that they are followed appropriately by an ophthalmologist. Specific treatment of ROP and RLF may be indicated, and associated problems of myopia and other refractive errors and strabismus with the possible development of amblyopia can be treated. Low-vision aids may be prescribed if necessary, and the ophthalmologist will make referrals to the appropriate social agencies and community organizations.

*230 Central Street, Auburndale, Massachusetts 02166 (617) 332-4014.

REFERENCES

Charles, S. Vitrectomy in the treatment of RLF. Presented to the American Academy of Ophthalmology, Chicago, Oct. 30 to Nov. 3, 1983.

Committee for the Classification of Retinopathy of Prematurity. An international classification of retinopathy of prematurity. *Arch. Ophthalmol.* 102 : 1130, 1984a.

Committee for the Classification of Retinopathy of Prematurity. An international classification of retinopathy of prematurity. *Pediatrics* 74 : 127, 1984b.

Faris, B., and Brockhurst, R. Retrolental fibroplasia in the cicatricial stage: The complication of rhegmatogenous retinal detachment. *Arch. Ophthalmol.* 82 : 60, 1969.

Flynn, J. T., O'Grady, G. E., Herrera, J., et al. Retrolental fibroplasia. I. Clinical observations. *Arch. Ophthalmol.* 95 : 217, 1977.

Fulton, A. B., Manning, K. A., and Dobson, V. A behavioral method for efficient screening of visual acuity in young infants. II. Clinical application. *Invest. Ophthalmol. Vis. Sci.* 17 : 1151, 1978.

Hirose, T. Open sky vitrectomy for cicatricial ROP. Presented to the New England Ophthalmological Society, Boston, May 1985.

Hittner, H. M., Godio, L. B., Rudolph, A. J., et al. Retrolental fibroplasia: Efficacy of vitamin E in a double-blind clinical study of preterm infants. *N. Engl. J. Med.* 305 : 1365, 1981.

Kinsey, V. E., Arnold, H. J., Kalina, R. E., et al. PaO_2 levels and retrolental fibroplasia: A report of the cooperative study. *Pediatrics* 60 : 655, 1977.

Manning, K. A., Fulton, A. B., Hanson, R. M., et al. Preferential looking vision testing: Application to evaluation of high-risk prematurely born infants and children. *J. Pediatr. Ophthalmol. Strabismus* 19 : 286, 1982.

McPearson, A., Hittner, H., and Kretzer, F. *Retinopathy of Prematurity: Current Concepts and Controversies.* Toronto: Decker, 1986.

Nagata, M., Yamagishi, N., and Ikeda, S. Summarized results of the treatment of acute proliferative retinopathy of prematurity during the past 15 years in Tenri Hospital. *Acta Soc. Ophthalmol. Jpn.* 86 : 1236, 1982.

Phelps, D. L., Rosenblaum, A. L., Isenberg, S., et al. Safety and efficacy of tocopherol in preventing retinopathy of prematurity. *Ophthalmology.* In press.

Reese, A. B., King, M. J., and Owens, W. C. A classification of retrolental fibroplasia. *Am. J. Ophthalmol.* 10 : 1331, 1953.

Sasaki, K., Yamashita, Y., Maekawa, T., and Adachi, T. Treatment of retinopathy of prematurity in active stage by cryocautery. *Jpn. J. Ophthalmol.* 20 : 384, 1976.

Schaffer, D. B., Johnson, L., Quinn, G. E., et al. Vitamin E and retinopathy of prematurity: Follow-up at one year. *Ophthalmology* 92 : 1005, 1985.

Sokol, D. Measurement of infant visual acuity from pattern reversal evoked potentials. *Vision Res.* 18 : 33, 1978.

21

Intracranial Hemorrhage

Allen J. Cherer

I. Introduction

Intracranial hemorrhage is the most common serious neurologic event of the neonatal period. Although forms of hemorrhage other than subependymal and intraventricular occur, especially in the full-term infant, the most frequently encountered sequelae affect those premature infants with the more severe grades of intraventricular hemorrhage (IVH). Issues relating to the management of seizures and hydrocephalus, as well as to long-term neurodevelopmental outcome frequently arise in the neonatal intensive care unit (NICU) and persist beyond discharge. Clearly for the primary care providers, general guidelines for management are both useful and necessary. Nevertheless, such guidelines should be followed in a flexible way when treating individual patients.

II. Background and major issues

Early postmortem studies suggested that the incidence of IVH in nonsurviving infants less than 1,500 g was between 30 and 50 percent (Larroche, 1972; Lorber and Bhat, 1974). The general belief was that (1) severe IVH in the newborn was nearly uniformly fatal, (2) posthemorrhagic hydrocephalus in surviving infants was inevitable, and (3) the ultimate developmental and neurologic status of survivors was poor. With the routine use of computed tomographic (CT) scanning as a screening and follow-up tool in the late 1970s, the natural history of intracranial hemorrhage in the newborn began to be delineated. Ahmann and coworkers (1980) showed that infants less than 35 weeks' gestation with subependymal hemorrhage (SEH) or IVH had a survival rate of 71 percent, an incidence of 22 percent of posthemorrhagic hydrocephalus (PHH), and spontaneous resolution of posthemorrhagic hydrocephalus in approximately 33 percent after 1 month of age. They also noted increasing ventricular size 2 to 3 weeks before the onset of accelerated head growth, bulging anterior fontanelle, and other signs suggesting increased intracranial pressure. The findings were consistent with those reported by Volpe and associates (1977) in an earlier study and formed the basis of a paper by Hill and Volpe (1981), which characterized the state of normal pressure hydrocephalus in the preterm infant after intracranial hemorrhage. That study suggested that a proportion of infants with all degrees of hemorrhage will develop PHH, and approximately half will exhibit arrest or resolution of their hydrocephalus by 4 weeks. More recent studies by Allan and coworkers (1984) have focused on the natural history of PHH. They distinguish between ventriculomegaly (i.e., ventricular dilatation not associated with accelerated head growth or signs or symptoms of increased intracranial pressure) and PHH, which they define as

229

increasing ventricular size associated with evidence of intracranial hypertension. They found a 61 percent resolution of ventriculomegaly and advocated a conservative approach to the infant with ventricular dilatation until PHH occurred. An important issue regarding ventricular dilatation and its management is the possible long-term neurologic morbidity (Palmer et al., 1982) associated with prolonged cerebral compression or other factors versus the known morbidity (e.g., shunt dependency, obstruction, infection) associated with permanent cerebrospinal fluid (CSF) diversion.

III. Posthemorrhagic hydrocephalus

The natural course of PHH has only recently been delineated with the advent of portable ultrasonography. Its management remains controversial. Based on current data, we have devised a management protocol (Fig. 21-1). Studies have demonstrated that a significant proportion of all infants less than 1,500 g or less than 35 weeks' gestation develop some degree of ventricular enlargement after an initial hemorrhage (Ahmann et al., 1980; Allan et al., 1984; Papile et al., 1980). The smaller the infant and the more extensive the hemorrhage, the more likely the development of PHH. With the mechanism involved believed to be disturbed CSF absorption on the basis of obstruction to flow or an obliterative arachnoiditis, early studies suggested lumbar puncture either at the time of hemorrhage or at the initial appearance of increasing ventricular enlargement (Mantovani, 1980; Papile et al., 1980). Neither management appeared to change the course, possibly because an insufficient quantity of CSF was removed. It was the finding that approximately one-third to one-half of such cases of PHH arrest or resolve spontaneously approximately 1 month after the hemorrhage, which led to a less aggressive approach in patients with enlarging ventricular size but without signs and symptoms of increased intracranial pressure (Hill and Volpe, 1981). Repeated lumbar punctures and the placement of either a temporary or permanent CSF diversion apparatus appeared inappropriate in fragile, already compromised, low-birth-weight infants soon after IVH.

On the other hand, in the infant who demonstrates evidence of raised intracranial pressure within the first month after hemorrhage, intervention is appropriate, although the mode is less clear. Generally, after verification of communicating hydrocephalus, serial lumbar punctures are effective in immediately decreasing raised intracranial pressure if adequate volumes of CSF (approximately 10–15 ml) are removed. Pharmacologic agents such as acetazolamide and furosemide are effective in decreasing CSF production. Although controlled studies are needed, we recommend empirical use of these drugs with serial lumbar punctures and close monitoring of electrolyte and acid-base status. Although the duration of lumbar punctures is generally limited to approximately 2 weeks, pharmacologic treatment may continue beyond discharge. Since progressive hydrocephalus may occur after a period of stable ventricular size but very rarely after 3 months, pharmacologic therapy should be tapered at that time. If at any time during management with serial lumbar punctures or pharmacologic therapy, progressive ventriculomegaly associated with accelerated head growth or signs and symptoms of increased intracranial pressure occurs, placement of an external ventricular drain is indicated. Generally, the duration of the drain is 10 to 14 days owing to the risks of infection. If progres-

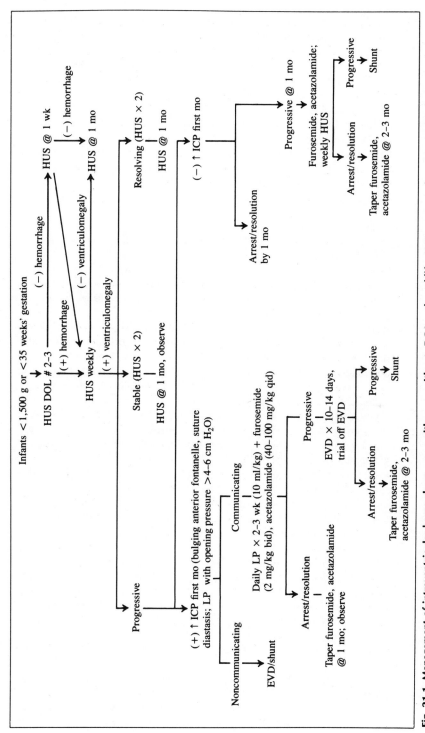

Fig. 21-1. Management of intraventricular hemorrhage. + = with; − = without; *DOL* = day of life; *EVD* = external ventricular drain; *HUS* = head ultrasound; *ICP* = intracranial pressure; *LP* = lumbar puncture.

sive hydrocephalus occurs after the drain is removed, a permanent CSF diversion procedure is generally performed.

Some infants have enlarged ventricles without evidence of previous SEH or IVH. The association between asphyxia and subsequent ischemic changes resulting in periventricular leukomalacia may well explain this ventriculomegaly. Because such anatomic changes occur by 1 to 2 months after birth and the ultrasonographic appearance rarely changes after 3 months, we recommend that all infants with complicated perinatal courses have cranial ultrasonography performed at 1 month of age. Those infants with abnormal scans should have follow-up ultrasonography at 3 months. In general, subsequent follow-up to 1 year of age with monthly head circumference measurements and bimonthly neurodevelopmental screening is adequate to detect the rare infant who requires further investigation.

IV. Shunts

As previously noted, the hydrocephalus that occurs after intracranial hemorrhage in the premature infant is often transient. However, when temporary diversion and pharmacologic management fail to control increasing ventriculomegaly and intracranial hypertension, permanent shunting of CSF is necessary. In the infant, the ventriculoperitoneal shunt has proved to be the most appropriate. The peritoneal cavity possesses a number of features that make it suitable for CSF diversion. Normal intestinal peristalsis keeps the abdominal tubing moving and allows for rapid and efficient absorption. The risk of obstruction of the shunt catheter is small. In addition, the long length of the abdominal catheter not only improves the siphonlike function of the diversionary catheter but also decreases the frequency of revision due to axial growth. When only 3 to 5 cm of the distal end of the catheter remains in the peritoneal cavity, elective lengthening is performed. On the average, approximately two revisions for distal catheter lengthening are required during the first 10 years of life. Valveless systems are frequently placed if the CSF protein concentration is greater than 200 mg per dl. The theoretic disadvantage of such a system is that excessive CSF drainage may result in obstruction of the proximal catheter by slitlike ventricles. Yet, this does not appear to be a major clinical problem during infancy, and no restrictions in body positioning are warranted. Nevertheless, placement of a low-pressure valve is frequently advocated as soon as possible. Once a shunt is placed, the overwhelming majority of patients remain shunt dependent.

The complications of ventriculoperitoneal shunts are well known. Obstruction of the apparatus may occur at any level. The most apparent signs in an infant are a bulging anterior fontanelle, feeding intolerance, lethargy, and increasing head circumference. Determination of shunt obstruction is best left to the neurosurgeon, who frequently uses a combination of history, examination, radiography, and observation to make the diagnosis.

The incidence of shunt infections has decreased as the experience of surgical teams and the use of antimicrobial prophylaxis have increased. In addition, shunt materials have changed, resulting in less risk of colonization by certain bacteria. Nevertheless, the incidence of infection remains between 10 and 20 percent. A recent review by Odio (1984) described 516 shunt procedures in 297 patients. Fifty-nine infections occurred in 50 patients, and more than one-half of the infections developed within 2 weeks of the procedures. Coagulase-negative *Staphylococcus epidermidis* and *S. aureus* account for approximately 75 percent of such infections, with gram-negative bacilli responsible for most of the remaining infections. The clinical symptoms are frequently nonspecific, with only a few patients presenting with such signs as wound infection, erythema and edema of the shunt track, or tense fontanelle (Table 21-1). Although some studies report a greater than 50 percent incidence of shunt malfunction, others do not substantiate this finding.

Although intravenous antibiotics alone are sometimes successful in treating mild shunt infections not complicated by distal symptoms (e.g., wound infection, peritonitis), the current recommendation for treatment is removal of the apparatus, placement of an external ventricular drain, and administration of intravenous antibiotics based on Gram's stain and CSF culture. In general, the advantages of the external ventricular drain are that normal intracranial pressures are maintained with ready access to CSF for monitoring sterilization and bacteriologic cure is more prompt with the shunt removed. The overall treatment success rate with shunt removal is 96 percent compared with only 36 percent when the shunt remains in place. Nafcillin or vancomycin with or without rifampin is suggested for infection caused by *Staphylococcus* species, and cefotaxime for gram-negative bacillary infections. Once the CSF is sterile, antibiotics are continued for a total of 10 days. Thereafter, serial CSF cultures are obtained for 3 days. If these remain sterile, the shunt may be replaced.

V. Neonatal seizures

A discussion of neonatal seizures is best prefaced with the statement that the majority of newborns with seizures have normal outcomes. Results of the National Collaborative Perinatal Project (NCPP) suggested that 70 percent of surviving infants will be normal at 7 years of age (Holden, 1982).

Accurate estimates of the incidence of neonatal seizures are lacking. The many manifestations, especially of the subtle forms of oral-buccal-lingual and oculomotor movements, make precise incidence figures impossible (Table 21-2). Clearly the more distinctive forms, such as the generalized tonic type characteristic of the premature infant and the multifocal clonic type often seen

Table 21-1. Signs and symptoms of central nervous system infections in shunted patients without evidence of wound infection

Sign or symptom	Percentage of patients
Fever (> 38.5° C)	92
Change in sensorium	94
Irritability	83
Shunt malfunction	65
Vomiting*	33
Abdominal pain*	19
Diarrhea*	6
Peritonitis*	4

*Abdominal symptoms are almost twice as common when there is evidence of wound infection.
Adapted from R. Yogev. Cerebrospinal fluid shunt infections: A personal view. *Pediatr. Infect. Dis.* 4 : 113, 1985.

Table 21-2. Types of neonatal seizures

Type	Description
Subtle	Constitutes approximately half of all neonatal seizures Often associated with other seizure types
Generalized tonic	Characteristic of the premature infant Frequently associated with intraventricular hemorrhage or diffuse central nervous system disease EEG often shows burst-suppression pattern or decreased amplitude Generally poor prognosis
Multifocal clonic	Characteristic of the full-term infant EEG shows multifocal abnormality
Focal clonic	Often associated with focal traumatic injury, subarachnoid hemorrhage, or metabolic disturbance EEG shows unifocal disturbance Generally good prognosis
Myoclonic	Often associated with diffuse central nervous system disorder EEG shows burst-suppression pattern that may evolve into a hypsarrhythmia pattern Generally poor prognosis

EEG = electroencephalogram.

in the more mature infant, allow for better estimates of incidence and, particularly, outcome.

The most frequent causes of seizures are perinatal asphyxia and intracranial hemorrhage; other less common causes include central nervous system infection, metabolic disturbances (especially hypoglycemia and hypocalcemia), drug intoxication or withdrawal, and central nervous system developmental abnormalities. Despite the varied causes, the long-term management of seizures during the neonatal period is based on a combination of factors and is similar whether the seizures are associated with asphyxia, IVH, or both.

A number of studies have examined the relationship between certain neonatal factors and outcome among infants with seizures. The NCPP included the largest cohort of such infants and followed them to 7 years of age (Holden, 1982). Outcome was judged in terms of the development of cerebral palsy, mental retardation, and afebrile seizure disorder. Neurologic sequelae were noted in approximately 30 percent of the survivors. A 5-minute Apgar score of less than 6, resuscitation longer than 5 minutes after birth, seizures lasting longer than 3 days, the early onset of seizures, and low birth weight were all associated with poor outcome. In a more recent study, Bergman (1983) was unable to demonstrate the predictive value of the 5-minute Apgar score but noted a correlation between late onset of seizures, long duration of seizures, and the presence of tonic seizures with adverse outcome. In his study of term infants with hypoxic-ischemic encephalopathy, Finer (1981) noted a relationship between time of onset of seizures and outcome. Almost half of infants with seizures in the first 24 hours demonstrated major handicap at later follow-up. Volpe (1981) has suggested that approximately 15 percent of neonatal seizures are associated with intracranial hemorrhage. Of those infants with seizures as manifestations of IVH, less than 10 percent are expected to have normal outcomes.

In the NCPP, the incidence of later seizure disorders in surviving infants was approximately 22 percent, similar to the findings of Bergman (1983). Predictors of later seizure disorder included duration of neonatal seizures and type of seizure (myoclonic and tonic seizures being most highly associated with later seizures). Neither the 5-minute Apgar score nor the electroencephalogram proved to be useful predictors of the development of a later seizure disorder. Ellison (1984), on the other hand, demonstrated the usefulness of the neonatal electroencephalogram as a predictor of later abnormal neurologic outcome and seizure disorder.

Decisions regarding the duration of anticonvulsant therapy for neonatal seizures must be based on a number of factors. Those neonatal factors predictive of both adverse neurologic outcome and the development of later seizure disorder have proved to be useful. Prolonged treatment hardly seems warranted in the great majority of infants, and a number of protocols suggest that management with a single anticonvulsant (generally, phenobarbital) maintaining therapeutic serum levels until the corrected age of 3 months is appropriate. Scoring systems as shown in Table 21-3 serve as practical guides in identifying

Table 21-3. Scoring system for evaluating seizures at 3 months' corrected age

Abnormality of EEG
  0 = Normal
  1 = Mildly abnormal (slow rate for age, mild hemispheric voltage asymmetry)
  2 = Markedly abnormal (epileptiform discharge)
Neurologic examination
  0 = Normal
  1 = Mildly abnormal (mild hyptonia)
  2 = Markedly abnormal (moderate or marked hypotonia or spasticity)
Etiology of initial seizure
  0 = Unknown, late hypocalcemia, electrolyte abnormalities
  1 = Early hypocalcemia, hypoglycemia, meconium aspiration, mild or chronic
      hypoxemia (5-min Apgar = 4–6), septicemia, drug withdrawal, subarachnoid
      hemorrhage, grade I or II IVH
  2 = Meningitis, severe hypoxemia (5-min Apgar < 3), cerebral malformation,
      grade III or IV IVH
Seizures since hospital discharge
  0 = None
  1 = Questionable
  2 = Definite
Birth weight
  0 = > 1,500 g
  1 = < 1,500 g
Scoring at 3 mo
  If 5 or less and on single anticonvulsant, discontinue the medication over 2–3 wk
  If 5 or less and on two anticonvulsants, continue one medication and reevaluate
    in 2 mo
  If 6 or more, continue anticonvulsants and reevaluate in 2 mo

EEG = electroencephalogram; IVH = intraventricular hemorrhage.
Adapted from P. H. Ellison. Management of seizures in the high-risk infant. *Clin. Perinatol.* 11 : 178, 1984.

infants whose anticonvulsant therapy should be extended beyond 3 months of age.

VI. Neurodevelopmental outcome

It is commonly accepted that infants with intracranial hemorrhage in the neonatal period do not fare as well as infants without hemorrhage. Results of early studies suggested notable impairments in both cognitive and motor function in infants with intracranial hemorrhage (Chaplin et al., 1980). With the more recent ability to detect lesser, asymptomatic hemorrhages and to follow the resolution of hemorrhage, the findings concerning outcome have been modified. Despite the difficulties encountered in comparing studies that have employed different grading systems for intracranial hemorrhage, infants with lesser grades of hemorrhage in general perform equally as well as infants without hemorrhage during the preschool years. It has become increasingly clear that hemorrhages associated with intraparenchymal involvement and hydrocephalus are most important in terms of neurodevelopmental morbidity (Dubowitz et al., 1984). Factors relating to ischemic changes in the germinal matrix and the periventricular white matter appear to be of major importance in identifying those infants with or without hemorrhage whose outcomes will be poor. The ultimate value of such identification lies in the appropriate utilization of services to maximize individual potential.

Because the most frequent impairments in infancy associated with major intracranial hemorrhage include vision and hearing loss, tone abnormalities, and cognitive defects, such infants should be screened with a complete ophthalmologic examination, as well as brainstem auditory evoked potentials, by 2 months of age. Serial neurologic examinations, looking specifically for evidence of increased flexor tone, hypertonia or hypotonia, poor head control, abnormal eye movements, or asymmetry may lead to early identification of infants who may benefit from a multidisciplinary intervention program. Neurodevelopmental assessments at 6 and 12 months' corrected age using formal tests such as the Bayley Scales of Infant Development may, in addition, identify infants in need of special services.

REFERENCES

Ahmann, P., Lazzara, A., Dykes, F., et al. Intraventricular hemorrhage in the high-risk preterm infant: Incidence and outcome. *Ann. Neurol.* 7 : 118, 1980.

Allan, W., Dransfield, D., and Tito, A. Ventricular dilatation following periventricular-intraventricular hemorrhage: Outcome at age one year. *Pediatrics* 73 : 158, 1984.

Bergman, I., Painter, M., Hirsch, R., et al. Outcome in neonates with convulsions treated in an intensive care unit. *Ann. Neurol.* 14 : 642, 1983.

Chaplin, E., Goldstein, G., Myerberg, D., et al. Posthemorrhagic hydrocephalus in the preterm infant. *Pediatrics* 65 : 901, 1980.

Dubowitz, L., Bydder, G., and Mushin, J. Developmental sequence of periventricular leucomalacia: Correlation of ultrasound, clinical, and NMR functions. *Arch. Dis. Child.* 60 : 349, 1985.

Dubowitz, L., Dubowitz, V., Palmer, P., et al. Correlation of neurologic assessment in the preterm infant with outcome at one year. *J. Pediatr.* 105 : 452, 1984.

Ellison, P. H. Management of seizures in the high-risk infant. *Clin. Perinatol.* 11 : 178, 1984.

Finer, N., Roberston, C., Richards, R., et al. Hypoxic-ischemic encephalopathy in term neonates: Perinatal factors and outcome. *J. Pediatr.* 98 : 112, 1981.

Haywood, R., Bryant, D., Payne, J., et al. Clinical NMR imaging of the brain in children: Normal and neurologic disease. *Am. J. Roentgenol.* 141 : 1005, 1983.

Hill, A., and Volpe, J. Normal pressure hydrocephalus in the newborn. *Pediatrics* 68 : 623, 1981.

Holden, K., Millits, E., and Freeman, J. Neonatal seizures. I. Correlation of prenatal and perinatal events with outcomes. *Pediatrics* 70 : 165, 1982.

Kruesser, L., Tarby, T., Kovnar, E., et al. Serial lumbar punctures for at least temporary amelioration of neonatal posthemorrhagic hydrocephalus. *Pediatrics* 75 : 719, 1985.

Lacey, D., and Terplan, K. Intraventricular hemorrhage in full-term neonates. *Dev. Med. Child Neurol.* 24 : 332, 1982.

Larroche, J. Post-haemorrhagic hydrocephalus in infancy: Anatomical study. *Biol. Neonate* 20 : 287, 1972.

Lorber, J., and Bhat, U. S. Posthemorrhagic hydrocephalus. *Arch. Dis. Child.* 20 : 287, 1972.

Mantovani, J., Pasternak, J., Mathew, D., et al. Failure of daily lumbar punctures to prevent the development of hydrocephalus following intraventricular hemorrhage. *J. Pediatr.* 97 : 278, 1980.

Ment, L., Scott, D., Ehrenkranz, R., and Duncan, C. Neurodevelopmental assessment of very low birthweight neonates: Effect of germinal matrix and intraventricular hemorrhage. *Pediatr. Neurol.* 1 : 164, 1985.

Odio, C., McCracken, G., Jr., and Nelson, J. CSF shunt infections in pediatrics. A seven-year experience. *Am. J. Dis. Child.* 138 : 1103, 1984.

Palmer, P., Dubowitz, L., Levene, M., and Dubowitz, V. Developmental and neurologic progress of preterm infants with intraventricular hemorrhage and ventricular dilatation. *Arch. Dis. Child.* 57 : 748, 1982.

Papile, L., Burstein, J., Burstein, R., et al. Posthemorrhagic hydrocephalus in low-birth-weight infants: Treatment by serial lumbar punctures. *J. Pediatr.* 97 : 273, 1980.

Papile, L., Munsick-Bruno, G., and Schaefer, A. Relationship of cerebral intraventricular hemorrhage and early childhood neurologic handicaps. *J. Pediatr.* 103 : 273, 1983.

Perlman, J., and Volpe, J. Intraventricular hemorrhage in extremely small premature infants. *Am. J. Dis. Child.* 140 : 1122, 1986.

Sauerbrei, E. Serial brain ultrasonography in two children with leucomalacia and cerebral palsy. *J. Can. Assoc. Radiol.* 35 : 164, 1984.

Shinnar, S., Gammon, K., Bergman, E., Jr., et al. Management of hydrocephalus in infancy: Use of acetazolamide and furosemide to avoid cerebrospinal fluid shunts. *J. Pediatr.* 107 : 31, 1985.

Tekolste, K., Bennett, F., and Mack, L. Follow-up of infants receiving cranial ultrasound for intracranial hemorrhage. *Am. J. Dis. Child.* 139 : 299, 1985.

Volpe, J. *Neurology of the Newborn.* Philadelphia: Saunders, 1987.

Volpe, J., Pasternak, J., and Allan, W. Ventricular dilatation preceding rapid head growth following neonatal intracranial hemorrhage. *Am. J. Dis. Child.* 131 : 1212, 1977.

22

Severe Perinatal Asphyxia

Mario Becker and H. William Taeusch

I. Introduction

Perinatal asphyxia accounts for more nonprogressive neurologic deficits seen in children than any other insult (Hill and Volpe, 1982). Although intrapartum asphyxia is established as an important cause of perinatal loss, there is nonetheless little consensus as to how much of the burden of neurologic handicap in the community can be attributed to intrapartum and neonatal asphyxia (Paneth and Stark, 1983). Best estimates of major neurologic handicap resulting from this condition are between 1 and 6 per 1,000 live births (Levene and Evans, 1985). Neonatal mortality from perinatal asphyxia is approximately 15 percent (Volpe et al., 1985).

II. Definition

There is little agreement on the definition of severe perinatal asphyxia (Table 22-1) (Brann, 1985). We define acute, severe perinatal asphyxia as a clinically evident hypoxic-ischemic episode in the perinatal period of sufficient severity to necessitate respiratory support and to be associated with nontrivial clinical problems in the week or so following the episode (i.e., post asphyxial encephalopathy). Common clinical and laboratory findings are listed in Table 22-2. Outcomes during early childhood after severe perinatal asphyxia have been described (Sarnat and Sarnat, 1976) and are listed in Table 22-3.

III. General management

Prevention of perinatal asphyxia by means of improving prediction of risk and use of tertiary perinatal services, fetal resuscitation, and immediate delivery is the primary goal but its discussion is beyond the scope of this chapter. Management after the fact is aimed at eliminating the underlying causes leading to asphyxia, reducing brain ischemia and edema, reducing the brain's metabolic requirements, and anticipating complications such as seizures, congestive heart failure, or inappropriate antidiuretic hormone secretion.

After discharge from the neonatal intensive care unit (NICU), the infant who has had an episode of asphyxia should be closely followed by a pediatrician who is aware of the infant's perinatal course and who is skilled in the organic, emotional, and social needs such an infant and family may present. Early detection of delayed progress should prompt early intervention. Depending on the specific needs of the child and family, management may include multiple professionals over the years (Table 22-4).

It is primarily the pediatrician who coordinates a multidisciplinary approach and makes it comprehensible for the family (Rubin, 1983a). Interdisciplinary evaluation processes vary in clinical settings, team composition, professional

Table 22-1. Asphyxia: Indicators and outcome

Indicators	Normal development (%)	Age at follow-up	Died (%)	Study
Prenatal, perinatal, and postnatal conditions associ- with asphyxia (e.g., maternal shock, neonatal respiratory disease) (n = 94)	26	21 mo	22	Brown et al., 1974
Fetal distress or Apgar score ≤ 5 at 1 or 5 min (n = 21)	57	6–12 mo	19	Sarnat and Sarnat, 1976
Apgar score 0 at 1 min or < 4 at 5 min (n = 31)	65	8 yr		Thomson et al., 1977
Abnormal neurologic examination and one or more of the following: intrapartum fetal distress, Apgar score < 5 at 1 or 5 min, immediate neonatal resuscitation (n = 95)	50	19 mo	7	Finer et al., 1981
Fetal distress; Apgar score <6 at 5 min; resuscitation; abnormal neurologic signs (n = 62)	43	18 mo	5	Fitzhardinge et al., 1981
Apgar score < 4 at 5 min (n = 116)	57[a], 45[b]	24 mo	21[a], 48[b]	Ergander et al., 1983
Abnormal neurologic examination and one or more of the following: intrapartum fetal distress, Apgar score ≤ 5 at 1 or 5 min, immediate neonatal resuscitation (n = 49)	57	12 mo	0	Finer et al., 1983
Abnormal neurologic examination and one or more of the following: intrapartum fetal distress, Apgar score < 5 at 1 or 5 min, immediate neonatal resuscitation (n = 167)	100[c], 79[d], 0[e]	44 mo	0[c], 5[d], 75[e]	Robertson and Finer, 1985
Intubation because of asphyxia; seizures; severe feeding problem; severe muscular tone abnormalities	23.5	4–7 yr	31.5	Becker et al. (in press)

[a]> 37 weeks' gestation.
[b]≤ 37 weeks' gestation.
[c]Mild hypoxic-ischemic encephalopathy.
[d]Moderate hypoxic-ischemic encephalopathy.
[e]Severe hypoxic-ischemic encephalopathy.

**Table 22-2. Clinical and laboratory findings
associated with perinatal asphyxia in the perinatal period**

Demography
  Family characteristics (mother's education, socioeconomic status, race)
Antepartum or intrapartum disorders
  Maternal cardiac arrest, shock, severe respiratory disease, or a combination of these
  Hemorrhage
  Placental insufficiency
  Cord tight around neck or occluded
  Fetal distress
Common clinical findings and diagnoses
  Low Apgar scores
  Seizures
  Abnormal reflexes
  Abnormal muscular tone
  Increased intracranial pressure
  Hydrocephalus
  Alterations of level of consciousness
  High-pitched "cerebral" cry
  Intracranial hemorrhage
  Abnormal pupillary reflex
  Hypothermia
  Apnea and/or hypoventilation often requiring ventilation
  Persistent fetal circulation
  Meconium aspiration syndrome
  Severe postpartum respiratory distress
  Increased secretion in respiratory pathways
  Cardiac dysfunction (failure, arrhythmia, tricuspid regurgitation)
  Feeding difficulties
  Necrotizing enterocolitis
  Persistent vomiting
  Gastrointestinal bleeding
  Increased gastrointestinal motility
  Diffuse intravascular coagulation
  Hearing loss
  Renal failure
Test results
  Abnormal electroencephalogram
  Abnormal brainstem auditory evoked potentials
  Abnormal brainstem visual evoked potentials
  Abnormal cerebral blood flow
  Abnormal acid-base and/or blood gas status
  Elevated enzymes (cardiac, hepatic, cerebrospinal fluid)
  Inappropriate secretion of antidiuretic hormone with hyponatremia
  Hypoglycemia
  Hyperglycemia
  Hypocalcemia
  Hematuria

Table 22-3. Possible clinical outcomes during early childhood after severe perinatal asphyxia

No abnormalities
Motor deficits (cerebral palsy)
  Spastic diplegia
  Spastic quadriplegia
  Spastic hemiplegia
  Choreoathetosis
  Ataxia
  Other dystonia
Behavioral issues
  Hyperactivity
  Attention deficit
  Self-injury
  Socialization disorders
  Emotional problems
  Sleep disorders
Intellectual disabilities
  Disorders of abstract reasoning
  Low IQ and DQ
Seizures
Sensory deficits
  Abnormal hearing
  Abnormal vision
Abnormal speech and language
Posthemorrhagic hydrocephalus
Microcephaly
Nutrition and gastrointestinal problems
  Feeding and eating difficulties
  Gastroesophageal reflux
  Recurrent vomiting
  Recurrent pneumonia and chronic aspiration
  Esophagitis
  Malnutrition
  Anemia
  Constipation
  Poor or excessive weight gain
  Sphincter control problems
Dental problems
Repeated urinary tract infections
Trauma

DQ = developmental quotient; IQ = intelligence quotient.

relationships among team members, and time interval between evaluations. Efficacy of different approaches has become increasingly difficult to evaluate. Consultants in psychology, physical therapy, or psychiatry, for example, usually believe (with some justification) that their services meet current primary management goals, are not intrusive or redundant, and certainly are cost-effective. For some families, the pediatrician, the neurologist, or the social worker must assume the role of "gate-keeper," so that the parents are not overwhelmed with interested, concerned, and expensive consultants. In some

Table 22-4. Assessments

Assessment	Professional
Child's general health	Pediatrician
Neurologic function	Neurologist, neurosurgeon
Motor function	Orthopedist, physical therapist, occupational therapist
Behavior	Developmental pediatrician, psychiatrist
Development	Psychologist
Sociofamilial situation	Social worker, psychiatrist
Community resources	Nurse, social worker
Vision	Ophthalmologist
Hearing	Audiologist
Speech and language	Speech-language pathologist
Dental health	Dentist
Education	Educator

areas of the United States and other countries, the opposite problem occurs: There is a paucity of professionals with special management expertise in the consequences of severe perinatal asphyxia, and the parents feel abandoned. The sum of the evaluations should be synthesized into an unified diagnosis and a long-term goal-oriented plan of management (Rubin, 1983a). This plan should be reviewed and updated periodically with the parents.

IV. Specific problems

A. Reflex abnormalities in the first year
Chronic central nervous system (CNS) dysfunction may become evident in the early months of life. Frequently noted are abnormally strong reflexes in the first 6 months of life and reflexes that persist beyond the time of their normal disappearance or inhibition (Palmer et al., 1983).
1. Moro reflex. The Moro reflex can be elicited by placing the infant in a supine position on a surface and allowing the head to fall back approximately 1 cm or by abruptly releasing both hands. The full response includes wide symmetric flinging of the arms, followed by symmetric flexion and adduction of the arms. There may be extension of the lower extremities. Normal infants frequently cry immediately after the response is provoked. An abnormally strong Moro reflex from perinatal asphyxia may interfere with almost all early motor achievements. The Moro reflex may be absent or asymmetric (related to hemiplegia, clavicular fracture or brachial plexus insult, or hypotonia) after severe perinatal asphyxia. In normal infants, the Moro reflex nearly disappears by 4 months of age.
2. Asymmetric tonic neck reflex (ATNR). The ATNR is easily elicited when the infant is supine. When the head is rotated 45 to 90 degrees to either side, there is active flexion of the extremities on the occipital side and extension on the chin side. The presence of a strong ATNR interferes with development of volitional rolling, sitting, and upper extremity midline activity. It may preclude development of propping ability of the infant (tripod sitting). Marked ATNR activity may give rise to falsely asym-

metric deep tendon reflexes and abnormal Babinski sign. The child's head should therefore be held in midline while evaluating these reflexes. The ATNR is normally most prominent from 4 to 6 months of age and rapidly decreases thereafter. Sustained obligatory responses are virtually never seen in normal children at any age (Palmer et al., 1983).

3. Tonic labyrinthine (TL) reflexes in supine and prone positions. To elicit the TL reflex in the supine position, the child's neck is hyperextended while he or she is held supine. The TL supine reflex consists of the trunk and lower extremities' tonic extension with tonic shoulder adduction, generally with elbow flexion. The TL reflex in the prone position is elicited by flexing the child's neck while he or she is held in the prone position. The TL prone reflex shows active flexion of trunk and lower extremities and active protraction of shoulders.

Strong TL reflexes interfere with the development of upper extremity weight bearing on extended arms in the prone position when head and neck are extended. The TL supine reflex has developmental patterns that are similar to the ATNR. Active flexion of trunk and lower extremities when the head is flexed in the prone position persists well into the second year of life. If the TL supine reflex is active, the infant is unable to roll over retracted shoulders (Palmer et al., 1983). Overlap with the symmetric tonic neck reflex and the Landau righting reaction makes TL prone reflex evaluation difficult. Tonic trunk extension interferes with development of segmental truncal derotation, a postural response (Palmer et al., 1983). The TL supine reflex may interfere with volitional rolling from the supine position, stable sitting, and propping reactions. True decerebrate posturing (truncal and lower extremity extension, shoulder retraction, upper extremity extension), not seen in normal children, may be related to TL supine reflex (Palmer et al., 1983).

4. Placing reflexes. The placing reflexes are elicited by holding the infant in vertical suspension and touching the dorsum of the extremities to the edge of a surface. The extremities will flex and then extend over the surface. The abnormal persistence of placing reflexes may interfere with volitional mediated behavior. Placing reflexes are normally present in lower extremities at birth and in upper extremities by 3 months of age; thereafter, they merge into visually mediated volitional behavior (Palmer et al., 1983).

5. Landau reaction. The Landau reaction is elicited when the child is held in prone suspension. Voluntary head and neck extension is followed by truncal extension. Hip and knee extension may also occur. An immature Landau reaction may interfere with volitional rolling and independent sitting. Reflexive flexion in the prone position seen with an obligatory TL prone reflex does not allow expression of this reaction. The Landau should always be present after 9 months of age (Menkes, 1984; Palmer et al., 1983).

B. Intellectual disabilities and early schooling

Assessing intellectual capacity after severe perinatal asphyxia is often complicated by motor problems and less often by hearing loss. Children with disabilities should be placed in the least restrictive environments consistent with their needs. Placement decisions should be made on the basis of multidimensional and nonbiased assessment. Evaluations of the preschool child can be difficult, particularly if home experiences have been limited. Available resources for these children are shown in Table 22-5.

Principles of management of intellectual disabilities have been summarized by Neuman (1983) and include avoiding preconceptions, recognizing the child's defense mechanisms, ensuring good communication, using standard measures for assessment, and considering both teaching and learning difficulties.

Infants warrant regular monitoring of development after any major perinatal insult. Bayley Scales of Infant Development are probably most frequently used in infants less than 2½ years of age. If a child shows delays after this age, more formal intelligence testing is required. Children with

Table 22-5. Resources for pupils with cerebral palsy or intellectual impairment

Appropriate pupils	Placement (from least to most restrictive)
Full, normal intelligence; no major specific learning disability or communication or sensory handicap (degree of motor involvement less important)	Regular class with adaptations and consultation
Normal or near-normal intelligence; mild, specific learning disability or mild-to-moderate communication, hearing, or visual handicap	As above, but with tutorial or resource room support for academics
Normal or near-normal IQ; moderate-to-severe learning disabilities or severe communication or sensory handicap (also mildly retarded)	Self-contained special class; some mainstreaming when appropriate
All cognitive levels; serious sensory or emotional handicap, unintelligible speech, poorly controlled seizure disorder	Self-contained class within public school; minimal interaction with normal peers
Needs that cannot be met in local district because district is small or pupil needs many specialized services	Regional or collaborative class or private day school program
All degrees of handicap; needs cannot be met at home	Combination of foster, group, or pediatric nursing home and day school in community
Severely multihandicapped children who need nursing care; short-term alternative for others	Private residential school, state institution, or pediatric home with stimulation program
Not appropriate except on interim basis	Home or hospital tutoring

IQ = intelligence quotient.
From J. M. Zadig, The Education of the Child with Cerebral Palsy. In G. H. Thompson, I. L. Rubin, and R. M. Bilenker (eds.), *Comprehensive Management of Cerebral Palsy*. New York: Grune & Stratton, 1983. Pp. 319–330. With permission.

developmental delay often have attention problems and behavior disorders. Table 22-6 lists nonverbal intelligence scales and tests used for children with communication difficulties.

Zadig writes:

If the error of other times was that handicapped infants were snatched from their families at an age when all children are helpless and placed in environments that could not meet their developmental needs, the error of these times may be that society assumes that every "good" parent will be able to cope indefinitely with a severely handicapped child. (Zadig, 1983)

C. Motor deficits
Cerebral palsy (CP) is a frequent outcome after severe perinatal asphyxia. Infants with orthopedic deformities such as instability, malalignment, contracture, and imbalance need the assistance of an orthopedist to preserve function, correct deformity, and relieve pain (Shapiro et al., 1983). A comprehensive treatise on the management of cerebral palsy from all causes has recently been published (Thompson, 1983).

D. Seizures
Management of the asphyxiated infant with seizures should include serial tests of CNS function, linked with family support and specific therapy. The infant's history; developmental, physical, and neurologic examinations; and special evaluations are most useful when carried out sequentially by the same professionals. The history should include family, gestational, perinatal, and postnatal factors. Review of development should include motor, social, language, and nonlanguage problem solving, with close attention to the nature and degree of delay, deficits, or both. Head circumference, weight, and height, considered together, deserve special attention for early detection of hydrocephalus or microcephaly. Neurologic examination should include close study of posture, gait, abnormal movements, muscle tone, bulk, and strength; primitive and deep tendon reflexes; postural responses; sensory evaluations; and cranial nerve function. Special evaluations include brain imaging (magnetic resonance imaging, computed tomography scan, or ultrasonography), angiography, skull radiographs, electroencephalogram, electromyogram, brainstem auditory evoked potentials, brainstem visual evoked potentials, nerve conduction time, and metabolic investigations. Complete blood count, studies of serum electrolytes and liver and kidney function, and urinalysis may be necessary for

Table 22-6. Standard measures: Nonverbal scales and tests

Scale or test	Appropriate mental age (yr)
Leiter International Performance Scale	2–7½
Columbia Mental Maturity Scale	3–9
Hiskey Nebraska Test of Learning Aptitude	3–16
Normed toys	At any age

Adapted from S. S. Neuman, Intellectual Disabilities. In G. H. Thompson, I. L. Rubin, and R. M. Bilenker (eds.), Comprehensive Management of Cerebral Palsy. New York: Grune & Stratton, 1983. Pp. 151–156.

monitoring adverse drug reactions. Once a child is started on antiseizure drugs, blood levels should be checked.

Length of treatment depends on the presence of neurologic signs and the results of the electroencephalogram. At the present time, barbiturates are the preferred first agents because of their "protective effect" (Brann, 1985).

Recurrent seizures that continue into childhood cause problems ranging from side effects of anticonvulsant drugs to prejudices that make it difficult for the child to adjust to the underlying disability. Long-term effects on behavior and learning from antiseizure drugs are unknown (Shapiro et al., 1983). The unpredictable nature of seizure episodes may cause anxiety and emotional difficulties in both child and parents.

E. Hearing loss

Hearing loss associated with CP is almost always sensorineural. Available data suggest that prevalence of marked hearing loss in children with CP is at least 20 times that in general pediatric population. Communication handicaps may be related to dysarthria, oral dyspraxia, voice production, or central language dysfunction (Yost and McMillan, 1983). Thorough hearing evaluation and appropriate hearing-aid fitting may extend over many months.

Observation of reflexive behavior and classic and operant conditioning techniques can usually be used for audiologic evaluation. Motor involvement may obscure subtle behavioral responses to sound in the infant and prevent the use of standard test techniques in older children. Impedance audiometry typically can be used although the child may exhibit uncontrolled movements. Visual problems or developmental delay may complicate the audiologic diagnosis and habilitation process. Auditory brainstem response audiometry can be used to estimate physiologic hearing threshold. Auditory brainstem responses are useful in the absence of or as a confirmation of responses obtained with behavioral audiometry. Because cooperation and sedation are necessary, measurements in some children with brain damage can be misleading. The presence of cortical auditory evoked responses indicate that the anatomic pathway is intact. Children with CP who are not deaf but are unable to speak present a special problem. They may have normal responses to behavioral impedance audiometry. In some severely impaired patients, early components of auditory evoked potentials, which reflect eighth nerve and brainstem activity, are normal, but late components, which reflect cortical activity, are abnormal (Alvarez, 1983).

Parents' acceptance of hearing loss and hearing aids is important for the child's adjustment to the hearing handicap and habilitation. Life span of hearing aids for active children approximates 3 to 5 years and auditory evoked potentials may be used to assess the benefits of the hearing aid. Annual audiologic reevaluation is generally indicated. Sign language can be used by hearing-impaired children with CP, although modification may be needed to maximize the ability to communicate of a child with major visual or motor problems. Altered signs, a tactile-manual sign language, and other communication systems, some involving electronic equipment, can be used (Yost and McMillan, 1983).

F. Abnormal vision

Management should include the infant's history, external eye examination, fundoscopy, determination of intraocular pressure, and screening tests. External eye examination should evaluate head posture, orbit symmetry, eyelids, conjunctiva, cornea, retina, eye position and movements, anterior chamber, iris, cataracts, pupillary response to light, accommodation, refraction, nystagmus, amblyopia, strabismus, stereoacuity, fusion potential, visual acuity, and binocular vision. Tests should include Allen Eye Chart, illiterate E or alphabet chart, communication board for the infant with impaired speech, Sheridan Test for Young Children and Retardates (STYCAR), preferential looking testing, and visual evoked potentials. Screening tests are aimed at evaluating ocular motor defects, corneal light reflexes, ocular rotation, and vision (Manning et al., 1982; Mayer et al., 1982; Mitchell, 1983).

G. Abnormal speech and language

Educating parents about normal speech, language auditory development, and expected development for cerebrally injured infants may be helpful. The speech-language pathologist's role may include assessment of attention span and eye contact, positioning for respiration and phonation, and speech quality. Palatal lifts may be helpful. In recent years, with nonverbal or severely unintelligible children, the trend has been to introduce nonverbal communication modes early (Yost et al., 1983).

H. Nutrition and gastrointestinal problems

The process of eating necessitates intact oral structures and oral motor control to ingest food and liquids as well as established hand-to-mouth pattern and utensil use for self-feeding. Oral-motor deficits can cause feeding and eating difficulties. An occupational therapist can assess self-feeding abilities and provide necessary equipment and training that make the child more independent (Lawlor and Zielinski, 1983).

Gastroesophageal reflux, a not uncommon source of recurrent vomiting, is more common in severely impaired children. It may result in aspiration pneumonia, chronic wheezing, esophagitis, malnutrition, anemia, and failure to thrive. If symptoms persist, diagnostic studies including barium swallow with upper gastrointestinal series technetium 99m gastric emptying scintiscan, overnight pH probe studies, esophagoscopy, and esophageal biopsy should be conducted. Even so, a single sensitive and specific diagnostic test to detect disorders of reflux and chronic aspiration is lacking. Medical management includes positioning the infant upright during waking hours, elevating the head of the bed 6 in., feeding four to six small meals daily (for infants), administering postprandial and bedtime antacids, withholding food or liquid 3 hours before bedtime, and placing the infant in the prone position for sleeping. The upright prone position may be most effective. Metoclopramide may be helpful if gastric emptying is inadequate or insufficiently rapid. The surgical technique most frequently used is Nissen gastroesophageal fundoplication (Sondheimer and Morris, 1979).

Constipation is common in infants with severe CP and retardation. For unclear reasons, they may have poor colonic motility. Stools positive for occult blood or of narrow caliber suggest injury possibly following necrotizing enterocolitis. Severe constipation can lead to bladder compression and subsequent stress incontinence (McNeal et al., 1983). Frequently, bowel function is improved with dietary changes—specifically, increased fiber. Attention should be directed to drugs that could cause constipation (e.g., aluminum-containing antacids).

I. Repeated urinary tract infections
Renal failure or neurogenic bladder or both associated with severe perinatal asphyxia may lead to repeated urinary tract infections.

J. Immunization
Infants with severe CNS damage should be routinely immunized at the usual ages. Pertussis immunization should be withheld if seizures are poorly controlled or if CNS signs and symptoms are changing (American Academy of Pediatrics, 1982).

V. Prognosis
Prognosis is uncertain after severe perinatal asphyxia. Although the assessment before age 2 years does not accurately predict late outcome, there are significant correlations between abnormalities at that age and later outcome (Amiel-Tison and Ellison, 1986). A variety of studies have attempted to correlate outcome with some measures of neonatal asphyxia (see Table 22-1).

Investigators have used indicators that may be *predictors* of asphyxia (e.g., abnormal fetal heart tracings), measurements that may *reflect* acute asphyxia (e.g., low Apgar scores or low cord blood pH), or measures that may indicate acute (serum and cerebrospinal fluid lactic dehydrogenase or serum creatine phosphokinase) or subacute (neonatal motor problems or seizures) *consequences* of asphyxia. Delineation of prognosis is hindered by difficulties in establishing factors that help define risk. We estimate that approximately 50 percent of infants who survive after meeting criteria for severe perinatal asphyxia will have one or more major problems attributable to asphyxia during the first years of life. Perinatal factors related to poor outcome include prolonged intrapartum asphyxia, persistence of abnormal neurologic signs, low socioeconomic status, administration of two or more anticonvulsant drugs, neonatal convulsions, mechanical ventilation, and lengthy NICU stay (Robertson and Finer, 1985). Favorable signs are rapid initial improvement in neurologic status, normal interictal electroencephalogram, or rapid return of electroencephalogram to normal (Hill and Volpe, 1981).

The prognosis following neonatal seizures associated with asphyxia of the fetus or newborn has been extensively documented and has improved in the past 15 years. Among more than 1,000 full-term infants in a composite series taken from reports published before and after 1969, the mortality of infants with neonatal seizures decreased from 40 to 15 percent, while the incidence of neurologic sequelae in survivors remained about 35 percent (Hill and Volpe, 1981). Some authors have suggested that the prognosis after asphyxia is improved for preterm infants compared with full-term infants (Volpe et al.,

1985). Evidence indicates that large discrepancies exist in incidence of severe asphyxia and the outcome of survivors, depending on the quality and sophistication of care (Rubin, 1983b).

Improved outcomes are related to improved prevention, recognition, and management of perinatal asphyxia, as well as optimal multidisciplinary follow-up care for infants with asphyxia.

REFERENCES

Allan, W. C., and Volpe, J. J. Periventricular-intraventricular hemorrhage. *Pediatr. Clin. North Am.* 33 : 47, 1986.

Alvarez, N. Neurologic Examination. In G. H. Thompson, I. L. Rubin, and R. M. Bilenker (eds.), *Comprehensive Management of Cerebral Palsy.* New York: Grune & Stratton, 1983. P. 113.

American Academy of Pediatrics. Report of the Committee on Infectious Diseases. Baltimore, 1982. Pp. 24, 202.

Amiel-Tison, C., and Ellison, P. Birth asphyxia in the fullterm newborn: Early assessment and outcome. *Dev. Med. Child Neurol.* 28 : 671, 1986.

Becker, M., Taeusch, H. W., Jr., Duffy, F. H., et al. Outcome at four to seven years after severe perinatal asphyxia. In press.

Brann, A. W., Jr. Factors During Neonatal Life That Influence Brain Disorders. In J. M. Freeman (ed.), *Prenatal and Perinatal Factors Associated with Brain Disorders.* Washington, D.C.: National Institutes of Health, 1985. Pp. 304, 305, 317, 318.

Brown, J. K., Purvis, R. J., Forfar, J. O., and Cockburn, F. Neurological aspects of perinatal asphyxia. *Dev. Med. Child Neurol.* 16 : 567, 1974.

Ergander, U., Eriksson, M., and Zetterstrom, R. Severe neonatal asphyxia. Incidence and prediction of outcome in the Stockholm area. *Acta Paediatr. Scand.* 72 : 321, 1983.

Finer, N. N., Robertson, C. M., Peters, K. L., and Coward, J. H. Factors affecting outcome in hypoxic-ischemic encephalopathy in term infants. *Am. J. Dis. Child.* 137 : 21, 1983.

Finer, N. N., Robertson, C. M., Richards, R. T., et al. Hypoxic-ischemic encephalopathy in term neonates: Perinatal factors and outcome. *J. Pediatr.* 98 : 112, 1981.

Fitzhardinge, P. M., Flodmark, O., Fitz, C. R., and Asby, S. The prognostic value of computed tomography as an adjunct to assessment of the term infant with postasphyxial encephalopathy. *J. Pediatr.* 99 : 777, 1981.

Gottfried, H. W. Intellectual consequences of perinatal anoxia. *Psychol. Bull.* 80 : 231, 1973.

Hall, R. T., Kulkarni, P. B., Sheehan, M. B., and Rhodes, P. G. Cerebrospinal fluid lactate dehydrogenase in infants with perinatal asphyxia. *Dev. Med. Child Neurol.* 22 : 300, 1980.

Hill, A., and Volpe, J. J. Seizures, hypoxic-ischemic brain injury, and intraventricular hemorrhage in the newborn. *Ann. Neurol.* 10 : 109, 1981.

Hill, A., and Volpe, J. J. Hypoxic-ischemic brain injury in the newborn. *Semin. Perinatol.* 6 : 25, 1982.

Jacobs, I. B. Epilepsy. In G. H. Thompson, I. L. Rubin, and R. M. Bilenker (eds.), *Comprehensive Management of Cerebral Palsy.* New York: Grune & Stratton, 1983. Pp. 131–137.

Lawlor, M. C., and Zielinski, A. Occupational Therapy. In G. H. Thompson, I. L. Rubin, and R. M. Bilenker (eds.), *Comprehensive Management of Cerebral Palsy.* New York: Grune & Stratton, 1983. Pp. 188–189, 203.

Levene, M. I., and Evans, D. H. Medical management of raised intracranial pressure after severe birth asphyxia. *Arch. Dis. Child.* 60 : 12, 1985.

Lipper, E. G., Voorhies, T. M., Ross, G., et al. Early predictors of one-year outcome for infants asphyxiated at birth. *Dev. Med. Child Neurol.* 28 : 303, 1986.

Manning, K. A., Fulton, A. B., Hansen, R. M., et al. Preferential looking vision testing: Application to evaluation of high-risk, prematurely born infants and children. *J. Pediatr. Ophthalmol. Strabismus* 19 : 286, 1982.

Mayer, D. L., Fulton, A. B., and Hansen, R. M. Preferential looking acuity obtained with a staircase procedure in pediatric patients. *Invest. Ophthalmol. Vis. Sci.* 23 : 538, 1982.

McNeal, D. M., Hawtrey, C. E., Wolraich, M. L., and Mapel, J. R. Symptomatic neurogenic bladder in a cerebral-palsied population. *Dev. Med. Child Neurol.* 25 : 612, 1983.

Menkes, J. H. Neurologic Evaluation of the Newborn Infant. In M. E. Avery and H. W. Taeusch (eds.), *Diseases of the Newborn*. Philadelphia: Saunders, 1984. Pp. 652–661.

Mitchell, P. R. Ophthalmologic Problems. In G. H. Thompson, I. L. Rubin, and R. M. Bilenker (eds.), *Comprehensive Management of Cerebral Palsy*. New York: Grune & Stratton, 1983. Pp. 139–150.

National Institutes of Health. Report on causes of mental retardation and cerebral palsy. Task Force on Joint Assessment of Prenatal and Perinatal Factors Associated with Brain Disorders. *Pediatrics* 76 : 457, 1985.

Neuman, S. S. Intellectual Disabilities. In G. H. Thompson, I. L. Rubin, and R. M. Bilenker (eds.), *Comprehensive Management of Cerebral Palsy*. New York: Grune & Stratton, 1983. Pp. 151–156.

Palmer, F. B., Shapiro, B. K., Wachtel, R. V., and Capute, A. J. Primitive Reflex Profile. In G. H. Thompson, I. L. Rubin, and R. M. Bilenker (eds.), *Comprehensive Management of Cerebral Palsy*. New York: Grune & Stratton, 1983. Pp. 171–179.

Paneth, N., and Stark, R. I. Cerebral palsy and mental retardation in relation to indicators of perinatal asphyxia. An epidemiologic overview. *Am. J. Obstet. Gynecol.* 147 : 960, 1983.

Robertson, C., and Finer, N. Term infants with hypoxic-ischemic encephalopathy: Outcome at 3.5 years. *Dev. Med. Child Neurol.* 27 : 473, 1985.

Rose, A. L., and Lombroso, C. T. Neonatal seizures: A study of clinical, pathological, and electroencephalographic features in 137 full-term babies with a long-term follow-up. *Pediatrics* 45 : 404, 1970.

Rubin, L. Perinatal Factors. In G. H. Thompson, I. L. Rubin, and R. M. Bilenker (eds), *Comprehensive Management of Cerebral Palsy*. New York: Grune & Stratton, 1983a. Pp. 57–58.

Rubin, L. The Role of the Pediatrician. In G. H. Thompson, I. L. Rubin, and R. M. Bilenker (eds.), *Comprehensive Management of Cerebral Palsy*. New York: Grune & Stratton, 1983b. Pp. 7–15.

Sarnat, H. B., and Sarnat, M. S. Neonatal encephalopathy following fetal distress. A clinical and electroencephalographic study. *Arch. Neurol.* 33 : 696, 1976.

Sattler, J. M. (ed.). Highlights of Assessment Management. *Assessment of Children's Intelligence and Special Abilities*. Boston: Allyn & Bacon, 1982. Pp. 608–622.

Shapiro, B. K., Palmer, F. B., Wachtel, R. C., and Capute, A. J. Associated Dysfunctions. In G. H. Thompson, I. L. Rubin, and R. M. Bilenker (eds), *Comprehensive Management of Cerebral Palsy*. New York: Grune & Stratton, 1983. Pp. 91–93.

Sondheimer, J. M., and Morris, B. A. Gastroesophageal reflux among severely retarded children. *J. Pediatr.* 94 : 710, 1979.

Thompson, G. H., Rubin, I. L., and Bilenker, R. M. (eds). *Comprehensive Management of Cerebral Palsy*. New York: Grune & Stratton, 1983.

Thomson, A. J., Searle, M., and Russell, G. Quality of survival after severe birth asphyxia. *Arch. Dis. Child.* 52 : 620, 1977.

Vohr, B. R., and Garcia Coll, C. T. Neurodevelopment and school performance of very-low-birth-weight infants: A seven-year longitudinal study. *Pediatrics* 76 : 345, 1985.

Volpe, J. J., Herscovitch, P., Perlman, J. M., et al. Positron emission tomography in the asphyxiated term newborn: Parasagittal impairment of cerebral blood flow. *Ann. Neurol.* 17 : 287, 1985.

Yost, J., and McMillan, P. Communication Disorders. In G. H. Thompson, I. L. Rubin, and R. M. Bilenker (eds.), *Comprehensive Management of Cerebral Palsy.* New York. Grune & Stratton, 1983. Pp. 160–166.

Zadig, J. M. The Education of the Child with Cerebral Palsy. In G. H. Thompson, I. L. Rubin, and R. M. Bilenker (eds.), *Comprehensive Management of Cerebral Palsy.* New York: Grune & Stratton, 1983. Pp. 319–330.

23

Communication Disorders

Anthony S. Bashir and Kristine E. Strand

I. Introduction: Aspects of normal speech and language development

The first 3 years of life are critical for the acquisition and development of speech and language abilities. These linguistic accomplishments parallel the development of cognitive and sensorimotor abilities. The child learns to see him- or herself as separate from the environment and capable of controlling it. The child learns about the independence of objects, the functions of objects, and the ways in which objects act on each other. This early learning forms the foundation for the development of language, a system through which the child represents what he or she knows about the world and intends to communicate.

The child participates actively in learning to speak. Initially, the child communicates through gazing, reaching, and vocalizing. Adults respond to these behaviors and help the child focus on the activity and communicate about the event. Interactions centered around activities are critical to the acquisition of communication skills.

An adult responds to what the child intends and helps the child by structuring the activity. An adult talks with a child using language to soothe, point out things, control, and explain. The adult often adapts his or her speech to the child by repeating, shortening the length of sentences, using words familiar to the child, and speaking slowly and with emphasis. An adult also provides information for the child by introducing and demonstrating new words and concepts.

The child must acquire a language system and a means for producing that system to become socially interactive and independent. The child learns words to mark events and entities in the environment as well as meaningful relationships between those events and entities (semantic learning). In addition, the child learns to order words into sentences that express relationships (syntactic learning). The child also learns to produce the sounds of the language (phonological or speech learning). The acquisition of language is developmental in nature, and individual variation in both acquisition and style exist. By 3 to 3½ years of age, children have learned the basic phonologic, syntactic, and semantic rules needed to communicate. Although the language system is still immature, 3-year-old children are generally intelligible and effective in questioning, challenging, reporting, and controlling the environment.

The acquisition and development of language occurs in a social context. Beginning in infancy, the child acquires the notion of conversation and turn-taking in dialogue. The child attempts to respond appropriately to conversations with others by selectively attending to the speaker's face, looking at the objects that are being talked about, smiling or laughing, and using simple gestures such as reaching, waving, and pointing. Gradually, words and sentences accompany and clarify these social responses. The child uses language to specify important events; request information, action, or clarification; make explanations; control the behavior of others and self; and assert his or her uniqueness and independence.

As part of language learning, the child develops the ability to alter his or her language styles from one situation to another. For example, the language of politeness is learned along with the appropriate situations in which to use such language. Similarly, a child learns to alter the choice of words and methods of presenting ideas to parents, grandparents, teachers, and peers. Learning to use language to accommodate social relationships continues throughout the school years.

Disorders of communication result from a wide variety of causes associated with acute and chronic medical, psychiatric, and developmental conditions. An impairment of communication is present when a person's speech deviates from what is acceptable to the social group. Communication is impaired when the manner of communication interferes with the speaker's ability to be understood or when attention is detracted from the intent of the message to the way in which the person is speaking. Disorders of communication have major effects on a child's social and emotional development. Also, the majority of children with notable preschool language disorders experience problems in later school learning, especially in reading and written language acquisition. This is not to say that aural-oral language deficits cause reading and writing disorders. Rather, it emphasizes that language deficits may occur along a continuum ranging from highly specific conditions to multiple handicapping conditions. For this reason and for the amelioration of the consequences of language impairment, early diagnosis and intervention are essential.

The presence of certain antecedent conditions may be used to determine the risk status of children for communication disorders. Predicting later developmental problems is difficult, however, because of the extended range of possible outcomes. For example, although advances in the treatment and management of children born prematurely have reduced severe developmental compromise, the developmental status of children who survive is variable. Because of the variability in developmental outcomes, assessment of sensory, cognitive, motor, and communicative abilities is essential for determining the child's status and needs.

The following is a discussion of the major communication disorders encountered in early childhood. In addition, suggestions for referral of children with suspected communication disorders are included.

II. Language disorders

A. Receptive language disorders
   1. *Receptive language* refers to the understanding of language—word meanings, word relationships, sentence structures (declarative, negative, interrogative)—and the social intent and context in which the message is heard. Underlying language comprehension is the ability to apply reasoning skills and to perceive presuppositional data assumed by the speaker, but not present in the message.

Disorders of receptive language are revealed in a wide array of deficits ranging from a complete inability to interpret any auditory stimulus to difficulty in extracting meaning from varying sentence forms. Thus, children with predominant disorders of receptive language have degrees of difficulty in symbol-object associations or relationships, in interpreting and distinguishing sentence types, and in interpreting social conversations.

2. Behaviors

The child with a receptive language disorder may exhibit some or all of the following:

a. The child appears to be hearing impaired but after repeated audiologic testing is found to have normal or near-normal hearing.

b. Affectively, the child relates and can enter into reciprocal relationships, but may appear shy and overdependent on his or her family.

c. Social skills are present, and the child, while employing social graces such as smiling and nodding, may give the erroneous impression of understanding what is said.

d. On psychologic assessment employing nonverbal instruments, the child generally demonstrates age-appropriate functioning. However, he or she may manifest problems in visual-motor, spatial, or integration abilities.

e. Variability is noted in the child's auditory processing skills (see III). These deficits are not viewed as causal to the symbolic language problem, but are seen as concomitant problems in the management of auditory information.

B. Disorders of auditory processing

As a child develops, he or she becomes increasingly skilled in activities such as attending to spoken messages, remembering what was said and in what order it was said, and in differentiating between sounds. Recent evidence suggests that the child's ability to attend to sound and to differentiate sounds and voices is present in infancy. This finding suggests an inherent organization of systems present innately that permits the child to sort and use acoustic information from the environment. The development of auditory skills is then dependent on the interaction of these innate abilities and the experiences the child has in his or her listening environment. The skills involved in organizing incoming auditory information are referred to as auditory processing or auditory perceptual skills.

Although there are many aspects to auditory processing, we discuss four areas of concern: attention, discrimination, figure-ground relationships, and sequential memory.

1. Auditory attention

Although some children demonstrate general attentional deficits, there are others for whom attending to auditory stimuli, verbal or nonverbal presents specific problems. A disruption of auditory attention should be described in terms of the task, the status of the child, and the desired behavioral outcome. One or more of the following may be seen in the child with a disorder in auditory attention:

   a. Distractible behaviors to irrelevant environmental stimuli
   b. Problems maintaining attending behavior
   c. Difficulty shifting from one task to another easily
   d. Rapid adaptation or inconsistent responses to auditory stimuli
2. Auditory discrimination
   The child becomes increasingly able to discriminate and categorize the similarities and differences between auditory stimuli as a function of experience with the sound environment and with maturation. This ability to discriminate and categorize acoustic events is referred to as *developmental auditory discrimination*. Children who demonstrate problems in auditory discrimination often have difficulty distinguishing sounds and may confuse words that are similar sounding (e.g., *milk* for *melt, grow* for *growl, knife* for *night*). Although deficits in the child's ability to discriminate between and among speech sounds has been regarded as a primary reason for articulation deficits and reading disabilities, recent research has questioned this assumption. Evaluation of auditory discrimination problems must realize the influence of factors such as

   The child's familiarity with the stimuli, either sounds or words
   The type of test and task presented to the child
   The child's knowledge of the language system
   The presence or absence of competing noise
   Auditory memory functions
   Hearing impairment

   The import of auditory discrimination problems is unclear, and the effects of auditory discrimination training are not clearly realized in improved speech or reading skills.
3. Auditory figure-ground relationships
   Persons developing normally are able to select the primary signal from a background of noise and to resist the distortion of that signal as the background noise increases or fluctuates.
   a. Some children, when placed in situations of increasing or fluctuating background noise, are unable (or evidence reduced abilities) to manage and understand speech signals.
   b. Auditory figure-ground difficulties in children are not necessarily evident under the normal one-to-one examination in a structured and quiet environment. Therefore, special on-site observations may be needed in addition to special auditory tests of speech perception in various noise conditions.
4. Auditory sequential memory deficits
   As a child develops, he or she is capable of remembering for short periods of time increased amounts of auditory information. Some children, however, have a specific deficit in their ability to retain auditory information on a short-term basis.
   A variety of different materials are used to assess immediate auditory sequential memory: digits, command series, and sentences. The child may perform differentially on these tasks. For example, a child may

have appropriate memory for digits but not for sentences. Such a child frequently reproduces the sentences in altered grammatic form that reflects his or her productive abilities to deal with the syntax. Other children may show equal reductions in all tasks. For some children, failure to recall data may be a function of their inability to preserve serial order. These children frequently replicate the original stimuli string but alter the order of elements. The importance of self-image, performance anxiety, and types of materials used in the assessment must be understood to evaluate performance accurately and plan remedial strategies.

C. Expressive language disabilities

Children with specific disorders of expressive language show a wide variety of oral language impairments. These deficits are described by considering the ways in which a child expresses ideas, feelings, and concepts in spoken verbal symbols.

In describing oral language skills in children, reference is made to the following areas:

Primary means of communication (i.e., signs, gestures, jargon, words, phrases, sentences)

The use of words for specification of objects and events and the relationships between them

The child's overall sentence-building and word-finding skills

Narrative appropriateness

Narrative elaboration and sequential organization

Deficits in sentence formulation, word-finding, and narrative are covered in the following discussions.

1. Sentence formulation deficits

Sentence formulation deficits are seen as a basic disruption in the child's ability to use the rules of syntax in a manner commensurate with mental age. The following behavioral profile is seen in children with sentence formulation deficits.

a. Hearing is normal or near normal.

b. Receptive language skills are usually within normal limits; depending on the tests used, however, specific areas of understanding (e.g., the language of time, the language of space, certain grammatic constructions) may be reduced.

c. The child relates and can be engaged in reciprocal activities.

d. The child uses a gestural, representational system, possibly in conjunction with attempts to communicate through words or phrases.

e. The child uses only single words or telegraphic syntax (e.g., "boy push girl truck"), has problems with the use of tense and number, has difficulty forming questions that begin with words such as what and why, and uses irregular forms of grammar.

f. Language milestones are frequently delayed.

g. On psychologic assessment employing nonverbal measurements of intellectual levels, the child functions within normal limits; problems in visual motor-spatial integration, however, may be present.

h. The child demonstrates an inability to adapt language to diverse social contexts and interactions.

i. Problems with word-finding skills and narrative organization and development are present.

2. Word-finding disorders

Word-finding disorders represent a momentary inability on the part of the child to recall the name of an object or event for which he or she has previous knowledge. It is most commonly observed under confrontation situations of naming, answering questions, or in prolonged explanations. One or more of the following behaviors may be associated with word-finding disorders.

Parents report, "He can't say what he wants," "I can't follow her stories," or "It's like it's on the tip of his tongue and he just can't get it out."

During confrontation naming of pictures or objects, the child evidences increased latencies of response time.

The child attempts to represent words using gestures that conform to the object's shape, features, or uses.

The child speaks in definitions, descriptions, or illusions.

The child uses associated labels (e.g., *rain* for *umbrella*, *fish scooper* for *pelican*, *smoke* for *pipe*).

The child uses a word that sounds similar to the one sought after (e.g., *slow* for *low*, *tornado* for *volcano*).

The child mixes the phonemic sequences (e.g., *donimo* for *domino*, *nirosus* for *rhinoceros*).

The child communicates in indefinite narratives in which only illusion is present.

The child may become dysfluent and needs to be carefully managed before true stuttering is established. Although word retrieval skills often improve with age, many of these children develop concomitant written language disorders in the middle and upper schools.

3. Narrative deficits

Children may show evidence of narrative deficits and may have difficulties in one or more of the following ways:

a. The child is unable to comment on content or shows reduced storytelling skills.

b. The child has difficulty elaborating on a story or speaks only in the most concrete and basic way about events.

c. The child has difficulty maintaining organizational features and seems to ramble and build incoherent narratives. Parents often comment, "If I didn't know what she was talking about, I wouldn't understand her."

d. The child has problems in word-finding, serial order development, coherency, and intention, which compound the problems of narrative organization.

D. Treatment

Management of language-impaired children varies depending on the degree and types of deficits present. For some children, cognitive play approaches may be used, in which symbolic play activities help the child acquire the abilities to represent events with objects and actions and from there use language. Some children may require behavioral approaches. Still others may require compensatory strategies for dealing with formulation problems or special self-contained classrooms for language learning.

The consequences of language impairments are grave. They significantly disrupt social growth and development, limit the child's adaptive skills, and interfere with the expression of emotions as well as with assertion of the self as a controlling agent in the environment. Many children with early language impairment develop additional problems in reading and written language in school. The need for early assessment and treatment is obvious.

III. Articulation disorders

Disorders of speech sound production or articulation disorders are the most common communication problem. Disorders of articulation are characterized by the following four types of error patterns:

Substitution errors (e.g., *wabbit* for *rabbit*)
Omission errors (e.g., *boo* for *book*)
Addition errors (an extra sound placed inappropriately in a word)
Distortion errors, such as a lateral lisp

The following is constructed on the work of Templin (1957) and provides an age-approximate schedule for the acquisition of speech sounds.

AGE (YR)	SPEECH SOUNDS
3*	m, n, ng, p, f, h, w
3.6	y as in *you*
4	k, b, d, g, r
4.6	s, sh, ch
6	t, th-voiced (as in *the*), v, l
7	th-voiceless (as in *thistle*), z, zh, dz

Speech sound production errors may vary from one speech sample to another: The child may be capable of producing a sound in one word context but not in another. The number of types of consonants and vowels that are misarticulated may vary. The child's production may be so limited as to preclude intelligible speech.

The causes of articulation deficits are heterogeneous. Indeed, one factor may not explain the disorder. A complex of interacting variables may be present and explain the child's inability to produce intelligible speech (e.g., cleft lip and palate; dysarthria associated with spastic-quadriplegia cerebral palsy). Factors contributing to disorders of articulation include

Chronic middle-ear disease
Sensorineural hearing impairment

*All vowels are 75 percent correct in production by age 3.

Structural disorders of the oral cavity
Central nervous system dysfunction as revealed in the dyspraxias
Central nervous system dysfunction as revealed in the dysarthrias
Peripheral nervous system dysfunction as seen in the dysarthrias
Mislearning of speech sounds
Oral sensory changes
Changes in the way speech sounds are perceptually managed

Factors such as deficient speech models in the environment, a lack of appropriate stimulation, reduced motivation to speak, and disruption in self-image also can contribute to disorders of articulation.

IV. Voice disorders
Voice disorders represent a deviation in the quality, pitch, or loudness of the voice. The basis of these deficits may be psychologic, physiologic, or both.

A. The most common causes of voice disorders in children are
   1. Vocal abuse from excessive talking, yelling, or singing, which most often leads to vocal nodules
   2. Vocal misuse (e.g., speaking at an inappropriate pitch or loudness level), which most often leads to vocal nodules
   3. Allergy, which most often leads to edema of the laryngeal tissue and membranes
   4. Nonmalignant growths (e.g., juvenile papillomas)

B. Not all voice disorders are the result of structural changes.
   1. Psychogenic explanations can also result in voice disorders. (Voice disorders are noted in psychogenic aphonia.)
   2. Anxiety can cause increased tension of the extrinsic and intrinsic laryngeal musculature; this may, in turn, lead to structural changes.
   3. A child's expression of aggression or anger may result in the use of an unusually high or low vocal intensity and may place a burden on the laryngeal structures.
   4. Persistence of prepubescent voice in the male adolescent may signal problems with emotional growth and development.

C. Management of voice disorders varies according to the underlying cause.
   1. Initially, referral should be made to an otolaryngologist for examination of the laryngeal structures and tissues.
   2. The voice itself should be assessed by a qualified speech and language pathologist.
   3. On the basis of these examinations, decisions regarding conservative management with medications or voice therapy or surgical management with subsequent vocal reeducation can be made. For example, allergies or juvenile papillomas are managed medically and surgically, with voice reeducation following. In contrast, vocal nodules are treated with noninvasive methods: Voice therapy and vocal reeducation bring about changes in the underlying tissue.

  D. The general goals of voice therapy include
    1. Monitoring and manipulating vocal use in varying speaking contexts
    2. Providing new methods of voice use and techniques for appropriate vocal behavior
    3. Preventing recurrence of the disorder

V. Resonance disorders
Resonance disorders are deficits arising from a disruption in the normal sound balance and are most commonly heard as hypernasality or hyponasality.

  The separation and coupling of the oral and nasal cavities is necessary for speech sound production. The relationships between the cavities are regulated through the effective functioning of the velopharyngeal mechanism. Varying degrees of velopharyngeal closure are needed to maintain appropriate production of the consonants and vowels, with the exception of *m*, *n*, and *ng*. For these three speech sounds, the oral and nasal cavities are coupled.

  A. The principal causes of disturbances in resonance are
    1. Incompetence of the velopharyngeal mechanism, giving rise to hypernasality
    2. Obstruction of the nasal passageways or nasopharyngeal space, giving rise to hyponasality

  B. A child with chronic hyponasality or sudden, unexplained hyponasality should be referred to an otolaryngologist for medical or surgical management. Speech therapy is not indicated for treatment of hyponasality. Hyponasality results from
    1. Nasal and nasopharyngeal obstructions
    2. Enlargement of the adenoids
    3. Chronic allergic conditions with subsequent edema of the mucosal linings

  C. Hypernasality results from velopharyngeal insufficiency or inefficiency caused by the following:

    Abnormal formation of the velum and palate as seen in complete and partial clefts of the palate, submucous clefts, or congenital foreshortening of the velum
    Injury or postsurgical complications
    Weakness or paralysis of the soft palate and pharyngeal functions owing to neurologic damage (e.g., as in pseudobulbar palsy, peripheral neuropathies, or acute myopathies)

    The primary results of the insufficiency are an increase in nasal tone or nasal emission of air, a decrease in ability to maintain intraoral breath pressure, and, in general, nasalized vowels and distorted or misarticulated consonants.

D. Management of velopharyngeal incompetence is best accomplished by an interdisciplinary team including surgeons, speech-language pathologists, otolaryngologists, nurses, and dentists. Management goals must consider both morphologic and psychologic developmental changes. Advantages and disadvantages of surgical management or more conservative management (i.e., speech therapy) must be carefully weighed before determining treatment.

VI. Disorders of fluency
Disorders of fluency are characterized by the presence of inappropriate rates of speech (too fast or too slow), disruption of flow of speech, and disturbance in rhythm of speech (tempo). The most common disorder of fluency is stuttering. Stuttering is a complex disorder of communication, characterized by alteration in the flow and production of speech as well as by the development of communication anxiety and fear. As the child develops, the child's beliefs and attitudes about his or her communication abilities change, and the extent and varieties of his or her social interactions change. Parents, peers, and others often will place undue stress on the child or create unreasonable performance expectations.

A. Parents' concern about the child's fluency occurs during the second or third year of life.
   1. Parents should be helped to understand the situations in which the child demonstrates dysfluent speech.
   2. Parents should be encouraged not to overrespond to the dysfluent speech and not to make suggestions to slow down, repeat the sentence without stuttering, or take a deep breath before talking.
   3. Parents should be assisted in providing both attention to their child as the child speaks and models of speaking that provide appropriate sentences.
   4. If dysfluencies persist for 2 to 3 weeks, the child and parents should be referred to a qualified speech-language pathologist for consultation.

B. The following are danger signs of stuttering behavior (Walle, 1985). They are ordered from least to most severe.
   1. Multiple repetitions of syllables, words, and phrases
   2. Unstressed vowel (e.g., "uh, uh, uh")
   3. Prolongation of sounds
   4. Tremor and arrhythmia in the voice
   5. Rises in pitch as child tries to "get unstuck"
   6. Struggle with muscle tension
   7. Fear
   8. Avoidance of speech

C. To understand and treat stuttering one must know the following:
   1. Underlying factors that contribute to dysfluencies (e.g., environmental stress, language competence, emotional adaptation)
   2. Situations that cause or maintain dysfluent speech
   3. Changes in the way speech is produced

D. Treatment for dysfluency varies depending on its severity and the child's age. Therapy includes varying emphasis on activities to alter
   1. Speech production
   2. Attitudes toward communication
   3. Patterns of interaction between the child and the child's environment

E. Dysfluent speech poses a major threat to a person's sense of self and comfort within the social group. Early referral to and treatment by a qualified speech-language pathologist are critical factors in success.

VII. Referral
When should a pediatrician be concerned and refer a child to the speech-language pathologist for speech and language assessment? The following are some guidelines:

A. An 18-month-old child should be referred if the child
   1. Does not appear to understand common words and commands, such as "Come here," "Where's your blanket?" or "Sit down."
   2. Does not use any true words
   3. Does not use any expressive jargon
   4. Uses only vowels or a single syllable (e.g., "da") when vocalizing
   5. Does not specifically indicate what he or she wants by pointing or gesturing with vocalization

B. A 2-year-old child should be referred if the child
   1. Does not use single words to ask for things
   2. Does not follow simple directions to get items that are out of sight

C. A 2½-year-old child should be referred if the child
   1. Does not have several true two-word combinations that combine two ideas (e.g., "no cookie," "more juice," "me go," "daddy car")
   2. Uses primarily gestures (possibly an elaborate gesture system) to communicate
   3. Is often misunderstood or not understood at all (these are children for whom verbal communication may be a specific source of frustration)

D. A 3-year-old child should be referred if the child
   1. Uses no simple sentences
   2. Cannot understand simple explanations or discussions of any past or future events (by age 3, a child understands certain aspects of expressed time)
   3. Is unintelligible

E. A child should be referred *at any age* if the child
   1. Shows no interest in communicating with others
   2. Speaks in a monotone, extremely loudly, or inaudibly
   3. Has a noticeable hypernasal, hyponasal, or other unusual voice quality
   4. Is embarrassed or frustrated by his or her speech

F. All children whose speech and language status is questioned should have a hearing assessment, preferably by a certified audiologist with specific pediatric experience and training.

REFERENCES

Berko-Gleason, J. *The Development of Language.* Columbus, Ohio: Merrill, 1985.

Dale, P. *Language Development* (2nd ed.). New York: Rinehart & Winston, 1976.

deVilliers, P., and deVilliers, J. *Early Language.* Cambridge, Mass.: Harvard University Press, 1979.

Graham, J. M., Bashir, A., and Stark, R. E. Communication Disorders. In M. D. Levine, W. B. Carey, A. C. Crocker, and R. T. Gross (eds.), *Developmental-Behavioral Pediatrics.* Philadelphia: Saunders, 1983.

Hixon, T. J., Shriberg, L. D., and Saxman, J. H. (eds.). *Introduction to Communication Disorders.* Englewood Cliffs, N.J.: Prentice-Hall, 1980.

Lass, N. J., McReynolds, L. V., Northern, J. L., and Yoder, D. E. (eds.). *Speech, Language, and Hearing. Vol. I: Normal Processes. Vol. II: Pathologies of Speech and Language.* Philadelphia: Saunders, 1982.

Liebergott, J. W., Bashir, A. S., and Schultz, M. C. Dancing Around and Making Strange Noises. Children at Risk. In A. L. Holland (ed.), *Language Disorders.* San Diego: College-Hill, 1984.

Martin, J. A. M. *Voice, Speech, and Language in the Child: Development and Disorder.* New York: Springer-Verlag, 1981.

McLean, J., and Snyder-McLean, L. *A Transactional Approach to Early Language Training.* Columbus, Ohio: Merrill, 1978.

Owens, R. *Language Development: An Introduction.* Columbus, Ohio: Merrill, 1984.

Prizant, B. M., and Schuler, A. L. Facilitating Communication: Language Approaches. In D. Cohen and A. Donnellan (eds.), *Handbook of Autism and Pervasive Developmental Disorders.* New York: Wiley, 1985.

Templin, M. *Certain Language Skills in Children.* Minneapolis: University of Minnesota Press, 1957.

Wallach, G. P., and Butler, K. G. (eds.). *Language Learning Disabilities in School-age Children.* Baltimore: Williams & Wilkins, 1984.

Walle, E. Prevention of Stuttering. I: Identifying Danger Signs (a film). Seven Oaks Productions, Silver Spring, Md., 1985.

Wiig, E., and Semel, E. *Language Assessment and Intervention.* Columbus, Ohio: Merrill, 1980.

Specific Handicaps Identified at Birth

Lawrence C. Kaplan and I. Leslie Rubin

I. Introduction

The treatment of the child with congenital anomalies requires medical management of multiple organ systems. This chapter discusses practical approaches to the care of these children.

II. Types of anomalies

Major anomalies result from errors in morphogenesis that have serious medical and surgical implications and typically involve the central nervous, cardiovascular, and renal systems (Table 24-1). They are present in 2 percent of all newborns and in 4 percent of all infants 1 year of age and account for 9 percent of perinatal deaths and 18 percent of deaths in the first year. Approximately 20 percent of deaths from major anomalies occur in the first day of life, 50 percent by 1 month, and 75 percent by the end of the first year.

Minor anomalies alone usually have no medical consequences and are usually detected by physical examination alone (Table 24-1). Infants with one or two minor anomalies have a low likelihood of having major anomalies, but when three or more minor anomalies are found, 90 percent of patients have one or more major anomalies (Holmes, 1985; Marden et al., 1964). Serious life-threatening defects must therefore be sought in any child with three or more minor anomalies regardless of the diagnosis.

Specific anomalies can be classified depending on their presumed pathogenesis, and based on these, certain predictions concerning growth and development may be possible. If they comprise individual syndromes (e.g., Down's syndrome, de Lange's syndrome), prognosis based on known natural history is frequently easier (Fig. 24-1).

Malformation implies abnormal formation of tissue or abnormal tissue interaction. Malformations frequently cause secondary defects (malformation sequence), for example, the hydrocephalus and myelomeningocele that result from the malformation of abnormal neural tube closure. They are frequently due to single gene or chromosome defects and usually do not improve in an extrauterine environment (Smith, 1982) (Table 24-2).

Deformation or deformation syndrome involves normal tissue altered by abnormal mechanical forces on an otherwise normally developing embryo or fetus. When deformation is from extrinsic forces, such as in the case of intrauterine crowding, extrauterine unconstrained growth and movement usually improve the defect (Clarren et al., 1979; Dunn, 1976). When the embryo or fetus is neurologically impaired or an internal structure impinges on otherwise normal structures, deformation is intrinsic and improves if neurologic status

Table 24-1. Examples of major and minor congenital anomalies and their significance

Physical feature	Origin and significance	Clinical clues to diagnosis
Major Anomalies		
Central nervous system: myelomeningocele	Defective closure of neural tube	Anencephaly, myelodysplasia
Craniofacial-orofacial: cleft palate	Failure of closure of maxillary palatine shelves	Trisomy 13
Cardiac: ventriculoseptal defect or atrioventricular canal defect	Abnormal closure of the ventricular septum or endocardial cushion	Down's syndrome (trisomy 21)
Gastrointestinal tract: duodenal atresia	Duodenal recanalization	Down's syndrome (trisomy 21)
Minor Anomalies		
Calvarium: small fontanelle	Insufficient brain growth	Cerebral dysgenesis
Upper third of face: ocular hypertelorism	Widely spaced eyes and orbits	Frontonasal dysplasia
Oral region: prominent lateral palatine ridges	Defective tongue thrust against hard palate	Neurologic disease
Auricular region: preauricular tags	Accessory hillocks of Hiss	Hemifacial microsomia
Limb: simian crease	Planes of folding of hands prior to 11 wk	Trisomy 18, Down's syndrome (trisomy 21)

Adapted from D. W. Smith, *Recognizable Patterns of Human Malformation.* Philadelphia: Saunders, 1981.

improves or if the deforming forces resolve (Hall, 1981). In the case of deformation, a careful review of gestational history and a thorough neurologic examination are critical.

Disruption or disruption sequences occur when an otherwise normal embryo or fetus undergoes destruction of normal tissue. This disruption may be mechanical such as tethering by amniotic bands, or it may involve vascular injury as hypothesized in some forms of hemifacial microsomia. Also, infections such as rubella or *Toxoplasma* virus may be involved (Cohen, 1982; Jones et al., 1974; Poswillo, 1976). The nature and timing of the disruption determine a large part of the subsequent growth and development.

The diagnosis of recognized multiple congenital anomaly syndromes is based on clinical suspicion and, where appropriate, confirmed by specific tests. For situations in which diagnosis is not apparent but prognosis must be considered, we use the following approach:

A. Attempt to classify the patient's anomalies as either minor or major, and predict from this the likelihood of finding multiple major anomalies that may be serious.

B. Evaluate each anomaly with reference to its being a malformation, deformation, or disruption, looking for a single cause for multiple problems

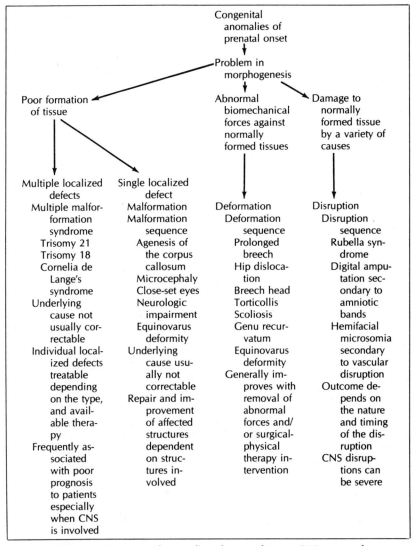

Fig. 24-1. Overview of congenital anomalies of prenatal onset. *CNS* = central nervous system. (Adapted from D. W. Smith, *Recognizable Patterns of Human Malformation*. Philadelphia: Saunders, 1981.)

(e.g., monogenic, chromosomal, teratogenic, maternal, intrauterine-mechanical). Abnormal development of earliest prenatal onset should prompt greatest suspicion of other major anomalies.

C. If no definitive diagnostic tests are possible, systematically evaluate and follow the child over time. Phenotype may change with age, and syndrome diagnosis may be evident later.

Table 24-2. Etiology of major anomalies (malformations) among 18,155 newborns at Boston Hospital for Women, 1972–1975

Cause	Incidence (%)
Genetic abnormalities	
Multifactorial inheritance	0.6
Single mutant genes	0.1
Chromosomal abnormalities*	0.1
Uncertain inheritance	0.3
Uterine factors	0.1
Drugs taken by mother	0.01
Maternal conditions	0.1
Unknown	1.1
Total	2.41

*Of these newborns, 0.14% had a clinically recognizable chromosomal abnormality. Most chromosomal abnormalities such as 47,XXX, 47,XXX cause no physical abnormalities that are apparent in newborn infants.
Adapted from L. B. Holmes. *The Malformed Newborn: Practical Perspectives.* Boston: Massachusetts Developmental Disabilities Council, 1976.

    D. If specific diagnosis cannot be given, explain defects in terms of likely mechanism of abnormal morphogenesis. This serves to allay parental guilt and helps parents remember relevant obstetric or perinatal history.

    E. In the older child, review history by examination of actual test reports and x rays. Interpretations vary, and tests may be repeated as improvements in medical technology occur (e.g., magnetic resonance imaging versus computed tomographic scan).

III. Long-term management
  The contribution of complex chronic medical conditions to medical practice has increased and now accounts for 10 percent of all office visits to primary care providers and 33 percent of visits to medical and surgical subspecialties (Gortmaker and Sappenfield, 1984). Among patients with myelodysplasia, for example, 63 percent received their primary care from specialists or specialty clinics, and 35 percent received care from other sources. The remainder had no primary care (Kanthor et al., 1974).

    A. Growth and nutrition
      One of the first issues for the primary care provider (usually the pediatrician) is to monitor growth and nutrition. Staged surgical procedures, difficult postoperative courses, the physical stresses of major surgery, and possible debilitating medical complications may interfere with a child's full growth potential. Careful nutrition is necessary, as caloric requirements in children with complex handicaps may greatly exceed those of normal children. Additional nutrition may be required in children who have potential for somatic catch-up growth, as, for example, in infants with the extrinsically deformed mandible seen in the Robin sequence.

The child whose normal development is interrupted by frequent medical and surgical intervention may fall behind in the acquisition of normal feeding skills or may not develop them at all. Although capable of normal metabolism, children who feed poorly have limited access to necessary calories and nutrients. It may be necessary to consider alternative feeding practices early, and if a child is able, solids should be introduced and self-feeding encouraged in as normal a manner as possible (Table 24-3). Many larger referral centers have feeding teams composed of persons who specialize in specific feeding problems to help the parents and physicians.

B. General health care plan

Regardless of complexity of a child's problems, or the number of consulting specialists involved, a plan must be devised for general health care, even if multiple hospitalizations interrupt this plan. A plan provides parents the opportunity to express their feelings and to ask questions on a regular basis. It can shorten visits by allowing more problems to be addressed individually over time rather than in clusters. A well-established relationship in the well-child-care format permits attention to immunizations, drug allergies, follow-up vision and hearing screenings, and communicable infectious diseases representative of the community in which the child lives.

The office medical record can benefit in complex cases by use of a problem-oriented medical record (POMR) format, presumably to parallel the problem list used in the patient's hospital care (Weed, 1969) (Fig. 24-2).

An interim summary can be used to track a patient's progress. The summary is updated at regular intervals and is designed to be distributed to any person involved in the patient's care, including physicians, nurses, physical therapists, and social service personnel (Fig. 24-3). These summaries can communicate recent information on medications and provide documentation to insurance companies, schools, social welfare agencies, hospital admitting offices, and house officers. They can also accompany the patient and family to other parts of the country should the patient require care in another office or hospital.

The development of comprehensive multidisciplinary clinical programs for children with congenital handicapping conditions has enhanced delivery of medical care. Rather than the patient making numerous visits to a variety of subspecialists and paramedical support staff, such multidisciplinary programs bring these professionals together to address each of the patient's problems in detail. Typical programs in the hospital and community for infants with anomalies include those for myelodysplasia, cerebral palsy, craniofacial anomalies, cleft lip and palate, limb anomalies, scoliosis, and Down's syndrome (Kaplan, 1986).

Usually the pediatric nurse-clinician serves as the first contact for the patient, performing triage of individual problems. An administrative coordinator arranges clinic appointments, test requisitions, and billing. The patients may have individualized schedules for each clinic meeting, and they are provided with these when they arrive at the clinic. Multidisciplinary programs work best when all members meet to update the total plan of care by reviewing each patient seen. The multidisciplinary program often

270 IV. Management of Specific Problems

Table 24-3. Nutritional concerns for representative congenital problems

Clinical entity	Significant nutritional issues	Suggestions
Congenital heart disease	Increased oxygen consumption Decreased body fat Risk of congestive heart failure with too much volume 21% of patients below 5th percentile for weight by 5 yr	Usual caloric needs 150–180 kcal/kg/day Range of formula caloric density: 20–30 cal/oz
Cleft lip	Infant usually learns to feed despite defect Certain feeding devices can interfere with surgical correction	Breck and Mead Johnson feeders Holding head above chest level minimizing regurgitation
Cleft palate	Child usually adapts to soft palate cleft; in hard palate clefts, the child may develop no suction	Same as for cleft lip
Robin sequence	Retrognathic jaw with U-shaped cleft palate places child at risk for tongue obstructing airway ? NG feedings until jaw grows	Introduce Breck or Mead Johnson feeder once breathing or swallowing becomes coordinated
Hemifacial microsomia	Cleft of corner of mouth, abnormal occlusal plane, and neurologic dysfunction of palate produce poor seal and coordination until repair	Hold cheek of affected side upward and face forward Lamb's nipple preferable
Choanal atresia	Frequent use of stents makes feeding difficult Obligate nose breathing may necessitate gavage if bilateral	Clear nasal airway of mucus Plastic airway through nipple useful to develop suck
Macroglossia	Attempt feeding if sucking and swallowing can coordinate without aspiration	Use long lamb's nipple Give water after feedings Oral hygiene important
TEF with esophageal atresia	Most patients need G tube High association with reflux Esophageal motility problems Stress oral feeding	Attempt to wean G tube Small feedings Encourage pacifier and oral feeding
Myelodysplasia	Any new feeding problem may indicate shunt malfunction Poor sucking may indicate spinal cord compression	Monitor for reflux and aspiration

Adapted from D. M. McDonald, The Child with Special Feeding Needs. In R. B. Howard and H. S. Winter, *Nutrition and Feeding of Infants and Toddlers*. Boston: Little, Brown, 1983. Pp. 309–336.
G = gastric; NG = nasogastric; TEF = tracheoesophageal fistula.

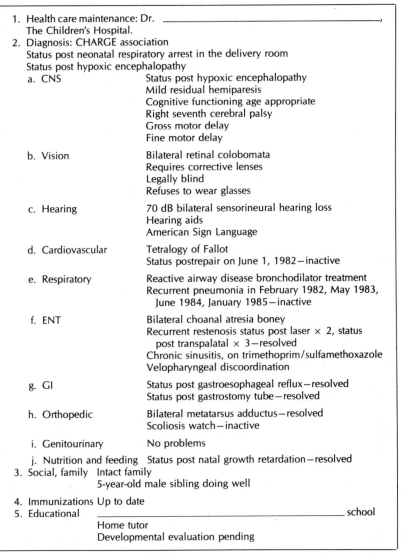

1. Health care maintenance: Dr. _____,
   The Children's Hospital.
2. Diagnosis: CHARGE association
   Status post neonatal respiratory arrest in the delivery room
   Status post hypoxic encephalopathy
   a. CNS   Status post hypoxic encephalopathy
                             Mild residual hemiparesis
                             Cognitive functioning age appropriate
                             Right seventh cerebral palsy
                             Gross motor delay
                             Fine motor delay

   b. Vision   Bilateral retinal colobomata
                             Requires corrective lenses
                             Legally blind
                             Refuses to wear glasses

   c. Hearing   70 dB bilateral sensorineural hearing loss
                             Hearing aids
                             American Sign Language

   d. Cardiovascular   Tetralogy of Fallot
                             Status postrepair on June 1, 1982—inactive

   e. Respiratory   Reactive airway disease bronchodilator treatment
                             Recurrent pneumonia in February 1982, May 1983,
                                June 1984, January 1985—inactive

   f. ENT   Bilateral choanal atresia boney
                             Recurrent restenosis status post laser × 2, status
                                post transpalatal × 3—resolved
                             Chronic sinusitis, on trimethoprim/sulfamethoxazole
                             Velopharyngeal discoordination

   g. GI   Status post gastroesophageal reflux—resolved
                             Status post gastrostomy tube—resolved

   h. Orthopedic   Bilateral metatarsus adductus—resolved
                             Scoliosis watch—inactive

   i. Genitourinary   No problems

   j. Nutrition and feeding Status post natal growth retardation—resolved
3. Social, family   Intact family
                     5-year-old male sibling doing well

4. Immunizations Up to date
5. Educational   _____ school
                     Home tutor
                     Developmental evaluation pending

Fig. 24-2. Example of a problem list generated for a child with CHARGE association (colobomata, *h*eart disease, choanal *a*tresia, *r*etarded growth and development, *g*enital renal abnormalities, and external *e*ar and hearing anomalies). *CNS* = central nervous system; *ENT* = ear, nose, and throat; *GI* = gastrointestinal.

This will summarize the past medical history and present clinical status of
_____, as of _____. The following individuals are involved
in _____'s care and should be contacted if you need further information.

1. Pediatrician (address)   5. Primary nurse
2. Neurologist   6. Social worker
3. Orthopedic surgeon   7. Physical therapist
4. Neurosurgeon   8. Other

I. Problem list
A. Health care maintenance (active, inactive, resolved, unresolved)
B. _____
C. _____

II. Medications
Medicine   Dose   Schedule   When started

III. Gestational/neonatal history

IV. Medical history (by problem)
A. Health care maintenance
B. _____
C. _____

V. Summary of hospitalizations
Problem   Treatment   Discharge diagnosis

VI. Allergies

VII. Immunization status

VIII. Transfusions

IX. Trauma

X. Relevant childhood illnesses

XI. Relevant family history

XII. Social history

XIII. Development/current developmental status

XIV. Current treatment plans
A. _____
B. _____
C. _____

XV. Legal status and guardianship

XVI. All copies of treatment records, agency reports, and correspondence should
be sent to _____

_____
Signature and title

Fig. 24-3. Interim summary worksheet.

does not provide primary care; therefore its success depends on communication with primary care providers. The multidisciplinary clinic also permits patients and their families to meet with one another, to participate in discussion groups, and to maintain a liaison with local, state, or national family support groups. Attended often by the social worker, these sessions can help identify deficient services in the hospital, clinic, or community.

IV. Developmental concerns for the congenitally handicapped

A number of priorities should be considered that are important for enhancing developmental outcomes. First, attention should be given to the receptive skills of hearing and vision. This is especially important for children with major motor handicaps who may have good cognitive function. A plan of vision and hearing testing should be devised, and speech and hearing therapy should be considered in the early intervention plans. During hospitalizations, especially if prolonged, early intervention or formal schooling should continue. Medical providers from various specialties should coordinate invasive tests and operations for the same hospital visit. This helps prevent missed school days.

We find that referral to an early intervention program is central to developmental follow-up and serves to extend the number of persons who may be able to recognize new problems. Parental participation in parent support groups can occur within and outside of multidisciplinary programs (Moore et al., 1983). Respite care can further provide parents with professional help in the day-to-day care of the child. Parents frequently do not request this resource and may be sensitive when the issue is raised. It may be helpful to let the parents know that temporary respite care can be an extension of their concern for the child and does not represent parental failure.

Finally, parental participation is a key element if supports for parents are in place and effective and, with the developmental and physical therapy, can facilitate the education of the child.

V. Down's syndrome: An illustration of management issues

The clinical, educational, and social issues that have been elucidated in the studies of infants, children, and adults with Down's syndrome have served as prototypes for other congenital syndromes that are associated with developmental delays and mental retardation.

Prior to the social revolution that encouraged the integration of children with developmental handicaps into the mainstream of social and educational life, little clinical awareness of Down's syndrome existed except for the listing of dysmorphic features for diagnostic identification and the fact that major congenital heart disease and duodenal atresia were common findings. Parents were encouraged to place their infants in institutions as soon as possible and forget about them. This practice has fortunately changed. Although informing parents that their newborn infant has Down's syndrome results in the well-documented responses of shock, grief, and mourning, it is clear that the manner in which they are told is extremely important and has important consequences for outcome, particularly in maintaining family stability. Providing emotional support and information about the disorder, outcome, and available services are invaluable.

A vast array of services exists for infants and children with developmental handicaps from congenital anomalies or birth trauma. Some examples are early intervention programs, hospital-based special clinics, and parent groups. Individuals with Down's syndrome have the widest representation with local, regional, and national Down's syndrome associations. A journal, *Trisomy 21,* is devoted solely to this condition. Active research on Down's syndrome involves the fields of genetics, immunology, molecular biology, and early developmental and clinical management.

A. Neonatal period

In the neonatal period, the first issues to evaluate are the cardiac status and patency of gastrointestinal tract. Severe congenital heart disease rapidly becomes evident; however, subtle cardiac diseases may also be present. For this reason, an electrocardiogram (ECG) and a chest radiograph should be obtained. If an axis deviation indicating endocardial cushion defect is suggested, an echocardiogram should be obtained. The chest radiograph helps determine whether there is cardiomegaly or a left-to-right shunt, which should show increased vascular markings in the lung fields. A radiograph of the abdomen can indicate the presence of duodenal atresia. The absence of duodenal atresia does not rule out duodenal stenosis or annular pancreas, and excessive vomiting should be investigated with radiographic contrast studies or ultrasonography. Screening for hypothyroidism is important, as congenital hypothyroidism can exist.

B. Infancy

After the neonatal period, monitoring cardiac status for congestive heart failure should continue. Close monitoring of heart size, murmur, liver size, tachypnea, and failure to thrive is important. In addition, the thyroid status should continue to be monitored as hypothyroidism can evolve. We recommend assessing thyroid status every 6 months for the first 2 years and annually thereafter.

Constipation is another common problem in infants with Down's syndrome. Occasionally during the first month it is associated with prolonged jaundice. If constipation persists and becomes severe, the diagnosis of Hirschsprung's disease should be considered, as this occurs with increased frequency in infants with Down's syndrome.

A number of eye problems occur. Cataracts can be apparent in the neonatal period. Some blockage of the tear ducts with tearing and stickiness of the eyes may develop into conjunctivitis. Refractory errors are extremely common, and strabismus may also be present. Cataracts are rare during infancy. Coarse nystagmus may be present during infancy and usually improves without treatment as the child grows. Routine ophthalmologic evaluations are therefore mandatory.

Recurrent otitis media is a frequent problem, and the diagnosis may be difficult because of the narrow external ear canals with resulting difficulty in visualizing the tympanic membrane. If fever and irritability are present and no other systemic causes of infection are identified, it is justifiable to administer antibiotics as if it were otitis media. Hearing tests should be conducted by experienced audiologists with frequent recourse to tympanometry, as fluid accumulation in the middle ear can be a problem that may not be clinically detected during the first years of life. Many infants and children require placement of tympanic membrane tubes.

A blocked nose with difficult breathing and tachypnea may also be a notable feature in infancy. Saline nose drops, suction, and humidification are the usual measures recommended. The other respiratory conditions that may be evident are congenital abnormalities of the respiratory tract (e.g., tracheomalacia).

Incoordination of swallowing and reflux with aspiration can occur and should be fully investigated. If recurrent pneumonias occur in infancy, gastroesophageal reflux with aspiration should be excluded, particularly when vomiting or gagging is present.

Infantile spasms occur more frequently in infants with Down's syndrome. Therefore, any sudden changes in behavior between 4 and 6 months of age should alert the pediatrician to this diagnosis. Prognostically, infantile spasms occurring in infants with Down's syndrome are generally more benign than those occurring in other infants, particularly infants with underlying central nervous system abnormalities. It is not unusual for infants to outgrow this seizure disorder.

A number of dermatologic conditions may require attention. Dry skin prominent on the cheeks, particularly in winter, can be treated with topical creams. Seborrheic dermatitis and cheilosis can also be troublesome.

Dentition may be delayed, irregular, and unusual; the teeth may be unusually shaped and some may be missing. Attention should be given to good dental hygiene, not so much because of cavities, but because of periodontal disease. After infancy, children with Down's syndrome frequently require orthodontic care.

The growth of infants with Down's syndrome differs from that of infants without Down's syndrome. Growth curves have been developed for these infants to appreciate more accurately deviations from the norm (Fig. 24-4).

Any symptom that concerns parents should receive thorough and detailed clinical evaluation, as relatively nonspecific signs and symptoms may turn out to have major pathologic consequences. Examples of this are tachypnea, pectus excavatum, and pectus carinatum, which may be attributed to a normal phenomenon of Down's syndrome, when in fact these signs may represent pulmonary or cardiac disorders.

C. Toddler

As the infant grows and begins walking by 2 to 3 years of age, attention should be paid to walking patterns. Orthopedic disorders may appear at this stage. These include hip dysplasia, talipes planus, and hallux varus, with some unusual patterns in the shape of the foot. Standard radiographs of the hips in the anteroposterior and frog-leg positions are helpful in diagnosing hip disorder if suspected. These disorders may merely involve acetabular dysplasia or may be more serious and be associated with subluxation, dislocation, or even Legg-Calvé-Perthes disease. Check routinely for scoliosis.

At between 2 and 3 years of age, we recommend a radiograph of the lateral cervical spine in flexion, neutral, and extension to evaluate the stability of the atlantoaxial joint. Atlantoaxial subluxation occurs with increased frequency in Down's syndrome patients more than 3 years of age. If subluxation is present, parents should be cautioned to prevent the child from engaging in activities that stress the atlantoaxial joint. The Committee on Special Olympics mandates that cervical spine radiographs of all Down's syndrome persons be reviewed before allowing them to participate in the games. Periodic evaluation of the neck (radiologic and neurologic) is important. Changes in the gait pattern are often clues to atlantoaxial subluxation with spinal cord compression.

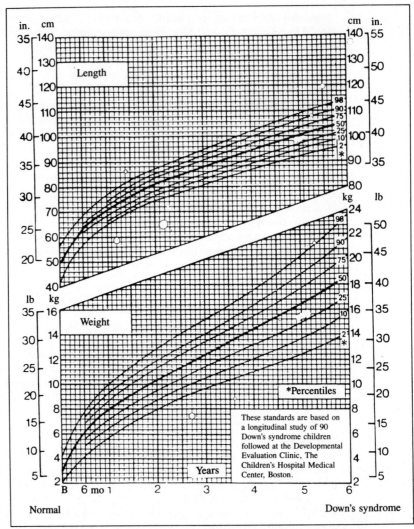

Fig. 24-4. Growth curves for children (combined sexes) with Down's syndrome.

D. Early childhood

Continued monitoring of cardiac status, thyroid status, constipation, dry skin, and the atlantoaxial joint, along with ophthalmologic and audiologic testing, should be part of routine health care of 3- to 5-year-old children with Down's syndrome.

Numerous other clinical associations occur in children with Down's syndrome, including increased incidences of leukemia, alopecia areata, and other skin conditions; mitral valve prolapse and aortic regurgitation; eye disorders (e.g., keratoconus); short stature; periodontal disease; and obesity.

Finally, these children should be screened for hepatitis, and we recommend immunization against hepatitis B. Hepatitis B is particularly a problem in institutionalized children as they have an increased susceptibility of developing a carrier state of hepatitis B surface antigen, and some may develop chronic or even lupoid hepatitis.

E. Development

The characteristic hypotonia of infants with Down's syndrome constitutes a delay in major motor milestones. For example, the infant may sit by 1 year of age and walk by 2 years of age (Table 24-4). The acquisition of speech also develops later than normal, toward the end of the second year. If there are any concerns about the development of speech, the child should be referred to a speech and language pathologist for speech therapy or the development of alternate communication systems. Cognitive development usually falls within the moderately retarded range. There is a wide variability in the achievement of developmental milestones, which can be adversely affected by the presence of uncorrected severe congenital heart lesions. Much recent research has been directed at the effects of early education as a means of affecting cognition development.

F. Behavior and learning

Behavioral problems have diverse manifestations and varied causes and

Table 24-4. Developmental milestones

	Children with Down's syndrome		Normal children	
	Average (mo)	Range (mo)	Average (mo)	Range (mo)
Milestone				
Smiling	2	1.5–4	1	0.5–3
Rolling over	8	4–22	5	2–10
Sitting alone	10	6–28	7	5–9
Crawling	12	7–21	8	6–11
Creeping	15	9–27	10	7–13
Standing	20	11–42	11	8–16
Walking	24	12–65	13	8–18
Talking, words	16	9–31	10	6–14
Talking, sentences	28	18–96	21	14–32
Self-help Skills				
Eating				
Finger feeding	12	8–28	8	6–16
Using spoon and fork	20	12–40	13	8–20
Toilet training				
Bladder	48	20–95	32	18–60
Bowel	42	28–90	29	16–48
Dressing				
Undressing	40	29–72	32	22–42
Putting clothes on	58	38–98	47	34–58

Adapted from S. M. Pueschel. Down's Syndrome. In M. D. Levine, W. B. Carey, A. C. Crocker, and R. T. Gross, (eds.), *Developmental Behavioral Pediatrics.* Philadelphia: Saunders, 1983. P. 359.

patterns of management. Attention should be given to these, and medical factors should be ruled out. For example, chronic constipation and hypothyroidism may cause disorders of behavior. Psychiatric disorders can occur, and depression is one that has been given special attention.

In addition to behavior problems, learning problems may also be brought to the attention of the pediatrician. These should be approached as are all educational problems, with a thorough medical examination that pays particular attention to hearing and vision and disorders of auditory and visual processing. The approach to learning disabilities in infants with Down's syndrome is the same as that for all children with learning disabilities.

It should be noted in conclusion that most infants with Down's syndrome grow up to live and work in semiindependent situations, and much of their success depends on successful management of the child and family during infancy and childhood.

REFERENCES

Clarren, S. K., Smith, D. W., and Hanson, J. W. Helmet treatment for plagiocephaly and congenital muscular torticollis. *J. Pediatr.* 94 : 43, 1979.

Cohen, M. M., Jr. *The Child with Multiple Birth Defects.* New York: Raven, 1982.

Dunn, P. M. Congenital postural deformities. *Br. Med. Bull.* 94 : 43, 1976.

Gortmaker, S., and Sappenfield, W. Chronic childhood disorders: Prevalence and impact. *Pediatr. Clin. North Am.* 31 : 3, 1984.

Hall, J. G. An approach to congenital contracture (arthrogryposis). *Pediatr. Ann.* 10 : 15, 1981.

Holmes, L. B. Congenital Malformation. In J. P. Cloherty and A. R. Stark (eds.), *Manual of Neonatal Care.* Boston: Little, Brown, 1985.

Jones, K. L., Smith, D. W., Hall, B. D., et al. A pattern of craniofacial and limb defects secondary to aberrant tissue bands. *J. Pediatr.* 84 : 90, 1974.

Kanthor, H., Pless, B., Satterwhite, B., et al. Areas of responsibility in the health care of multiply handicapped children. *Pediatrics* 56 : 779, 1974.

Kaplan, L. C. Assessment and Management of the Infant and Child with Multiple Congenital Anomalies. In L. Rubin, and A. Crocker (eds.), *Developmental Disabilities: Medical Care for Children and Adults.* Orlando: Grune & Stratton, 1986.

Keele, D. K. Counseling parents of handicapped infants. *Contemp. Pediatr.* 3(2) : 101, 1986.

Marden, P. M., Smith, D. W., and McDonald, M. J. Congenital anomalies in the newborn infant, including minor variations. *J. Pediatr.* 64 : 358–371, 1964.

McDonald, D. M. The Child with Special Feeding Needs. In R. B. Howard and H. S. Winter (eds.), *Nutrition and Feeding in Infants and Toddlers.* Boston: Little, Brown, 1983. Pp. 309–336.

Moore, C., Morton, K., and Southard, A. *A Readers Guide to Children with Mental, Physical, or Emotional Disabilities.* Baltimore: The Maryland State Planning Council on Developmental Disabilities, 1983.

Poswillo, D. Mechanisms and pathogenesis of malformation. *Br. Med. Bull.* 32 : 59, 1976.

Pueschel, S. M. *The Young Child with Down Syndrome.* New York: Human Sciences, 1984.

Pueschel, S. M., and Rynders, T. E. *Down Syndrome: Advances in Biomedicine and the Behavioral Sciences.* Cambridge, Mass.: Ware, 1982.

Smith, D. W. *Recognizable Patterns of Human Malformation.* Philadelphia: Saunders, 1982.

Weed, L. L. *Medical Records, Medical Education, and Patient Care.* Cleveland: Press of Case Western Reserve University, 1969.

25

Behavioral Problems

Michael W. Yogman, Kim Wilson, and Daniel J. Kindlon

I. Introduction

Adverse social and biologic conditions place preterm infants at risk for later developmental delays, learning disabilities, and behavioral problems, especially by school age. Historically, the increased incidence of behavior disorders among children born prematurely was attributed to the biologic (maternal and neonatal) complications accompanying prematurity. In a retrospective epidemiologic study, Lillienfeld et al. (1955) documented an increased frequency of confused, disorganized, or hyperactive behavior disorders in children born prematurely. Based on these studies, Lillienfeld and colleagues suggested a "continuum of reproductive casualty," leading to outcomes ranging from cerebral palsy, epilepsy, and mental deficiency to minor behavior disorders. More recently, in a longitudinal sample of low-birth-weight infants notable behavioral and emotional disturbances were found in over 30 percent by 4 years of age. This percentage was the same in each social class (Escalona, 1982). Other recent studies, however, have implicated socioeconomic conditions as having an equal, if not synergistic, influence on the behavior of preterm children. Evidence correlates low family income and education with an increased frequency of premature births (Garns et al., 1977; Keller, 1981). Two longitudinal studies suggested that the cumulative effect of neonatal stresses and poverty is associated with later behavioral problems in premature children. Premature infants from low-income families were more likely to exhibit behavior problems and to come from families with parenting problems than were preterm infants from high-income families or full-term infants (Drillien, 1964). Further, studies of the children of Kauai showed that premature birth alone did not increase a child's chance of developing mental health problems (Werner et al., 1971; Werner and Smith, 1977, 1982). However, preterm infants who were also from socially disadvantaged families exhibited a higher incidence of mental health problems at ages 10 and 18. Based on recent reviews of longitudinal studies with high-risk infants, the term *continuum of caretaking casualty* was coined to describe environmental influences on outcomes. Transactions between biologic factors and environmental influences were postulated to best predict outcome (Sameroff and Chandler, 1976). Thus, medical complications and social disadvantage place preterm infants at double jeopardy for developing behavior problems.

Despite these correlations between preterm birth and behavioral problems in later childhood, relatively few studies have looked at preterm behavior or problems during infancy and early childhood. Most studies of the infant focus on cognitive or neurologic outcome. The early behavioral literature is often difficult to interpret, often has methodologic problems, and is hampered by

279

contradictory findings, largely owing to the heterogeneity of the preterm populations included in the studies. Many older studies do not distinguish between small-for-gestational-age and preterm infants. More recent studies often do not differentiate between healthy preterm infants and those with serious neonatal complications or control for socioeconomic conditions.

Despite these drawbacks, we have summarized research in three areas of behavioral development in preterm infants during the first year of life: state organization, crying, and sleep. When possible, we have indicated management strategies for behavioral problems in these areas. Our approach to understanding the cause and management of these problems emphasizes the interactions between maturational forces within the infant (modified by perinatal complications, illness, and temperament) and interactions with parents who influence and shape the infant's behavior once at home. The most common behavioral problems in premature infants during the first year of life are in the areas of state organization, crying, and sleep as well as in feeding (discussed in Chap. 16). Common complaints include night crying, colic, difficulty falling asleep, night waking, sleeping too much, difficulty in feeding, frequent spitting, and inadequate or excess weight gain.

II. Neonatal state organization
Neonatal behavior during the final weeks prior to hospital discharge and during the early months at home can be described by the degree of state organization and coherence of response to stimulation. A *state* is a cluster of recognizable physiologic and behavioral variables that repeatedly occur together. By organization of state behavior, we mean the functional and adaptive use of state. This includes the degree of differentiation of each of the individual states, the degree of integration of state behavior with the environment (entrainment with light-dark cycles and feeding schedules), and the capacity to regulate transitions between states and to sustain long periods of selective state inhibition when it seems adaptive.

A. State in full-term infants
Wolff (1966) introduced the concept of "state of arousal" and designed the first descriptive rating scale for the term infant, which consists of six organized patterns of behavior: quiet sleep, active sleep, drowsiness, quiet awake, active awake, and crying. In the full-term infant, distinctions have been made between two major categories of sleep: deep or quiet, regular sleep, characterized by a lack of motor movement, eyes closed with absence of eye movements, and regular respiration; and active or light sleep, with irregular respiration, low muscle tone, body movements, and rapid eye movements visible under closed eyelids. Awake states have been separated into three states: a drowsy state with eyelids often fluttering and eyes glazed; a wide awake state with an alert, bright look and suppressed motor activity; and an active awake state with open eyes and considerable motor activity. The final state is a crying state with eyes open or closed and jerky motor activity. Brazelton (1984) used similar categories in the Neonatal Assessment Scale, and Prechtl (1974) defined only five states, omitting drowsy (considering it transitional), and required that the behavior consti-

tuting a state be present for at least 3 minutes. These states are relatively stable and constitute the basic rest-activity cycles of the infant.

B. State in preterm infants
Fetal rest-activity cycles have been demonstrated by recording fetal movements as early as 21 weeks' gestation (Sterman and Hoppenbrouwers, 1972). In the very young premature infant, it has proved difficult to classify states, in part because they are transient. While an atypical, undifferentiated sleep state (eyes closed, no gross movements) has been noted as early as 24 to 27 weeks, electroencephalographic (EEG) patterns more characteristic of active and quiet sleep appear by 32 weeks, and true differentiation of sleep states begins at 35 weeks (Dreyfus-Brisac, 1970). Most sleep (75%) prior to 34 weeks is called *unclassifiable* or *transitional* (Parmelee, 1975; Stern et al., 1973). Active sleep first appears as a separate state at about 30 weeks; thereafter the amount of quiet sleep gradually increases, and first transitional and then active sleep decreases (Parmelee, 1975). Roffwarg and colleagues (1966) have postulated that the increased active sleep present in a premature infant may provide a source of endogenous stimulation needed for central nervous system growth. Quiet sleep develops after 36 weeks and rapidly increases in amount to 3 months postterm. The behavioral indices of active sleep (e.g., eye movements, body movements) are well correlated by 34 to 36 weeks, while for quiet sleep this occurs 2 weeks later. By 40 weeks' postconceptional age, the distribution of sleep states is the same for preterm and full-term infants; active sleep occupies about 50 percent of total sleep time.

A primitive cycling of the sleep states appears at about 32 weeks' gestation. The periods for each cycle (active and quiet sleep) are short but increase with age (i.e., 40 minutes at 36 weeks, 60 minutes at term, 90 minutes in the adult).

The waking state with eyes open has been noted as early as 30 weeks' gestation but occurs spontaneously and for longer periods after 32 weeks. The awake state is poorly organized at 30 weeks as evidenced by uncoordinated, rolling eye movements. By 35 weeks, the quiet awake state is accompanied by improved visual attention and alertness (Hack et al., 1976). At 40 weeks postconception, alertness may occupy as much as 20 to 30 minutes of each 4-hour feeding cycle. Finally, the crying state occurs spontaneously as early as 32 weeks' gestation.

While state behavior for the preterm infant by 36 weeks is similar to that of the term infant, differences in stability and organization of state indices and EEG differences in state maturation persist for sick preterm infants reaching mature "term" values after many weeks in intensive care. While the healthy full-term infant has achieved smooth transitions between states and is differentiating the alert state to include attention, social interaction, and organized responses to stimuli, the preterm infant has not.

C. Responses to stimulation
Preterm state organization at 40 weeks postconception differs from that of full-term infants, particularly in the areas of alertness and response to stimu-

lation. When compared with day-old full-term infants, healthy preterm infants at 40 weeks postconception exhibited a more heterogeneous and poorer behavioral organization, reflected by lower scores in all the categories on the Neonatal Behavioral Assessment Scale (Paludetto et al., 1984). Other types of behavioral tests substantiate these findings. Preterm infants were reported to be less alert (DiVitto and Goldberg, 1979; Saint-Anne Dargassies, 1972); to maintain their alert state for a shorter time (McGehee and Eckerman, 1983); and to be more irritable, excitable, and difficult to console (Friedman et al., 1982a; Hatcher, 1977). Because state behavior is known to be influenced by many environmental factors (e.g., stimulation, diet, light, stress, medications, and most perinatal complications), such differences are not surprising. In explanation of these findings, Field (1979) suggested that preterm infants have a very narrow range of "appropriate" stimulation. They may respond poorly or not at all to low-intensity stimulation and overrespond in a disorganized manner to high-intensity stimulation. Premature infants seem to have a less well-developed attentional system; they tend to focus on individual environmental stimuli only briefly and are easily distracted. Some infants may not focus on the stimulus at all. It is not known how painful procedures such as repeated blood drawing and intubations in the NICU influence infants, but perhaps some infants develop a defensive barrier to stimuli, which interferes with visual attention to appropriate stimuli. Because of these differences in alertness and arousability, the caretaker may find it difficult to discover the optimally appropriate stimulus for the infant and may become frustrated with the infant's unpredictability and unreadability (McGehee and Eckerman, 1983). When parents try to calm their hyperactive infant with increasing stimulation, the infant may respond by averting his or her gaze and body (Field, 1979). These differences in both infant responsiveness and caretaker interaction may persist throughout the first year (Crnic et al., 1983).

Recently, longitudinal studies of state behavior in preterm infants have attempted to determine state characteristics influenced by biologic versus environmental factors. The proportion of quiet sleep and of the longest uninterrupted sleep period was most purely related to biologic factors (gestational age and birth weight), whereas active sleep and wakefulness were most purely related to environmental factors. Infant behavior that results in being taken from the crib at night (probably irritability) and the course of sleep between midnight and 5:00 A.M. were related to both environmental and biologic influences (Anders et al., 1985).

D. Management of state difficulties

Clinicians can help parents prepare for the infant's discharge and first few weeks at home by assessing the state organization of the infant with the parents and discussing parental expectations and the implications for caretaking. Discussing the infant's difficulties with alertness and visual orientation or the need for swaddling and self-consoling maneuvers such as nonnutritive sucking (pacifier or thumb) may help the parents interact successfully with their infant by finding the appropriate level of stimulation. This may reduce their anxiety about reading the infant's cues and enable them to avoid contributing to a vicious cycle of overstimulation and infant avoidance and aversion. Special groups of neonates such as those with bronchopulmo-nary dysplasia may have even less state flexibility than healthy preterm in-fants. It may be necessary for parents of these infants to cluster all feeding and caretaking activities when the newborn is spontaneously alert, rather than to attempt to manipulate the infant's state.

III. Crying

The difficulties with state organization manifested by premature infants may set the stage for interactional problems with parents and should influence the clinical management of crying and sleep problems in these infants.

In a sample of healthy, full-term infants, crying increased between 6 and 12 weeks of age (peaking at 2.75 hours/day at 6 weeks), and then decreased for reasons that seemed related to maturational changes rather than to environ-mental influences (Brazelton, 1962). While the pattern for preterm infants is more variable, similar increases in fussiness between 6 and 12 weeks' cor-rected age are common.

Severe, intermittent, unexplained crying leading to marked parental concern has often been termed *colic*. Both the definition and the syndrome are impre-cise, but most excessive crying represents an interaction of at least two contrib-uting factors: an infant who cries longer, louder, or in a more piercing way than other infants and a parent or caretaker who is unable to console the in-fant. Although incidence figures vary depending on definition, about 10 to 15 percent of parents are concerned about excessive crying, and the incidence is about the same in premature as in term infants (Schmitt, 1985a).

There appears to be a strong maturational component to crying because the onset occurs at a comparable age when corrected age is used. Although the in-cidence of parental report of colic may not differ in preterm and full-term in-fants, the character of infant crying and the effect on parent-infant interaction differ. Parents of premature infants may be so relieved to have their infants home from the NICU that they are less likely to express concerns spontaneous-ly about crying, and a clinician may need to ask specific questions about the infant's crying.

Infant cries vary in intensity, duration, frequency, and quality. Characteristic variations in the cry features have been associated with high-risk, neurological-ly impaired, small-for-gestational-age, malnourished, and other specific groups of infants (Lester and Zeskind, 1979; Michelsson, 1971). These differences in infant cries have both physiologic and social implications. Crying may reflect the functional organization of the infant's central nervous system during its re-sponse to external and internal stimuli (Lester and Zeskind, 1982; Parmelee, 1962). Further, different types of cries evoke different responses in the caretak-er (Zeskind, 1980).

Studies describing crying in preterm infants have yielded conflicting results. Elmer and Gregg (1967) and Friedman and coworkers (1982a) reported that preterm infants cry more than full-term infants. Conversely, other studies found that preterm infants cried less than full-term infants (DeVitto and Goldberg, 1979; Parmelee, 1975) and had cries of lower intensity and shorter duration (Brown and Bakeman, 1982). Despite these variable reports on the amount a preterm infant cries, spectral analysis indicates that preterm infants' cries have a characteristic quality, distinct from the cries of small-for-gestational-age or full-term infants. Preterm infants' cries have a higher frequency, more frequent pitch shift, lower glottal plosives, and fewer harmonics (Lester and Zeskind, 1979; Michelsson, 1971). Further, infants with the highest pitched cries exhibited the poorest performance on the Brazelton Neonatal Behavior Assessment Scale (Lester and Zeskind, 1978).

These variations in the crying of preterm infants may adversely affect the interaction of the preterm infant with the caretaker. DeVitto and Goldberg (1979) suggested that preterm infants do not give clear distress signals in the form of cries; consequently, their cries are more difficult for the caretaker to interpret. Further, the intrinsic quality of the preterm infant's cry is more disturbing to the caretaker. Preterm infants' cries are perceived as more adverse and elicit a greater autonomic response in the listener than cries of full-term infants (Frodi et al., 1978). This effect was especially pronounced for the crying of preterm infants with neonatal complications (Friedman et al., 1982b).

Managing excessive crying in premature infants requires consideration of organic causes and a careful physical examination, particularly if the onset is sudden and the crying continuous. Special complications of prematurity, such as hypertension, should be considered. Abdominal discomfort from gas is not a cause of colic, and cow's milk allergy as a cause is quite rare (Schmitt, 1985a). Medications, formula changes, and rectal dilatation are therefore of little value.

Clarifying behavioral factors in the infant and parents by observation during the physical examination can be helpful. For example, a hypersensitive infant with a low threshold for stimulation, a particularly aversive cry, an anxious or depressed mother, marital discord, or disorganized, chaotic caretaking may be observed. Parents should be informed that infants normally increase crying at about 6 weeks' corrected age and that gentle, soothing, vestibular stimulation is valuable when consoling an infant. Carrying infants has been shown to reduce crying markedly (Hunziker and Barr, 1986). Parents can help their particularly fussy infant learn how to console him- or herself. Nonnutritive sucking may console many infants, and parents can facilitate either thumb sucking or use of a pacifier, depending on their preference. Swaddling and rhythmic, entraining stimulation may help some infants. If the parents are anxious about their premature infant's fragility, they may be helped by discussing their concerns openly. Other parents may need help with modifying their style of interaction to be more soothing and less arousing, perhaps by using only one mode of stimulation (e.g., voice alone). Most important of all in managing excessive crying is that parents get support from family, friends, and professionals. Close follow-up, even daily telephone contact, is often required.

IV. Sleep

Infant sleep consists of two distinct states: active sleep and quiet sleep. In the full-term infant, a sleep cycle consists of an epoch of active sleep followed by quiet sleep. There are two to four such cycles between each feeding period, occasionally interrupted by periods of indeterminate sleep (Anders et al., 1971; Rose, 1983).

Prior to 45 weeks postconception, preterm infants' sleep differs notably from that of full-term infants. Sleep behavior characteristic of active sleep appears at 35 weeks, and quiet sleep exists as early as 37 weeks (Dreyfus-Brisac, 1970).

After 37 weeks, the two sleep cycles alternate as in the full-term infant. How-ever, preterm infants exhibit a greater latency period before entering quiet sleep and remain in quiet sleep for a shorter duration (Rose, 1983). By 45 weeks, these differences in sleep cycle periodicity between preterm and full-term infants have attenuated (Stern et al., 1973). However, preterm infants' sleep states remain less organized. Specifically, periods of irregular respiration and increased heart rate are often observed during quiet sleep (Dreyfus-Brisac, 1970; Rose, 1983).

Despite these early differences in sleeping patterns, little evidence suggests that behavior of preterm infants sleep differs from that of the full-term infant after the neonatal period. During the first 4 months of life, sleep state organiza-tion changes markedly for the term and the preterm infant (using corrected age). Quiet sleep increases to a plateau of about 70 percent, and active sleep correspondingly decreases from 50 percent eventually to the adult 20 percent. Furthermore, EEG sleep spindles appear at this time, and sleep onset shifts from the newborn mode of entry through active sleep to the adult mode through quiet sleep (Anders, 1978). Furthermore, by 10 to 12 weeks' corrected age (50–52 weeks postconception), infants at home in the normal light-dark cycle are predominantly awake during the day and asleep at night in contrast to the newborn period. Infants by this age can usually sleep through the night.

Given the similarities in neurophysiologic development of sleep states, it is hardly surprising that sleep disorders and problems are similar in preterm and full-term infants. In a recent longitudinal study we conducted with 20 preterm and 20 full-term infants from birth to 18 months' corrected age, there were no significant group differences in the number of hours of sleep at night or num-ber of night-waking bouts at 1, 5, 9, and 18 months' corrected age. However, the preterm infants showed a trend to have more night waking at 1 month and more bedtime problems at 9 months. An association between perinatal com-plications such as prematurity and the onset of night waking between 9 and 14 months of age has been noted but unexplained in previous studies (Bernal, 1973; Blurton-Jones et al., 1978).

Parents of preterm infants may be more concerned about their infant's sleep than parents of full-term infants, however. Ungerer and coworkers (1983) com-pared sleeping problems (e.g., sleep latency, night waking, fear) at 3 and 5 years of age in children born prematurely with those in children born full term. The preterm children were no more likely to have sleeping problems than full-term children. However, the parents of preterm children were more likely to perceive their children's sleep behavior as problematic.

Managing sleep problems for premature infants involves helping the parents learn to change some child care habits so that their infants can learn to sleep through the night (Schmitt, 1985b). Parents can begin to shape sleep-wake cycles of their infants from the first few weeks after the infant is at home so that the longest periods of sleep occur during the night hours (i.e., by about 3 months of age, infants are able to sleep 6–8 hours without interruption). Re-stricting the duration of sleep during the day and giving the last feeding at a late hour (between 10 and 11 P.M.) may be helpful. Calming presleep rituals such as a bath or a story are often useful. Most important, infants need to learn to fall asleep on their own in their crib. Parents need to place the baby in the crib, sleepy but awake; infants should not become accustomed to falling asleep in their parents' arms. During the normal sleep cycle, an infant cycles between active sleep and quiet sleep every 60 minutes, often entering the waking state, and must learn to reenter sleep on his or her own without being held or rocked. Parents of premature infants may need special reassurance about the adequacy of their infant's growth in order to eliminate a nighttime feeding and about the infant's robustness in order to avoid responding to the normal movements and rustlings of an infant during active sleep. If feedings are necessary at night, they should be brief and boring, and the infant should be allowed to fall asleep on his or her own in the crib. By 6 months of age, parents can provide a friendly, soft toy in bed as a transitional object to help the infant cope with separation anxiety and to provide comfort when he or she awakens during the night.

V. Conclusion

In managing the common behavioral problems of crying and sleep, a premature infant needs sensitive caretaking by parents to help the infant better organize state behavior. Professionals can support parents in two ways. First, they can assuage parental anxiety about the continuing vulnerability or fragility of their infant (Green and Solnit, 1964). Second, they can help parents understand the individual developmental needs of their infant so that they can in turn facilitate the optimal organization of the infant's behavior.

During the second year of life, problems with eating behavior (not eating enough) and sleep (resisting bedtime, night waking) continue to be common, and new concerns arise about delayed and difficult-to-understand speech. The behavioral problems of most concern to parents of premature infants include manifestations of negativism or the "terrible twos": stubbornness, temper tantrums, head banging, excessive activity, and curiosity. In our longitudinal study with 20 preterm and 20 full-term infants, almost two-thirds of the premature infants had daily tantrums by 18 months' corrected age compared with only one-fifth of the full-term infants. These problems during the second year may be considered disorders of autonomy, which reflect a conflict between the child's efforts to achieve independence and the parents' efforts to set consistent limits. Parents of premature infants may still perceive their infants as fragile or vulnerable during this second year and may have greater difficulty tolerating independent behavior. Management of many second-year behavior problems consists of discussing parents' fears about and perceptions of their child's prematurity and encouraging parents to set consistent limits. Given the high incidence of behavioral problems in older premature infants in previous studies, one hopes that preventive intervention during the first 2 years will decrease the incidence of later behavioral disorders.

REFERENCES

Als, H., Lester, B., and Brazelton, T. B. Dynamics of the Behavioral Organization of the Premature Infant. In T. Field (ed.), *Infants Born at Risk: Behavior and Development*. New York: Spectrum, 1979.

Anders, T. State and rhythmic processes. *J. Am. Acad. Child Psychol.* 17 : 401, 1978.

Anders, T., Emde, R., and Parmelee, E. *A Manual of Standardized Terminology, Techniques, and Criteria for Scoring States of Sleep and Wakefulness in Newborn Infants.* Los Angeles: University of California Brain Information, 1971.

Anders, T., Keener, M. A., and Kraemer, H. Sleep-wake state organization, neonatal assessment and development in premature infants during the first year of life. II. *Sleep* 8 : 193, 1985.

Bernal, J. Night waking in infants during the first 14 months. *Dev. Med. Child Neurol.* 15 : 760, 1973.

Blurton-Jones, N., Rossetti-Ferreira, M. C., Farquar Brown, M., and MacDonald, L. The association between perinatal factors and later night waking. *Dev. Med. Child Neurol.* 20 : 427, 1978.

Brazelton, T. B. Crying in infancy. *Pediatrics* 29 : 579, 1962.

Brazelton, T. B. Neonatal Behavioral Assessment Scale. *Clin. Dev. Med.* No. 50, 1984.

Brown, J., and Bakeman, R. Relationships of Mothers with Their Infants During the First Year of Life: Effects of Prematurity. In R. W. Bell and W. P. Smotherman (eds.), *Maternal Influences and Early Behavior.* Holliswood, N.Y.: Spectrum, 1982.

Crnic, K., Ragozin, A., Greenburg, M., et al. Social interaction and developmental competence of preterm and full-term infants during the first year of life. *Child Dev.* 54 : 1199, 1983.

DiVitto, B., and Goldberg, S. The Effects of Newborn Medical Status on Early Parent-Infant Interaction. In T. Field (ed.), *Infants Born at Risk: Behavior and Development.* New York: Spectrum, 1979.

Dreyfus-Brisac, C. Ontogenesis of human sleep in human prematures after thirty-two weeks of conceptional age. *Dev. Psychobiol.* 3 : 91, 1970.

Drillien, C. M. *The Growth and Development of the Prematurely Born Infant.* Edinburgh: Livingstone, 1964.

Elmer, E., and Gregg, G. S. Developmental characteristics of abused children. *Pediatrics* 40 : 596, 1967.

Escalona, S. Babies at double hazard: Early development of infants at biologic and social risk. *Pediatrics* 70 : 670, 1982.

Ferrari, F., Grosoli, M., Fontana, G., and Cavazzuti, G. Neurobehavioral comparisons of low-risk preterm and full-term infants at term conceptional age. *Dev. Med. Child Neurol.* 25 : 450, 1983.

Field, T. (ed.). Interaction Patterns of Preterm and Term Infants. In *Infants Born at Risk: Behavior and Development.* New York: Spectrum, 1979.

Friedman, S., Jacobs, B., and Werthmann, M. Preterms of low medical risk: Behavior and soothability. *Infant Behav. Dev.* 5 : 3, 1982a.

Friedman, S., Zahn-Waxler, C., and Radke-Yarrow, M. Perceptions of cries of full-term and preterm infants. *Infant Behav. Dev.* 5 : 161, 1982b.

Frodi, A., Lamb, M., Leavitt, L., and Donovan, W. Fathers' and mothers' responses to infant smiles and cries. *Infant Behav. Dev.* 1 : 187, 1978.

Gardner, J., and Karmel, B. Attention and Arousal in Preterm and Full-term Neonates. In T. Field and A. Sostek (eds.), *Infants Born at Risk: Physiological, Perceptual, and Cognitive Processes.* New York: Grune & Stratton, 1983.

Garns, S. M., Shaw, H., and McCabe, K. Effects of Socioeconomic Status and Race on Weight-Defined and Gestational Prematurity in the United States. In D. Reed and R. Stanley (eds.), *The Epidemiology of Prematurity.* Baltimore: Urban, 1977.

Green, M., and Solnit, A. Reactions to the threatened loss of a child: A vulnerable child syndrome. *Pediatrics* 34 : 58, 1964.

Hack, M., Mostow, A., and Miranda, S. Development of attention in preterm infants. *Pediatrics* 5 : 669, 1976.

Hatcher, R. The neurophysiological examination of the preterm infant. *Acta Med. Auxologica* 9 : 95, 1977.

Hunziker, U. A., and Barr, R. G. Increased carrying reduces infant crying: A randomized controlled trial. *Pediatrics* 77 : 641, 1986.

Keller, C. Epidemiological Characteristics of Preterm Births. In S. Friedman and M. Sigman (eds.), *Preterm Birth and Psychological Development.* New York: Academic, 1981.

Lester, B., and Zeskind, P. S. Brazelton scale and physical size correlates of the neonatal cry. *Infant Behav. Dev.* 1 : 393, 1978.

Lester, B., and Zeskind, P. S. The Organization and Assessment of Crying in the Infant Born at Risk. In T. Field (ed.), *Infants Born at Risk: Behavior and Development*. New York: Spectrum, 1979.

Lester, B., and Zeskind, P. S. A Biobehavioral Perspective on Crying in Early Infancy. In H. Fitzgerald, B. Lester, and M. Yogman (eds.), *Theory and Research in Behavioral Pediatrics*. New York: Plenum, 1982. Vol. 1.

Lillienfeld, A., Pasamanick, B., and Rogers, M. Relationship between pregnancy experience and the development of certain neuropsychiatric disorders in childhood. *Am. J. Public Health* May 1955. P. 637.

McGehee, L., and Eckerman, C. The preterm infant as a social partner: Responsive but unreadable. *Infant Behav. Dev.* 6 : 461, 1983.

Michelsson, K. Cry analysis of symptomless low birthweight neonates and of asphyxiated newborn infants. *Acta Paediatr. Scand. [Suppl.]* 216 : 1, 1971.

Paludetto, R., Rinaldi, P., Mansi, G., et al. Early behavioral development of preterm infants. *Dev. Med. Child Neurol.* 26 : 4, 1984.

Parmelee, A. Infant crying and neurological diagnosis. *J. Pediatr.* 61 : 801, 1962.

Parmelee, A. Neurophysiological and behavioral organization of premature infants in the first months of life. *Biol. Psychol.* 10 : 501, 1975.

Prechtl, H. F. R. The behavioral states of the newborn infant: A review. *Brain Res.* 76 : 185, 1974.

Roffwarg, H. P., Muzio, J. N., and Dement, W. C. Ontogenetic development of the human sleep-dream cycle. *Science* 152 : 604, 1966.

Rose, S. Behavioral and Psychophysiological Sequelae of Preterm Birth: The Neonatal Period. In T. Field and A. Sostek (eds.), *Infants Born at Risk: Physiological, Perceptual, and Cognitive Processes*. New York: Grune & Stratton, 1983.

Saint-Anne Dargassies, S. Neurodevelopmental symptoms during the first year of life. *Dev. Med. Child Neurol.* 14 : 235, 1972.

Sameroff, A., and Chandler, M. Reproductive Risk and the Continuum of Caretaking Casualty. In F. Horowitz, M. Hetherington, S. Scarr-Salapatek, and G. Siegel (eds.), *Review of Child Development Research*. Chicago: University of Chicago Press, 1976. Vol. 3.

Schmitt, B. D. Colic: Excessive crying in newborns. *Clin. Perinatol.* 12 : 441, 1985a.

Schmitt, B. D. Prevention of sleep problems. *Clin. Perinatol.* 12 : 453, 1985b.

Sterman, M. B., and Hoppenbrouwers, T. The Development of Sleep-Waking and Rest-Activity Patterns from Fetus to Adult in Man. In C. D. Clemente, D. P. Purpura, and F. E. Mayer (eds.), *Sleep and the Maturing Nervous System*. New York: Academic, 1972.

Stern, E., Parmelee, A., and Harris, M. Sleep state periodicity in premature and young infants. *Dev. Psychobiol.* 6 : 357, 1973.

Ungerer, J., Sigman, M., Beckwith, L., et al. Sleep behavior of preterm children at 3 years of age. *Dev. Med. Child Neurol.* 25 : 297, 1983.

Werner, E. E., Bierman, J. M., and French, F. E. *The Children of Kauai: A Longitudinal Study from the Prenatal Period to Age 10*. Honolulu: University of Hawaii Press, 1971.

Werner, E. E., and Smith, R. S. *Kauai's Children Come of Age*. Honolulu: University of Hawaii Press, 1977.

Werner, E. E., and Smith, R. S. *Vulnerable but Invincible*. New York: McGraw-Hill, 1982.

Wolff, P. The causes, controls and organization of behavior in the newborn. *Psychol. Issues* 5 : 1, 1966.

Zeskind, P. S. Production and Spectral Analysis of Neonatal Crying and its Relation to Other Biobehavioral Systems in the Infant at Risk. In T. Field and A. Sostek (eds.), *Infants Born at Risk: Physiological, Perceptual, and Cognitive Processes*. New York: Grune & Stratton, 1983.

26

Language and Visual Deficits

Marian Sigman

I. Introduction

This chapter suggests certain measurement techniques for assessing the developmental progress of preterm infants in the first years of life and the school-age period. Preterm infants appear to have delays in some language and visual attention skills. These potential deficits, methods of assessment, and possible therapies are briefly reviewed in this chapter.

II. Specific deficits in infancy

The strongest evidence for specific deficits has emerged from studies of visual fixation and visual preferences in preterm and full-term infants. In a number of studies, preterm infants appear to process visual information more slowly than full-term infants. For example, at expected date of birth, preterm infants show longer fixation to stimuli than full-term infants (Sigman et al., 1977; Spungen et al., 1985). Given a fixed familiarization time, preterm infants are less likely to show preferential looking at novel stimuli when these are contrasted with repeatedly presented stimuli, and this difference is particularly strong for high-risk preterm infants (Sigman, 1976; Sigman and Parmelee, 1974). If the preterm infants are given longer periods of time to process the visual stimuli, they are then likely to show preference for novel stimuli such as that demonstrated by full-term infants (Rose, 1983).

Preterm infants also seem less able to transfer information from one sensory channel to another. In a series of studies, Rose (1981) demonstrated that preterm infants show less preference for novel visual stimuli when the familiar stimulus has been presented in the tactual modality for a fixed period of time.

Deficits in preterm infants' abilities to categorize and form representations have been identified but are less consistent. Caron and Caron (1981) reported that preterm infants tend to use relational information less than full-term infants. Differences in sensorimotor skills emerged in comparisons of preterm and full-term infants at 13½ months postconception, but these differences were minimal by 22 months (Ungerer and Sigman, 1983). The same study showed that preterm and full-term infants did not differ in terms of their play skills at either age. Thus, high-risk infants seem most impaired in their abilities to take in information and transfer it across modalities and somewhat less deficient in their representational abilities as manifested in sensorimotor and play skills.

III. Specific deficits in the preschool and school years

Most follow-up studies have been designed to document the developmental progress of infants sampled from high-risk groups. In the studies without control groups, the authors frequently report that the majority of children perform well within the normal range (Davis and Stewart, 1975; Drillien et al., 1980; Wallace et al., 1982). Occasionally, the children are reported to have a surprisingly high incidence of school problems despite average intelligence quotients (IQs) (O'Dougherty et al., 1983). When preterm infants are compared with control samples, they almost universally have lower scores on outcome measures. For example, in one study of 23 infants born weighing 1,500 g or less matched with 23 controls on age, sex, and socioeconomic status, the low-birth-weight infants had lower verbal, performance, and full-scale IQs (Noble-Jamieson et al., 1982). In a follow-up of children who had respiratory distress syndrome, the high-risk group performed worse than the low-risk group on all of the McCarthy Scales at 5 years of age (Field et al., 1983). In another study, 151 low-birth-weight infants had lower scores on the Wechsler Intelligence Scale for Children Revised (WISC-R) on all scales than 43 children of normal birth weight (Kitchen et al., 1980). Generally, the outcome of high-risk infants seems more compromised in studies that contain control groups. One interpretation is that the control groups are self-selected to represent children of higher ability levels. Parents of control children may be more interested in participating if their children are progressing well. Another interpretation is that children in high-risk groups are performing within the average range but show subtle deficits, and the groups contain a greater number of children with serious intellectual limitations. However, the incidence of severe disorders and subtle deficits is not sufficiently frequent for these disorders to be obvious in the absence of control data.

In most investigations in which high-risk infants are performing at levels below low-risk infants, high-risk infants are deficient in all areas. For example, in a study that compared high-risk infants with their siblings, the average IQ difference was 14.6 points. Of 67 children seen at 6 years of age in this study, half had one or more problems with an equal distribution of language comprehension and visual-motor integration difficulties (Hunt et al., 1982).

Specific deficits are most consistently reported in visual-motor integration. A clear example is from a study by Siegel (1982). When 42 full-term infants were compared with 42 preterm infants at 5 years of age, the groups differed on their scores on the Beery Buktenica Developmental Test of Visual Motor Integration but did not differ on the Peabody Picture Vocabulary Test. There had been earlier differences on the Reynell Language Scales, but these were not apparent on the 5-year language measures, although some differences in syntax emerged in the school years (Siegel, 1983, 1985). In another study that carefully matched 5-year-old full-term children to a preterm group, the groups differed on a spatial-relations test and the Beery Buktenica Test but did not differ on IQ tests or subtests measuring auditory and verbal skills, such as memory for sentences and picture vocabulary (Klein et al., 1985). In a comparison of full-term and preterm infants in which preterm children who had normal development at the start of the study were selected, only transient deficiencies in language appeared. However, the preterm children performed more poorly than the full-term children on visual processing and perceptual motor skills at 36 months' corrected age (Ungerer and Sigman, 1983). In the only study in which perceptual problems did not differentiate high-risk and low-risk infants at 3 and 4 years of age, group differences did appear at 5 years (Field et al.,

1983). Although many studies have found a higher incidence of visual-motor problems in 4- to 9-year-old children than might be expected for their intelligence levels (Fitzhardinge and Ramsay, 1973; Francis-Williams and Davies, 1974; Hunt, 1981; Taub et al., 1977), many follow-up studies have also identified deficiencies in language abilities (DeHirsch et al., 1966; Hunt, 1985; Rubin et al., 1973).

IV. Methods of assessment

Because preterm infants are likely to have specific deficits in particular areas of perceptual and cognitive functioning and are at particular risk of school learning problems, cognitive assessments should be used that allow the differentiation of various functions. For this reason, the McCarthy Scales may be particularly useful at the young ages. Similarly, the WISC-R may be a more useful outcome measure than the Stanford-Binet because of the 12 separate subscales on the WISC-R.

Perceptual-motor abilities can be assessed only by standardized testing measures, some of which are listed in Table 26-1. The choice of test depends on the purposes of the assessment. The Beery Buktenica Developmental Test of Visual Motor Integration may be preferable for research studies, the Bender Visual-Motor Gestalt Test preferable as a screening technique, and the Frostig Developmental Test of Visual Perception preferable for more extensive investigations of visual-motor deficits.

Table 26-1. Assessments of specific areas of functioning in young children

Test	Measures derived
Visual Motor Tests	
Bender Visual-Motor Gestalt Test (5–12 yr)	Raw score and mental age (Koppitz scoring method)
Beery Buktenica Developmental Test of Visual Motor Integration (3–16 yr)	Visual-motor index in yr and mo
Graham Kendall Memory for Design Test (5–12 yr)	Raw score (norms available)
Frostig Developmental Test of Visual Perception (3–10 yr)	Perceptual ages: eye-motor coordination, figure-ground discrimination, form constancy, position in space, spatial relations
Language Tests	
Reynell Scales (1–7 yr)	Receptive and expressive language abilities; raw scores and age equivalents
Peabody Picture Vocabulary Test (2½ yr–adulthood)	Receptive language; mental age score and IQ
Test for auditory comprehension of language–Carrow (3–7 yr)	Language comprehension: vocabulary, morphology, grammar, and syntax; raw score, age score, and percentile rank
Illinois Test of Psycholinguistic Ability (2–9½ yr)	Receptive, expressive, and associative language processes; 9 subscales; raw score, language age, standard score, and total score

IQ = intelligence quotient.

Language assessments can be either formal or informal, depending on whether the assessment is carried out for clinical or research purposes. The pediatrician can evaluate language skills by attempting to elicit verbalization by (1) asking the child to respond to "who," "what," "when," and "where" questions; (2) requesting the child to tell a story; (3) asking the child to repeat a sentence; or (4) engaging the child in conversation. Comprehension can be evaluated by requesting that the child point to objects or pictures, follow commands, or answer questions. The pediatrician can simultaneously monitor the child's capacity for nonverbal communication. This informal assessment is probably adequate for screening purposes.

Formal assessments of language can be carried out as well (see Table 26-1 for a list of language tests). A test is chosen according to the purposes of the assessment as well as the age of the child. In scoring assessments of children, corrections for the degree of prematurity must be made through the fifth year of life because developmental lags, as a function of conceptional age, continue at least through that time (Siegel, 1983). Besides the formal tests listed in Table 26-1, language can be evaluated with a scale in which information is gathered from observation and parent interview. Two examples of such scales are the Receptive and Expressive Emergent Language Scale (Bzoch and League, 1971) and the Communicative Evaluation Chart (Anderson et al., 1963).

V. Approaches to remediation

While a number of programs exist for intervention in infants with early perceptual-motor problems, validation of these remediation programs is lacking. Some visual-motor problems in learning-disabled children have been amenable to intervention (Reynolds et al., 1983).

Language dysfunctions in childhood are treated with considerable success by linguists and speech therapists. As with perceptual-motor problems, specific interventions with language disorders of infancy have been used. Language delay presents a unique problem for intervention because the aim is often to create verbal behaviors rather than to modify existing behaviors. Evidence from studies of normal and high-risk infants suggests that certain precursors to language development exist. The development of representational play skills seems critical for language acquisition in normal and developmentally delayed children (Bates et al., 1979; McCune-Nicolich, 1981; Ungerer and Sigman, 1984). In addition, language acquisition also seems closely tied to the acquisition of interaction patterns that are structurally analogous to syntactic patterns (Bates et al., 1979; Bruner, 1975). Rocissano and Yatchmink (1983) showed that the caretaker-child interaction patterns of preterm infants with high language skills were more synchronous than the interactions of preterm infants with low language skills. Generally, mothers of infants in the low language group were more asynchronous and directive, and their children were uninvolved, although the opposite pattern of directive infants and uninvolved mothers also occurred. Based on this literature, attempts to encourage language should emphasize the infant's development of presymbolic play and joint attention skills as well as the formation of cognitive categories. Furthermore, interventions may be needed to encourage mothers to assume more of the interactive burden by monitoring the child's attention and using it to guide their own verbalizations.

REFERENCES

Anderson, R. M., Miles, M., and Matheny, P. A. *Communicative Evaluation Chart from Infancy to 5 Years.* Cambridge, Mass.: Educators Publishing Service, 1963.

Bates, E., Benigni, L., Bretherton, I., et al. *The Emergence of Symbols.* New York: Academic, 1979.

Bruner, J. S. The ontogenesis of speech acts. *J. Child Lang.* 2 : 1, 1975.

Bzoch, K. R., and League, R. Assessing Language Skills in Infancy. *Handbook for the Receptive-Expressive Emergent Language Scale.* Gainesville, Fla.: Tree of Life, 1971.

Caron, A. J., and Caron, R. E. Processing of Relational Information as an Index of Infant Risk. In S. Friedman and M. Sigman (eds.), *Preterm Birth and Psychological Development.* San Francisco: Academic, 1981.

Davis, P. A., and Stewart, A. L. Low-birth-weight infants: Neurological sequelae and later intelligence. *Br. Med. Bull.* 31 : 85, 1975.

DeHirsch, K., Jarsky, J., and Langford, W. S. Comparison between prematurely and maturely born children at three age levels. *Am. J. Orthopsychiatry* 36 : 616, 1966.

Drillien, C. M., Thomson, A. J. M., and Burgoyne, K. Low-birthweight children at early school age: A longitudinal study. *Dev. Med. Child Neurol.* 22 : 26, 1980.

Field, T., Dempsey, J., and Shuman, H. H. Five-year Follow-up of Preterm Respiratory Distress Syndrome Infants. In T. Field and A. Sostek (eds.), *Infants Born at Risk: Physiological, Perceptual, and Cognitive Processes.* New York: Grune & Stratton, 1983.

Fitzhardinge, P. M., and Ramsay, M. The improving outlook for the small prematurely born infant. *Dev. Med. Child Neurol.* 15 : 447, 1973.

Francis-Williams, J., and Davies, P. A. Very low birthweight and later intelligence. *Dev. Med. Child Neurol.* 16 : 707, 1974.

Hunt, J. V. Predicting Intellectual Disorders in Childhood for Preterm Infants with Birthweights Below 1501 Grams. In S. Friedman and M. Sigman (eds.), *Preterm Birth and Psychological Development.* San Francisco: Academic, 1981.

Hunt, J. V. Intellectual status of high-risk infants at 8 years. Presented to the Biennial Meeting of the Society for Research in Child Development, Toronto, Canada, April 1985.

Hunt, J. V., Tooley, W. H., and Harvin, D. Learning disabilities in children with birthweights less than 1500 grams. *Semin. Perinatol.* 6 : 280, 1982.

Kitchen, W. H., Ryan, M. M., and Richards, A. A longitudinal study of very low birth weight infants. IV. An overview of performance at eight years of age. *Dev. Med. Child Neurol.* 22 : 172, 1980.

Klein, N., Hack, M., Gallagher, J., and Fanaroff, A. Preschool performance of children with normal intelligence who were very low birth weight infants. *Pediatrics* 75 : 531, 1985.

McCune-Nicolich, L. Towards symbolic functioning: Structure of early pretend games and potential parallels with language. *Child Dev.* 52 : 785, 1981.

Noble-Jamieson, C. M., Lukenan, D., Silverman, M., and Davies, P. Low birthweight children at school age: Neurological, psychological and pulmonary functions. *Semin. Perinatol.* 6 : 266, 1982.

O'Dougherty, M., Wright, F. S., Garmezy, N., et al. Later competence and adaptation in infants who survive severe heart deficits. *Child Dev.* 54 : 1129, 1983.

Reynolds, L., Egan, R., and Lerner, J. Efficacy of early intervention on preacademic deficits: A review of the literatures. *Top. Early Child Spec. Educ.* 3 : 47, 1983.

Rocissano, L., and Yatchmink, Y. Language skill and interactive patterns in prematurely born toddlers. *Child Dev.* 54 : 1229, 1983.

Rose, S. A. Lags in the Cognitive Competence of Prematurely Born Infants. In S. Friedman and M. Sigman (eds.), *Preterm Birth and Psychological Development.* San Francisco: Academic, 1981.

Rose, S. A. Differential rates of visual information processing in full-term and preterm infants. *Child Dev.* 54 : 1176, 1983.

Rubin, R. A., Rosenblatt, L., and Balow, B. Psychological and educational sequelae of prematurity. *Pediatrics* 52 : 352, 1973.

Siegel, L. S. Reproductive, perinatal, and environmental variables as predictors of development of preterm (< 1501 grams) and full-term children at 5 years. *Semin. Perinatol.* 6 : 274, 1982.

Siegel, L. S. Correction for prematurity and its consequences for the assessment of the very low birthweight infant. *Child Dev.* 54 : 1217, 1983.

Siegel, L. S. Linguistic, visual-spatial, and attentional processes in school-age prematurely born children. Presented to the Biennial Meeting of the Society for Research in Child Development, Toronto, Canada, April 1985.

Sigman, M. Early development of preterm and full-term infants: Exploratory behavior in eight-month olds. *Child Dev.* 47 : 607, 1976.

Sigman, M., Kopp, C. B., Littman, B., and Parmelee, A. H. Infant visual attentiveness in relation to birth condition. *Dev. Psychol.* 13 : 431, 1977.

Sigman, M., and Parmelee, A. H. Visual preferences of four-month-old preterm and full-term infants. *Child Dev.* 45 : 959, 1974.

Spungen, L. B., Kurtzberg, D., and Vaughan, H. G. Patterns of looking behavior in full-term and low birthweight infants at 40 weeks post-conceptional age. *J. Dev. Behav. Pediatr.* 6 : 287, 1985.

Taub, H. B., Goldstein, K. M., and Caputo, D. V. Indices of prematurity as discriminators of development in middle childhood. *Child Dev.* 48 : 797, 1977.

Ungerer, J. A., and Sigman, M. Developmental lags in preterm infants from one to three years of age. *Child Dev.* 54 : 1217, 1983.

Ungerer, J. A., and Sigman, M. The relation of play and sensorimotor behavior to language in the second year. *Child Dev.* 55 : 1448, 1984.

Wallace, I. F., Escalona, S. K., McCarton-Daum, C., and Vaughan, H. G., Jr. Neonatal precursors of cognitive development in low birth-weight children. *Semin. Perinatol.* 6 : 327, 1982.

Environmental Interventions

Craig T. Ramey and Donna M. Bryant

I. Introduction

Risk for health and developmental problems is a function not only of birth weight per se but of other medical complications and environmental circumstances frequently associated with low birth weight (LBW). Two examples illustrate this point: First, for a given weight category the degree of prematurity (as measured by gestational age) is likely to be associated with poor health and developmental outcomes (Hardy et al., 1979); second, birth weight and maternal education are independent and additive contributors to developmental outcome as measured by intelligence quotient (IQ) tests administered in first grade (Ramey et al., 1984). Thus other medical complications and the quality of postnatal environments modify the impact of LBW on developmental outcome. A major clinical and scientific question currently being addressed by much research is whether early environmental interventions can reduce the deleterious impact of LBW on cognitive, social, and physical outcomes.

Currently, LBW infants (< 2,500 g) comprise about 7 percent of live births in the United States (Lee et al., 1980). The causes of LBW are complex and only partially understood. It is clear, however, that LBW infants are at elevated risk for increased mortality and morbidity compared with normal-birth-weight infants (McCormick, 1985).

II. Rationale for early environmental interventions

From the mid-1970s, the interplay of biology and environment as codeterminants of developmental outcome has been increasingly appreciated. Building on the work of Sameroff and Chandler (1975), Ramey and Finkelstein (1981) proposed a bioenvironmental model of development, which is summarized in Fig. 27-1.

The essential features of this model are that environment is perceived clinically as either supportive or nonsupportive for normal intellectual and social development within a particular culture, and further, the child's biology at the time of conception clinically is considered to be either typical or abnormal. With respect to biology at conception, Hunt (1961) noted that the interaction of the organism and environment begins at the moment of fertilization. Furthermore, the interaction is dynamic. Hunt quotes Sinnott and coworkers (1958), who contended that the phenotype of the organism is "determined not only by the environment that prevails at any particular moment but also by the whole succession of environments he has experienced during the life time" (Hunt, 1961).

Nor should it be overlooked that the conceptual biology is, in itself, a product of transacting biologic and environmental forces. Gruenwald (1968) pre-

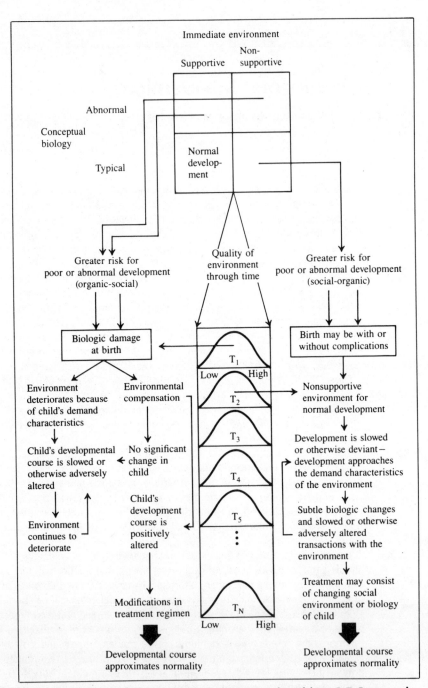

Fig. 27-1. A bioenvironmental model of development. (Adapted from C. T. Ramey and N. W. Finkelstein. Psychosocial Mental Retardation: A Biological and Social Coalescence. In M. Begab [ed.], *Psychosocial Influences and Retarded Performance: Strategies for Improving Social Competence*. Baltimore: University Park, 1981.)

sented studies over 4 decades that linked socioeconomic status, good prenatal care, and adequate nutrition during pregnancy with birth weight. He suggested that even when economic conditions improve, the full manifestations of such economic improvements may not be seen for two or three generations. However, our bioenvironmental model suggests that even abnormal biology can result in normal outcomes depending on the quality of the environment that the child encounters through time. More specifically, especially supportive environments may compensate for the biologic damage that is frequently associated with LBW.

III. Environmental interventions

Consistent with the premises of this model, several early intervention programs have been conducted to test the proposition that carefully delivered, developmentally appropriate educational programs could have a positive influence on the cognitive and social development of LBW infants. These programs have been referred to by such terms as *early stimulation, early intervention,* and more recently, *early education.* As we note elsewhere, the goal of intervention is to provide an optimal set of conditions in which the infant and environment can adapt to one another (Ramey et al., 1981). Ultimately, we are concerned with the LBW infant's capacity to respond to different environmental qualities or, in other words, with the ability to benefit from intervention. Because physical and social aspects of the infant's environment are known to be causally related to subsequent development, these factors have received considerable empirical attention.

To summarize reports of environmental interventions with LBW infants, we classified them in two ways. First, intervention programs were categorized based on who was the direct recipient of the intervention efforts: (1) infant only, (2) parents only, or (3) both infant *and* parents, either individually or together. Second, the interventions were classified by location of treatment: (1) in the hospital, (2) in the home, or (3) in both settings.

In this chapter, we have been selective in our choice of studies. The reader is referred to a recent article by Ramey and associates (1984) for a more comprehensive review.

A. Hospital-based, infant-focused interventions

It is noteworthy that the category with the most studies is that of hospital-based, infant-only interventions. This finding fits with the physical needs of LBW infants and with the prevailing theories of the past decade that focused on the need to provide special stimulation to the premature infant. Most environmental intervention research with LBW infants has been conducted in the neonatal intensive care unit (NICU). The history of such research can be traced to Hasselmeyer (1964), who increased the handling of one group of premature infants and did not increase the handling of another. The research showed that the group receiving increased sensory, tactile, and kinesthetic stimulation showed more quiescent behavior, especially before feedings, whereas the less-handled group exhibited more crying behavior before feedings. Freedman and colleagues (1966) studied a group of five pairs of twins: Five of the twins were rocked in a chair for 30 minutes twice daily beginning 7 to 10 days after they regained birth weight and the control twins were not. The rocked twins gained weight at a greater rate than did the control twins. Again, working from an extra-handling hypothesis, Solkoff and coworkers (1969) reported results when five infants were stroked in their incubators 5 minutes of every hour for 10 days, while five control infants were provided with routine nursery care. The infants who received the extra handling were reported to be more active and physically healthier than the controls. They also regained their initial birth weights faster and, at 7 to 8 months of age (at least by maternal report), received more intense and varied stimulation.

More recently, Rose and associates (1980) evaluated cardiac and behavioral responses of preterm infants who received tactile stimulation, visual contact, and vocalizations from the same person for 60 minutes per day. Compared with control infants, the infants who received the intervention showed cardiac and behavioral responses similar to those of full-term infants. Rausch (1981) also investigated the effects of tactile and kinesthetic stimulation on twenty 1,000 to 2,000 g infants. Compared with a control group that did not receive extra stimulation, treated infants increased their feeding and gained weight more quickly, although the group differences did not reach traditional levels of statistical significance.

Other environmental interventions conducted with infants still in the hospital have used extra stimulation as provided by waterbed movements. Waterbed flotation may reduce the apnea of preterm infants and increase their sleeping time (Korner et al., 1975). Infants also seem to fuss and cry considerably less when waterbeds are provided. It would be interesting to know if these early interventions, which seem to have a soothing effect on the infant, are associated with changes in the perceptions or behaviors of the caregivers (both NICU nurses and parents of the child) and if these early temperament changes persist. In summary, most of the hospital-based tactile, auditory, or kinesthetic stimulation programs have shown beneficial effects. It is true that the results—weight gain, visual alerting, or more regular sleep—were usually short-term, but the interventions themselves were usually short-term as well.

B. Hospital-based, parent-focused interventions

Other hospital-based interventions for LBW infants have focused on the parents. Schwartz (1977) randomly assigned 21 preterm infants to either an experimental or a control group. Parents of experimental group infants were trained in infant stimulation techniques while their infants remained in the NICU. Experimental group parents visited their infants more often, the infants had higher Brazelton Neonatal Behavioral Assessment Scale (NBAS) scores at hospital discharge, and the parents scored significantly higher on five of six subscales of Caldwell and Bradley's Home Observation for Measurement of the Environment (HOME).

Widmayer (1979) provided a one-time intervention for 15 mothers of preterm infants who had been randomly assigned to an experimental group. The treatment consisted of having the mothers watch the administration of the Brazelton NBAS. When the infants were 1 month of age, the demonstration-group mothers received better scores in feeding, face-to-face interactions with their infants, and their assessment of their infants' behaviors. Widmayer suggested that mother-child interactions can be facilitated, at least during the first month of infancy, by an intervention as modest as watching an assessment of the child.

Minde and colleagues (1980) reported on the positive effects of providing support and discussion groups for parents of hospitalized preterm babies. The purpose of the group was to be an informative, educational, and supportive forum for the parents to meet and talk about their infants. Results showed that these parents visited their infants more in the hospital and talked, touched, and looked at their infants more often than parents who did not attend the groups. After hospital discharge, mothers in the parents group were rated as being more involved with their infants, and they spent more time feeding their infants than did control mothers. They also felt more competent in their caretaking role. No long-term data were presented, but the authors suggested that the effects of the early self-help group meetings may be noticed in the later development of the infants.

C. Hospital-based, parent- and infant-focused interventions

Brown and coworkers (1980) conducted a multitreatment comparison study in which 41 premature infants and their mothers were randomly assigned to one of three treatment groups: an infant stimulation group, a maternal training group, and a group that received both infant stimulation and maternal training. An additional 26 preterm infants were assigned to a comparison group. The infant stimulation was similar to the tactile, auditory, and visual stimulation regimens that have been previously described. The mothers were trained by a nurse who demonstrated the stimulation program and helped the mothers perform it as well as observe the responses of their infants. Once the mothers were discharged, the groups did not differ in the frequency of the mother's visits to the hospital to see the baby. At hospital discharge, the infants did not differ on the Brazelton scoring, weight gain, or length of hospital stay. There were no long-term effects on the quality of the home at 9 months or in 12 -month Bayley scores. All scores were within normal limits. This study failed to find either short- or long-term effects of child- or parent-focused early intervention. Because the sample was composed of disadvantaged mothers with low levels of education and income (50% supported by welfare), the authors of the study hypothesized that the enormity of the other problems in the family environment was likely to have overshadowed any benefits that might otherwise have resulted from the early intervention program.

In another parent- and infant-focused study, Klaus and Kennell (1982) provided the opportunity for early physical contact between mothers and their LBW newborns by placing the infants in bed with the mothers for 1 hour on each of the first 3 days after birth. They were able to do this by placing a radiant heat panel over the mother's bed and by having a research nurse present during the entire visit to answer questions, monitor the infant, and observe the mother-infant interactions. They found that the mothers touched, looked at, and talked to their infants significantly more than mothers who only visited their newborns in the NICU. However, no follow-up of these infants has been reported to date.

An earlier study by Klaus and Kennell (1976) also tried to maximize the attachment of parents to their premature infants during the first 2 weeks of the infants' hospitalization by bringing the parents into the nursery for contact and caretaking of their infants. However, 1 month after the infants' discharge, mothers in the experimental and the control groups behaved similarly toward their infants and reported similar perceptions and attitudes about their premature infants.

D. Home-based, infant-focused interventions

In our review of the literature, we found very few home-based interventions for LBW infants or their parents. Only one was focused primarily on the infant. Williams and Scarr (1971) conducted an intervention program with 120 singletons and sole survivors of multiple births. All infants had birth weights less than 2,500 g, with 75 percent of the birth weights less than 1,500 g. Random assignment was employed to constitute an experimental and control group. Within each group, children ranged in age from less than 1 to 4 years. In the experimental groups, children were tutored for 4 months, except that infants less than 1 year were not tutored directly—rather, home visitors worked with their mothers. A comprehensive assessment battery found that intervention with toys alone (i.e., without tutoring) had no measured treatment effect. Performance on tests measuring motor functions, social maturity, and intellectual ability at the end of the 4-month period revealed that in all infants, the tutored group was superior to the untutored control group. Further, children with no neurologic damage made greater gains than those who were impaired.

E. Home-based and parent-focused interventions

Some studies have attempted to get the caregiver to continue at home with stimulation programs that the LBW infants received in the hospital. Rice Infant Sensorimotor Stimulation (a massage-type treatment) was taught to mothers by visiting nurses, and the mothers administered this stimulation 25 minutes, 4 times a day, for 1 month beginning the first day the infant arrived home. At 4 months of age, the infants had made marked gains in neurologic development, weight gain, and mental development. Rice (1977) concluded that this parent-provided treatment improved the infant's development and suggested that it also enhanced the mother-infant relationship.

A major home-based, parent-training intervention program focused on teenage, low-income black mothers and their preterm infants was conducted by Field and colleagues (1980). Intervention consisted of providing parent training in infant stimulation techniques, education about infant developmental milestones, and ways to increase communication skills and positive mother-infant relationships. Intervention efforts for the preterm infants of the teenage mothers resulted in more optimal growth, higher Denver Developmental Screening Test scores, and more face-to-face interactions at 4 months. At 8 months, superior Bayley mental scores, home environment ratings, and infant temperament scores were obtained. Positive gains were also noted for the mothers who rated their children more positively and had more realistic knowledge of developmental milestones.

F. Hospital- and home-based, parent- and infant-focused interventions

Two studies we reviewed took place in both the hospital and the home. In a study by Scarr-Salapatek and Williams (1973), infants less than 1,800 g born to low socioeconomic status mothers were alternately assigned to an experimental or a control group as they entered the NICU. Working from a sensory deprivation hypothesis, these investigators instructed nurses in an experimental nursery area to provide special visual, tactile, and kinesthetic stimulation that was thought to approximate good home care for newborn infants. The control group infants received standard pediatric care for LBW infants, which consisted of maintaining them in their Isolettes and feeding and changing them with minimal disturbance. After discharge from the hospital, mothers of infants in the experimental group received weekly visits for 1 year from a social worker who implemented a stimulation program developed by Gordon and Lally (1967) for disadvantaged normal-birth-weight infants and their mothers. Control infants received no home visits. During the neonatal period, the experimental group gained weight significantly faster than did the control group, although their scores on the Brazelton examination were not significantly different. At 1 year of age, experimental infants had higher scores on the Cattell Infant Intelligence Scale. It is especially important to note that the mean scores for the treated infants approximated those expected of normally developing children. Because the experimental group infants received both hospital treatment and home visits, it is impossible to assess the effects of either treatment alone.

The UCLA Infant Studies Project (Bromwich and Parmelee, 1979) is the longest-lasting educational intervention program that we are aware of. Thirty premature infants received free medical and nursing care from birth to age 2 and educational home visits from 10 months to 2 years of age. A control group of 33 infants received only medical and nursing care. The main purpose of the intervention was to enhance the quality of the parent-infant interaction through a home visit program that was essentially individually tailored for each family. Results showed that the intervention and nonintervention groups did not differ significantly on any physiologic measures, cognitive tests, or early mother-child interaction. Only the 24-month home observation of the mother-child interaction significantly favored the treatment group. One possible reason for lack of group differences in this study is that the control group did receive substantial treatment in the form of medical care and home visits from nurses.

IV. The Infant Health and Development Program

To date, there have been promising but preliminary results suggesting that the health and developmental outcomes of LBW infants may be considerably improved by providing high-quality medical and comprehensive services. No large-scale longitudinal study has, however, been conducted to pursue these issues adequately using national representative samples of LBW infants.

A national collaborative study, funded by the Robert Wood Johnson Foundation, is currently underway to test the efficacy of combining early child development services with pediatric care in reducing the incidence of health and development problems among LBW infants. This endeavor, known as the

Infant Health and Development Program, has enrolled approximately 1,000 infants born weighing less than 2,500 g.

Under this program, eight medical schools have received grants for a period of 4 years, beginning in 1984. The eight sites follow specific research protocols for health and development services and data collection. At each site, LBW infants have been enrolled and randomly assigned to one of two treatment groups. In both groups, infants receive pediatric care and developmental assessments. In addition, infants and parents in one of the groups receive special child and family development services both in the home and in a child development center. This protocol is followed until the children reach 3 years of age.

The Infant Health and Development Program will thereby determine the effects and the value of the two treatments. In addition, children and families with the greatest likelihood of benefiting from these services should be identified.

V. Conclusions from previous studies

Although this chapter reviews a limited number of intervention programs with LBW infants, we find that most work has been done with hospitalized infants. Several of these studies show positive results such as increased food intake, increased weight gain, more visual alertness or activity, and increased sleeping times. Rarely, however, has long-range follow-up been conducted or have measures been collected on cognitive processes or social development.

Studies in which parents have been the target of intervention suggest positive benefits of such efforts, but there have been so few studies that it is difficult to make any definitive statements on specific parent-intervention procedures. In general, however, parent intervention does appear to have positive benefits on parent-child interactions and on infant behavior.

Clearly, more emphasis needs to be placed on the role of parents if we believe that they are important for later development. Because parents typically make a major contribution to the quality of the infant's environment, the parents' role in interacting with LBW children must be closely documented and systematically incorporated into future intervention efforts.

VI. Clinical implications

Given that LBW and, particularly, disadvantaged LBW infants are at elevated risk for cognitive and social impairments, several clinical implications can be derived from evidence and current theory.

A. Systematic attention to the developmental needs of LBW infants is warranted.

B. High-quality education programs have produced some positive evidence to suggest their effectiveness.

C. Active and regular parent and, indeed, family participation in early education should be encouraged.

D. Additional long-term research is urgently needed to determine the changing need for intensive early intervention and its efficacy for the increasingly small infants who are surviving to be discharged from the NICU.

REFERENCES

Bromwich, R. M., and Parmelee, A. H. An Intervention Program for Pre-term Infants. In T. M. Field, A. M. Sostek, S. Goldberg, and H. H. Shuman (eds.), *Infants Born at Risk.* New York: S. P. Medical and Scientific Books, 1979.

Brown, J., LaRossa, M., Aylward, G., et al. Nursery-based intervention with prematurely born babies and their mothers: Are there effects? *J. Pediatr.* 97 : 487, 1980.

Caldwell, B., and Bradley, R. *Home Observation for Measurement of the Environment.* Little Rock, Ark.: Center for Child Development and Education, University of Arkansas.

Field, T., Widmayer, S., Stringer, S., and Ignatoff, E. Teenage, lower-class, black mothers and their preterm infants: An intervention and developmental follow-up. *Child Dev.* 51 : 526, 1980.

Freedman, D. G., Boverman, H., and Freedman, N. Effects of kinesthetic stimulation on weight gain and on smiling in premature infants. Presented to the annual meeting of the American Orthopsychiatric Association, San Francisco, 1966.

Gordon, I. J., and Lally, R. *Intellectual Stimulation for Infants and Toddlers.* Gainesville, Fla.: Institute for Development of Human Resources, 1967.

Gruenwald, P. Fetal growth as an indicator of socio-economic change. *Public Health Rep.* 83 : 867, 1968.

Hardy, J. M. B., Drage, J. S., and Jackson, E. C. *The First Year of Life: The Collaborative Perinatal Study of the National Institute of Neurological and Communicative Disorders and Stroke.* Baltimore: Johns Hopkins University Press, 1979.

Hasselmeyer, E. G. The premature neonate's response to handling. *American Nurses' Association* 11 : 15, 1964.

Hunt, J. McV. *Intelligence and Experience.* New York: Ronald Press, 1961. P. 41.

Klaus, M., and Kennell, J. Interventions in the premature nursery: Impact on development. *Pediatr. Clin. North Am.* 29 : 1263, 1982.

Klaus, M. H., and Kennell, J. H. *Maternal-infant Bonding.* St. Louis: Mosby, 1976.

Korner, A. F., Kraemer, H. C., Haffner, M. E., and Cosper, L. M. Effects of waterbed flotation on premature infants: A pilot study. *Pediatrics* 56 : 361, 1975.

Lee, K. S., Paneth, N., and Gartner, L. M. Neonatal mortality: An analysis of the recent improvement in the United States. *Public Health* 70 : 15, 1980.

McCormick, M. C. The contribution of low birth weight to infant mortality and childhood morbidity. *N. Engl. J. Med.* 312 : 82, 1985.

Minde, K., Shosenberg, N., Marton, P., et al. Self-help groups in a premature nursery: A controlled evaluation. *J. Pediatr.* 96 : 933, 1980.

Ramey, C. T., Bryant, D. M., Sparling, J. J., and Wasik, B. H. A biosocial systems perspective on environmental interventions for low birthweight infants. *Clin. Obstet. Gynecol.* 27 : 672, 1984.

Ramey, C. T., and Finkelstein, N. W. Psychosocial Mental Retardation: A Biological and Social Coalescence. In M. Begab (ed.), *Psychosocial Influences and Retarded Performance: Strategies for Improving Social Competence.* Baltimore: University Park, 1981. Vol. 1, pp. 65–92.

Ramey, C. T., Zeskind, P. S., and Hunter, R. Biomedical and Psychosocial Interventions for Preterm Infants. In S. L. Friedman and M. Sigman (eds.), *Preterm Birth and Psychological Development.* New York: Academic, 1981.

Rausch, P. Effects of tactile and kinesthetic stimulation on premature infants. *J. Obstet. Gynecol. Neonatal Nurs.* 34, 1981.

Rice, R. D. Neurophysiological development in premature infants following stimulation. *Dev. Psychol.* 13 : 69, 1977.

Rose, S., Schmidt, K., Riese, M., and Bridger, W. Effects of prematurity and early intervention on responsivity to actual stimuli: A comparison of preterm and full-term infants. *Child Dev.* 51 : 416, 1980.

Sameroff, A. J., and Chandler, M. J. Reproductive Risk and the Continuum of Caretaking

Casualty. In F. D. Horowitz (ed.), *Review of Child Development Research.* Chicago: University of Chicago Press, 1975. Vol. 4.

Scarr-Salapatek, S., and Williams, M. The effects of early stimulation on low-birthweight infants. *Child Dev.* 44 : 94, 1973.

Schwartz, S. The effects of supplementary social stimulation on preterm infants and their parents. *Dissertation Abstracts Int.* 38(12B) : 6173, 1977.

Sinnott, E. W., Dunn, L. C., and Dobzhansky, T. *Principles of Genetics.* New York: McGraw-Hill, 1958.

Solkoff, N., Jaffe, S., Weintraub, D., and Blase, B. Effects of handling on the subsequent development of premature infants. *Dev. Psychol.* 1 : 765, 1969.

Widmayer, S. An intervention for mothers and their preterm infants. *Dissertation Abstracts Int.* 40(4B) : 1947, 1979.

Williams, M., and Scarr, S. Effects of short-term intervention on performance in low-birthweight, disadvantaged children. *Pediatrics* 47 : 289, 1971.

V

Parents and Infants

Parental Grieving

F. Sessions Cole

I. Introduction

Clinical studies of the grief process are a fairly recent phenomenon. In the 1940s, Lindemann studied survivors of World War II and the Coconut Grove fire in Boston (Lindemann, 1944). His studies suggested survivors undergo a consistent series of feelings and reactions after the death of a friend or family member. The loss of a fetus or a newborn infant has long been recognized to invoke similar feelings in parents and siblings. Since the implications of infant-parent bonding for perinatal loss were noted and maternal reactions after a stillborn infant were described, the unique responsibility of caretakers for management of the grieving process has been recognized (Giles, 1970; Kennell et al., 1970; Kowalski and Bowes, 1976; Parkes, 1971). Lindemann's work identified the importance of memory of the deceased individual in facilitating the grieving process. After the death of an older child or adult, he or she is traditionally recalled at gatherings of persons who have known the deceased (e.g., wakes and funerals). In the death of a newborn infant, the caretakers from the neonatal intensive care unit (NICU) are frequently the only persons besides the parents who have known and seen the child. They therefore are the only persons who can help create a memory of the infant for the parents. This chapter summarizes strategies that have been used for managing the grieving process of families who sustain perinatal loss.

II. Stages of grieving

On the basis of Lindemann's early work and subsequent redefinition by Kübler-Ross of the grieving process, an understanding of the stages of this process has proved helpful for caretakers anticipating reactions of families to perinatal loss (Bruhn and Bruhn, 1984; Friel, 1982; Kübler-Ross, 1973; Sahu, 1981; Schulman and Rehm, 1983). The first stage is *denial,* which represents the period when a family repudiates the meaning of the anticipated loss of the fetus or newborn infant to minimize fear and anxiety. In the NICU, this stage is characterized by statements such as "He will be all right" or "She will come back soon." Frequently this attitude occasions the NICU staff's concern because the parents do not appear to understand the reality of the infant's imminent death. This stage is followed by *anger,* during which the focus may be on NICU caretakers, those associated with the delivery or other medical personnel, or other family members. Of concern is the potential vulnerability of surviving siblings during the anger stage. Parents frequently progress to a stage of *bargaining* during which the family attempts to understand the loss in terms that might bring the infant back to life. After bargaining, parents encounter a stage of *depression.* Finally, parents enter a stage of *acceptance* or of *resignation* to the loss.

The entire grieving process usually requires between 6 and 18 months, although successful resolution of perinatal loss is affected by parental age, previous childbearing experience, religion, and cultural attitudes. Although caretaker outreach and availability are essential in facilitating progress through the process, involvement of culturally or family-identified persons is critical for long-term establishment and sharing of the memory of the lost infant.

Important in the management of a family whose infant has died is the recognition that mothers and fathers cope with loss in distinctly different ways, so that each parent may pass through the stages at different rates. A simple partial explanation for this observation is that the mother has felt the infant grow for 6 to 9 months within the uterus, an experience not available to the father.

III. Goals and strategies of management

A. A major goal for the management of any family whose child is admitted to the NICU is to establish and maintain a non-outcome-dependent alliance between caretakers and family. This alliance is frequently difficult to generate because many caretakers are themselves overwhelmed by the emotional pain of the experience and thus cannot acknowledge the positive long-term therapeutic implications of providing "bad news" to a family. In addition, caretakers frequently underestimate the psychologic resilience of parents during periods of extreme stress. Information necessary to initiate an alliance with a family includes the following:

1. The family's previous experiences with losses of other children, family members, or friends, and especially with previous perinatal losses
2. The availability to the parents of one or more support figures who can share the loss (e.g., family members, friends, or an important religious or medical counselor)
3. The circumstances surrounding the pregnancy (e.g., planned or unplanned)
4. The family's religious, political, or cultural beliefs

Much of this information is available from caretakers who have long-term relationships with the family (e.g., obstetrician, midwife, pediatrician, pediatric nurse-practitioner, or social worker).

B. When death is anticipated as an inevitable outcome of the medical condition of an infant, two goals of care become important: first, to establish a memory of the child by encouraging and supporting parents' touching and holding their child and, second, to consider all necessary medical diagnostic tests that should be obtained prior to the death of the infant (Duff and Campbell, 1973). These tests include rigorous examination for infectious, metabolic, and genetic causes of death. While an autopsy is critical, the availability of tissue or blood specimens obtained before death may be necessary for diagnosis. Encouragement and support for parents to be present at the time of death may be complicated by anxiety and anger of parents concerning their child and initial parental ambivalence and fear about seeing the child, who is so ill. We suggest an aggressively supportive approach: Parents almost unanimously appreciate being with their children before and at the time of death. Because of legal problems in transporting an infant who has died to his or her parents if they are in another city or at a different hospital, caretakers in the NICU should be prepared to assist transport of a postpartum mother from an outside hospital to be with her infant and the father at the time of the death as long as the mother's medical condition is stable.

At the time of death, caretakers should offer remembrances of the infant, including hat, name bracelet, name card, and pictures to the parents. Frequently, parents will not want to accept these mementos. In this situation, caretakers should carefully put these items aside because parents will almost invariably request these items at the follow-up meetings some months after the death.

Autopsy permission should be sought from parents of all stillborn infants and newborn infants who die, regardless of the apparently obvious cause(s) of death. Again, parents will frequently need aggressive support and direction from caretakers to help make this decision. They should be informed that an autopsy might provide considerable unanticipated information concerning the cause of death and complications during future pregnancies.

Finally, parents should be given a bereavement booklet and the names and telephone numbers of caretakers (physician and nurse) who will coordinate their follow-up. The bereavement booklet is designed to validate early feelings of denial, anger, and depression, as well as provide a source of information concerning practical issues such as holding a funeral, telling friends and family about the death, and giving autopsy permission.

To provide a record of accountability and a reference source, we maintain information concerning the family, the infant, referral sources, and the physician and nurse responsible for follow-up in a loose-leaf notebook in the NICU (Figs. 28-1 and 28-2). The physician and nurse then determine who will contact the parents and at what intervals. Generally, telephone contact initiated by the medical team is recommended every 2 to 4 weeks for the first 8 to 10 weeks after the death. The content of these telephone calls should be briefly recorded in the follow-up notebook in the NICU. Approximately 8 weeks after the death, the caretakers should arrange to see the family to review their questions concerning the child, the preliminary autopsy results, and their progress in the grieving process. Prior to this meeting, physician and nurse should review in detail the infant's chart, available test results (e.g., chromosomes, cultures), and preliminary autopsy results and agree on the approach required for communication of these data. Identification of pathologic reactions is another important function of this meeting (Brown and Stoudemire, 1983; Canadian Pediatric Society, 1983). Specifically, drug or alcohol abuse, physical abuse of family members, inability to reintegrate into previous life activities, and disabling somatic complaints are signals that might prompt caretakers to refer one or both parents for more intensive psychiatric intervention. Severe sibling reactions should also be investigated and may also require referral (Reilly et

Infant Follow-up Meeting Record

Meeting # Date Location Persons present	Review of medical events	Review of autopsy	Need for genetic counseling	Implications for future pregnancies	Referral to bereavement group	JPN MD notified if not present	Plan next meeting	Assessment of meeting

Parental reaction	Mother	Father	Mother	Father	Mother	Father
Sleep disorders						
Spontaneous crying						
Recurrent dreams						
Difficulty eating						
Anniversary reactions						
Use of drugs/alcohol						
Inability to discuss infant with family						
Inability to return to normal activities (job, housework)						
Somatic symptoms (backaches, chest pain, etc.)						
Guilt						
Anger						
Anxiety						
Absence of grief						
Loneliness/isolation						
Other						

Parental interaction	Mother	Father	Mother	Father	Mother	Father
Shared feelings about death						
Father attempting to protect mother						
Mother feeling too weak relative to father, not wanting to burden him						
Father blaming mother						
Mother blaming father						
Parents blaming health care delivery for death						
Parents' interactions during meeting do/do not correlate with stated behavior						

Sibling reaction	Sibling #1	Sibling #2	Sibling #3	Sibling #4	Sibling #5	Sibling #6
Enuresis/encopresis						
Violent or angry behavior						
Falling school performance						
Withdrawal						
Onset of organic symptoms						
Avoidance of foods						
Sleep disorders						
Separation anxiety						
Other						

Fig. 28-1. Infant follow-up meeting record. *JPN* = Joint Program in Neonatology. (From S. J. Skoolicas, F. S. Cole, and D. Maguire. Bereavement and Infant Death Follow-up. In J. P. Cloherty and A. R. Stark [eds.], *Manual of Neonatal Care* [2nd ed.]. Boston: Little, Brown, 1985. Pp. 480–481. With permission.)

Infant Death Form 1984

Medical

Infant's name: _____ record # _____

Date of birth: _____

Date of death: _____

Gestational age: _____

Age at time of death: _____ hrs

Route of delivery: _____ C/S _____ NVD

Amniocentesis: _____ no _____ yes

Abdominal ultrasound: _____ no _____ yes

Intend to breast-feed? _____ no _____ yes

Actually breast-fed? _____ no _____ yes

Language used to describe death to family: _____

Diagnosis: _____

Parents' names: mother   _____

father _____

Parents' address: _____

_____

Parents' telephone: _____

Marital status: _____ S _____ M _____ W _____ D _____ SEP

Mother's age: _____

Mother's occupation: _____

Para: _____ Gravida: _____

Number of living children: _____

Mother's ethnic origin: _____

Mother's religion: _____

Father's age: _____

Father's occupation: _____

Father's ethnic origin: _____

Father's religion: _____

Siblings name(s) and age(s) _____

_____

Primary nurse: _____ ID# _____

RN ethnic origin: _____

RN previous involvement with death follow-up? _____ no _____ yes

Length of RN employment: _____ yrs

Primary doctor: _____

CHMC identification #: _____

MD ethnic origin: _____

MD previous involvement with death follow-up? _____ no _____ yes

Social worker? _____ no _____ yes

Community referrals _____ none _____ RN/MD _____ Social worker

CHMC referrals: _____ none _____ RN/MD _____ Social worker

Family involvement at time of death: _____

_____

Predeath conference? _____ no _____ yes

Postdeath conference? _____ no _____ yes

Did mother hold baby? _____ no _____ yes

Did father hold baby? _____ no _____ yes

Autopsy permission? _____ no _____ yes

Bereavement pkg. given? _____ no _____ yes

Pictures of baby taken? _____ no _____ yes

Record of telephone contact		
Date	Call initiated by	Purpose of call

Fig. 28-2. Infant death form (1984). *CHMC* = The Children's Hospital Medical Center (Boston); *C/S* = cesarean section; *D* = divorced; *M* = married; *NVD* = normal vaginal delivery; *pkg.* = package; *S* = single; *SEP* = separated; *W* = widowed. (From S. J. Skoolicas, F. S. Cole, and D. Maguire. Bereavement and Infant Death Follow-up. In J. P. Cloherty and A. R. Stark [eds.], *Manual of Neonatal Care* [2nd ed.]. Boston: Little, Brown, 1985. PP. 478–479. With permission.)

al., 1983; Rowe et al., 1978). Frequently, however, validating differences in grieving stages between mother and father is the most important function of this meeting. In addition, interpretation by caretakers of feelings and reactions unfamiliar to the parents (e.g., crying at specific times of the day or on certain days of the week, inability to concentrate at work, recurrent dreams, or visiting the grave site frequently) as normal is critical for progress through the grieving process. Parents frequently have no prior experience with which to understand that their feelings may persist for months. Parents usually require additional meetings as further data concerning the child become available or as issues concerning their grieving process require further attention.

IV. Conclusion

These recommendations are meant to be guidelines. The major goal is to afford each family who sustains a perinatal loss the opportunity for follow-up that is individually designed and coordinated by a physician and nurse team. To support caretakers who carry out these responsibilities, senior members of the nursing and medicine faculty should be identified as resource persons from whom help may be sought. In addition, regular (e.g., monthly) review of deaths and presentations and discussions of interesting or problem cases are helpful in establishing and maintaining the expectations for caretakers to perform these functions. Available data suggest that these interventions provide parents with improved capacity to cope with perinatal loss and to resolve their grief successfully (Forrest et al., 1982).

REFERENCES

Brown, J. T., and Stoudemire, G. A. Normal and pathological grief. *J.A.M.A.* 259 : 378, 1983.
Bruhn, D. F., and Bruhn, P. Stillbirth. A humanistic response. *J. Reprod. Med.* 29 : 107, 1984.

Canadian Pediatric Society, Fetus and Newborn Committee. Support for parents experiencing perinatal loss. *Can. Med. Assoc.* 129 : 335, 1983.

Duff, R. S., and Campbell, A. G. M. Moral and ethical dilemmas in the special care nursery. *N. Engl. J. Med.* 289 : 890, 1973.

Forrest, G. O., Standish, E., and Baum, J. D. Support after perinatal death: A study of support and counseling after perinatal bereavement. *Br. Med. J.* 285 : 1475, 1982.

Friel, P. B. Death and dying. *Ann. Intern. Med.* 97 : 767, 1982.

Giles, P. Reactions of women to perinatal death. *Aust. N.Z. J. Obstet. Gynaecol.* 10 : 207, 1970.

Hodge, D. S., and Graham, P. L. Supporting bereaved parents: A program for the NICU. *Neonatal Network* 4 : 11, 1985.

Kennell, J. H., Slyter, H., and Klaus, M. H. The mourning response of parents to the death of a newborn. *N. Engl. J. Med.* 283 : 344, 1970.

Kowalski, K., and Bowes, W. A. Parent's response to a stillborn baby. *Contemp. Obstet. Gynecol.* 8 : 53, 1976.

Kübler-Ross, E. *On Death and Dying.* New York: Macmillan, 1973. Pp. 34–121.

Lindemann, E. Symptomatology and management of acute grief. *Am. J. Psychol.* 101 : 141, 1944.

Parkes, C. M. Determination of outcome following bereavement. *Proc. R. Soc. Med.* 64 : 279, 1971.

Reilly, T. P., Hasazi, J. E., and Bond, L. A. Children's conceptions of death and personal mortality. *J. Pediatr. Psychol.* 8 : 21, 1983.

Rowe, J., Clyman, R., Green, C., et al. Follow-up families who experience a perinatal death. *Pediatrics* 62 : 166, 1978.

Sahu, S. Coping with perinatal death. *J. Reprod. Med.* 26 : 129, 1981.

Schulman, J. L., and Rehm, J. L. Assisting the bereaved. *J. Pediatr.* 108 : 998, 1983.

Parenting the Premature Infant: Problems and Opportunities

Klaus K. Minde

I. Introduction

Studies investigating the growth and development of prematurely born infants have usually focused on the infant's later height and weight, intelligence, and general neurologic or cognitive development (Fitzhardinge and Pape, 1981; Knobloch et al., 1982). However, there is an increasing amount of information for the professional and lay audiences that draws attention to the behavioral sequelae of prematurity, both in the infants and their caretakers (Goldberg and DiVitto, 1983; Minde, 1984; Shosenberg et al., 1980).

This chapter considers the impact of prematurity on parents by examining the challenges a premature infant presents to his or her caretakers during the first year of life. I first describe the reactions and feelings parents normally show when their infant is born prematurely and go on to discuss the most common caretaking difficulties the clinician encounters in parents of such infants. Finally, I review remedial actions that have been found useful in this population.

II. Reactions frequently encountered in parents of premature infants

A recent review of the clinical literature suggests that parents of an infant who is born with a handicap or who violates their expectations in any other way pass through three distinct stages of adjustment (Blacher, 1984). Although these stages have been given different names by different authors, Blacher calls them *initial crisis responses, feelings of emotional disorganization,* and *acceptance.* Blacher acknowledges the absence of empirical data confirming the validity of these stages and points out that there are studies that do not show parents going through an ordered sequence of stages or indeed ever attaining a final stage of acceptance of their child's handicap (Featherstone, 1980).

While the birth of a premature infant is clearly an unexpected and frightening event for most parents, no good clinical or research evidence suggests that parents experience stagelike reactions in the wake of such an event. Nevertheless, from both my clinical experience and a study of 60 very small premature infants (birth weight $< 1,501$ g) that examined interview data obtained 4 weeks after birth, and conducted home visits at 6 weeks, 3, 6, 9, and 12 months after discharge (Minde et al., 1985), I have identified specific reactions of parents of premature infants. These reactions can be best divided into (1) immediate hospital reactions (first 2 weeks after birth), (2) later hospital reactions (occurring up to the discharge from hospital) and (3) problems characteristic of the first year of life.

A. Immediate reactions

The most immediate reaction after the birth of a premature infant in virtual-ly all parents is a fear that the infant may die. Because approximately 50 percent of the mothers have had one or more previous miscarriages or abortions (Minde et al., 1980a), premature infants are often long and anx-iously awaited and especially precious to their parents. Fear with respect to the infant's survival is especially pronounced when the infant is delivered in a general obstetric unit and then transferred to a neonatal intensive care unit (NICU) at another hospital. The mother's inability to be with her infant during these first days and help him or her fight for survival may be agoniz-ingly painful. Approximately 10 percent of mothers demand an early dis-charge from their obstetric ward, which can lead to difficulties between the obstetrician and the infant's parents when the physician wants the mother to remain in the hospital longer.

Only after survival seems ensured do other concerns and feelings sur-face. Most commonly, the mother may be almost totally preoccupied with the infant. For example, 40 to 60 percent of all mothers think only about their infant for weeks on end. They visit the hospital every day for many hours, yet call the ward again to inquire about the infant's progress as soon as they get home. They sleep poorly, eat little, are disinterested in talking to relatives or friends about their infant's progress, and show quick mood changes toward both strangers and family members. Thus, small things such as a burnt potato at supper cause tears. To cope with these feelings, some read extensively about prematurity and its long-term consequences. Others are satisfied to sit with their infant, talk or sing, or simply touch and caress him or her for hours on end.

In the majority of cases, these feelings recede after 4 to 6 weeks, but about 10 percent of parents translate their concerns and preoccupations in-to a heightened vigilance over the medical staff caring for their infant. Thus, they may read the infant's chart several times per day or count the drops of the IV and complain if the infant gets 32 rather than the prescribed 35 drops per minute. In general, they seem to want to find fault with the nurs-ing or medical staff of the unit. On close examination, such parents often believe that they are relegated to the status of visitors rather than parents, and they feel they need to take control of their infant's day-to-day activities.

This concern about being a peripheral rather than central figure in the life of the infant is evident in almost 60 percent of all parents. It is especial-ly prominent if the infant's medical condition remains problematic for a long time and there is a realistic fear that the infant may be handicapped. To enhance their role as parents they may demand to have other relatives or siblings visit the infant, bring play material or clothing for the infant, or insist on reading the chart regularly. Although all these requests and coping strategies are eminently reasonable, they can at times be interpreted as un-warranted challenges by the hospital staff and can create mutual distrust and unhappiness.

Financial and other management issues also arise during the second month as not only medical bills and gasoline and hospital parking fees must be paid but also other children must be looked after during parental visits. Long-distance calls to hospitals or frequent meals away from home and the accompanying fatigue are also severe stresses that can lead to crying spells and temper outbursts toward the staff or other family members.

While all of these symptoms are more common in mothers, they are also seen in fathers. However, in our experience, approximately 70 percent of all fathers cope with the stress of having such a small infant by being especially helpful in the house and by visiting the infant frequently. Yet 25 percent do not talk to the infant's mother about their feelings, nor do they share their fears or hopes but battle them in isolation. This can lead to marital strain and can exacerbate the mother's grieving response (Marton et al., 1981).

B. Later reactions: Pre- and posthospital discharge

Once discharge from the hospital approaches, parents may become especially anxious as they now face the fact that they alone are responsible for their infant. This anxiety may be expressed in frequent inquiries about apnea, infections, or other minor disturbances that their infant may suffer. Once the infant is home, the parents may not dare to sleep for days for fear of missing an episode of apnea. As premature infants have a somewhat different behavioral repertoire than full-term infants have, even routine care and feedings may be more difficult than the parents expect. In fact, the whole first year with such an infant can be quite stressful. Some of this stress may come from the parents' overconcern for their infant's health and welfare and may be expressed in their unwillingness to take him or her out of the house or in their continuing unnecessary night feedings. Other stress, however, may be related to the early interactional deficiencies frequently present in these infants, as described by Als and coworkers (1982) and Goldberg and DiVitto (1983). A mother often attempts to overcome these deficiencies by being more active and intrusive in her interactions with her infant. Thus she may try to calm her hyperreactive and poorly regulated infant by providing him or her with ever increasing stimulation. As the immature infant cannot cope with the additional stimulation, he or she may react by trembling, crying, or extending the limbs in an uncontrollable, almost spastic fashion. This reaction in turn creates yet new parental fears and sets up a cycle of painful mutual misreadings of interactional cues.

III. Common difficulties encountered in parents of premature infants

Problems that are specific to the behavior of parents with an infant in an NICU and that go beyond the difficulties previously described are best divided into the following categories: (1) abnormal parental grieving, (2) parental anger or guilt, and (3) parental insensitivity to the premature infant's behavior and biologic cues.

A. Abnormal parental grieving

A small number of parents (about 5% in our sample) develop a severe or abnormal grief reaction following the birth of their premature infant. Such parents may refuse to visit the infant, claiming that they must prepare themselves for the infant's death, and may also show severe sleep and appetite disturbances. When forced to be with their infant they may initially feel a "lack of bonding" and may show more interest in other infants than in their own. A substantial number of these parents in our clinical experience have immigrated from countries with less sophisticated neonatal care and still assess the chance of their infant's survival on a scale appropriate for their country of origin.

Ongoing depression, with the accompanying psychologic unavailability of a mother during the first year of life, can have very powerful implications for the behavior and development of the young child, at least up to age 4 (Ghodsian et al., 1984). The early diagnosis and treatment of depression is therefore critical for the psychologic health of the infant. It is especially important to be aware of minor depressive episodes that last longer than 3 weeks because family members often consider these to be "normal" and see no need to assist such a mother.

B. Parental anger and guilt

Parents who cannot express their anger or guilt appropriately may be excessively critical of the staff in all or most of its functions. They may denigrate specific nurses in front of other parents, use the complex and multi-faceted communication patterns of an NICU to split the ward staff into several factions, and be unwilling to attend follow-up appointments.

Some parents (about 2%) project their anger or guilt toward their partner or other family members onto the baby or the NICU staff. Thus, rather than express anger at the infant's father who accuses her of being at fault for the early birth of the infant, a mother may blame unfriendly nurses for her refusal to visit her infant. Likewise, a father in need of total control of his life may rage at the restrictions the special care and needs of his infant impose on his interactions with his infant.

As such critical interchanges between staff and parent can lead to a mutual disengagement of the parties, which in turn may compromise the treatment of the infant, a rapid diagnosis and settling of such issues must be attempted.

C. Parental insensitivity to the premature infant's developmental needs

Parental insensitivity can be associated with any of the previously mentioned conditions and often is the most difficult to detect and treat. One reason for this difficulty may be that we do not usually observe the mother's interaction with her infant in the nursery. For example, we rarely record obscure and obviously incorrect attributions a parent may make about his or her infant's behavior (e.g., a mother saying "You really look as if you hate me today" or "Don't look so mean"). We seldom find out why a parent may have such thoughts and ideas.

1. What are the clinical symptoms identifying a parent who is insensitive to the needs of his or her infant? We consider parents exhibiting the following characteristics as possibly showing difficulties in this area:

    a. Any parents who either constantly stimulate or never touch or talk to their infant in the nursery and seem unable to respond in their ministrations to changes in the infant's state or alertness.

    b. Any parents who, during a follow-up visit, relate motives and intentions to the child that are outside the infant's developmental abilities (e.g., the attribution of hate, revenge, or "being spoiled" to a child less than 12 months of age).

   c. Any parents whose infant has not achieved a regular sleeping or eating pattern by 6 to 9 months.

   d. Any parents who do not appreciate or perceive the social cues an infant sends out from age 6 to 8 weeks onward. This would include parents who have failed to develop private games with their infants, have no sense of their infant's uniqueness, and are unable to appreciate when their infant may be frustrated, angry, or unhappy.

2. Although the sources for parents' difficulties in "reading" their infant's state or needs are obviously complex and multidetermined, differentiating these three groups of parents can often be done by sensitive nurses or during the psychosocial interview. In addition, it is important to assess if parents are

   a. Aware of their difficulties but seem unable to change them

   b. Oblivious to the distorted image they have of their infant

   c. Temporarily "out of phase" with their infant because of fatigue or other acutely stressful life events

IV. Assisting parents with premature infants

A. Premature infants, at least during their early lives, are more difficult to look after than are full-term infants. The adequacy of parental caretaking is as powerful a predictor of the final cognitive and behavioral outcome of these infants as many physiologic insults during the prenatal and postnatal period (Werner and Smith, 1982). Therefore, the physician is clearly obligated to provide parents and other primary caretakers with emotional support and optimal opportunities to learn adequate parenting skills. This can be done by creating a milieu that

1. Promotes parental visiting and contact with the infant in the NICU

2. Fosters communication between caretakers and nursery staff

3. Provides experiences for parents that increase the chances of their mastering the crisis associated with having such a small infant and thus augment their feeling of self-worth and personal autonomy

B. Our specific recommendations are similar to those we have outlined in an earlier review (Minde, 1984):

1. An NICU should be limited to 20 beds because larger units require so much personnel that meaningful personal interactions between staff, parents, and their families are extremely difficult.

2. Each NICU should have facilities that encourage comfortable visits. For example, there should be rocking chairs, the opportunity for breastfeeding or pumping, and a special area in which parents can be alone with their infant.

3. All professionals who work in an NICU should be carefully selected and provided with opportunities for regular in-service training. The physician in charge of the infant should be identified to the parents, and the physician should actively approach the parents and tell them of the in-

fant's progress. Each unit of 20 beds should also have at least one full-time social worker on staff who can assess individual families when indicated.

4. Each infant should be assigned a primary nurse for the total hospitalization. A primary nurse usually looks after a small number of patients for a prolonged period of time and, in this fashion, provides true continuity of care. As he or she is with the patients many hours every day, the nurse can monitor the parents' visiting patterns regularly and can also learn about the family's personal and social background. This may provide important clues about parenting abilities and alert other professionals if additional support is needed.

5. Parents who have not visited their infant within 2 weeks after admission to an NICU should be asked to meet formally with the neonatologist. The primary aim of this meeting is to inform the parents about the medical status of their infant, but it also allows the physician to address his or her wish to have the parents actively participate in the care of their infant. After the meeting, both the neonatologist and the parents can visit the infant together; this visit makes it easier for the parents to get over the initial hurdle of seeing and touching their infant. If such a consultation visit does not stimulate parental visits the family should be referred to a social worker or interested physician for a more detailed investigation. If such a consultation does not reveal specific psychosocial difficulties in the family in question, the physician need not be unduly alarmed about the future emotional health of the infant. In fact, it has recently been established that parents who do not visit their infants frequently in the NICU or who have been separated from them during this time for other reasons do not abuse or reject their children more often later on than do parents who did not experience an early separation (Egeland and Vaughn, 1981).

6. All parents should receive literature on prematurity (e.g., *The Premature Infant: A Handbook for Parents,* by Shosenberg et al., 1980) right after the delivery or during their initial visit to the nursery. They should also be given every opportunity to participate in the care of their infant. Parental and sibling visits should not be limited, and parents should be encouraged to get involved early in caretaking routines. Breast-feeding should also be encouraged. Physicians and other health care professionals should recognize, however, that the opportunity to participate in the initial care of the infant will not be sufficient to allay the anxieties or fears of all parents. Allowing the parents of a premature infant to develop a feeling that their infant has a life ahead of him or her that is worthwhile, therefore, is an important first step in connecting parents with their newborn infant. The perception that these infants are completely different from normal infants or the feeling of not knowing what is ahead often makes it difficult for parents to conceptualize their proper role in the caretaking process and consequently makes them unsure of how to deal with their infant. One way to increase the feeling of competence in parents is through group meetings with other parents of premature infants. These meetings may be led by a mother or father who has had personal experiences with a premature infant within the last 12

months. Such experienced parents invariably establish rapid and good relationships with new parents and allow them to come to terms with some of their grief within 2 or 3 weeks. Once this has been achieved, the new parents feel that they can participate more actively in caretaking routines, and as they now focus more on the present, they also retain information more readily that can assist them in their later caretaking tasks (Minde et al., 1980b).

7. Parents of premature infants should have the opportunity to sleep 1 or 2 nights with their infant, in a room separate from the nursery, prior to the infant's discharge from the hospital. This opportunity will familiarize them with the infant's night and will diminish the parental fears so commonly encountered after an infant's transfer from hospital to home.

C. Once the premature infant is discharged home, the following supportive measures have been found useful for the parents:

1. Parents with high-risk neonates must have access to a comprehensive follow-up program in which physicians, in addition to monitoring the infant's growth and development, can also provide information and counselling about the emotional and cognitive development of the infant and family. Visits should be scheduled to last 30 minutes and begin within 2 weeks after discharge.

2. Inform the parents that during the first months after discharge from the hospital, premature infants frequently develop feeding, crying, and sleeping difficulties and are hard to calm; day-to-day behavior is also difficult to regulate. Reassure parents that these phenomena are not unusual and encourage them to avoid overstimulating the infant. One way to do this is to hold the infant snugly during a feeding and to develop distinctive presleep rituals (e.g., a bath, a special song before bedtime to calm the infant).

3. Reassure parents about the development of their infant. Many parents worry about their infant despite outwardly good development. For example, they worry that the infant will never sit up. When the infant has achieved this task at an appropriate age, they are not consoled. Instead they worry that the infant will never walk or talk. It is not always possible to reassure parents about all these concerns. Physicians should accept limits of persuasion without getting angry with the family or discouraged with themselves. Likewise, parents will often refuse to leave the infant at any time despite the capability and experience of the babysitter. While this approach is contrary to my beliefs about optimal parenting, some parents simply cannot enjoy themselves away from their infant and should not be pushed to do so.

4. Parents who have been poorly parented, have an inadequate support system, and live in poor social circumstances are less likely to be attuned to their infant's developmental needs and may require one or more interventions (e.g., follow-up visits, contacts with public health nurses, community occupational therapists, infant stimulation programs, visiting homemakers, or a good daycare program). While these services may be delivered by a variety of agencies and professionals, it is important to select one professional during this first year who can pro-

vide the continuity of care so crucial for the establishment of parental trust and confidence.

5. Acknowledge to the parents that looking after a premature infant requires a great deal of time and effort, especially during the first year of life. Parents appreciate those physicians and other professionals most who readily acknowledge this in a positive manner and are available to talk with them about the problems and challenges associated with raising such a special infant. All professionals must have a special sensitivity to the total needs of the child and family.

REFERENCES

Als, H., Lester, B. M., Tronick, E. Z., and Brazelton, T. B. Towards a Research Instrument for the Assessment of Preterm Infant's Behavior (APIB). In H. Fitzgerald, B. M. Lester, and M. W. Yogman (eds.), *Theory and Research in Behavioral Paediatrics.* New York: Plenum, 1982. Vol. 1, pp. 35–63.

Blacher, J. Sequential stages of parental adjustment to the birth of a child with handicaps: Fact or artifact? *Ment. Retard.* 22 : 55, 1984.

Egeland, B., and Vaughn, B. Failure of "bond formation" as a cause of abuse, neglect and maltreatment. *Am. J. Orthopsychiatry* 51 : 78, 1981.

Featherstone, H. *A Difference in the Family: Life with a Disabled Child.* New York: Basic Books, 1980.

Fitzhardinge, P. M. Follow-up Studies on Infants. In H. Winick (ed.), *Mother and Infant.* New York: Wiley, 1985. Pp. 147–161.

Fitzhardinge, P. M., and Pape, K. E. Follow-up Studies of the High Risk Newborn. In G. B. Avery (ed.), *Neurology Pathophysiology and Management of the Newborn* (2nd ed.). Toronto: Lippincott, 1981. Pp. 350–367.

Ghodsian, M., Zajicek, E., and Wolkin, S. Maternal depression and child behavior problems. *J. Child Psychol. Psychiatry* 25 : 91, 1984.

Goldberg, S., and DiVitto, B. *Born Too Soon.* San Francisco: Freeman, 1983.

Knobloch, H., Malone, A., Ellison, P. H., et al. Considerations in evaluating changes in outcome for infants weighing less than 1501 grams. *Pediatrics* 69 : 285, 1982.

Linn, P. L., Horowitz, F. D., and Fox, H. A. Stimulation in the NICU: Is more necessarily better? *Clin. Perinatol.* 2 : 407, 1985.

Marton, P., Minde, K., and Perrotta, M. The role of the father in the infant at risk. *Am. J. Orthopsychiatry* 51 : 672, 1981.

Minde, K. The impact of prematurity on the later behavior of children and on their families. *Perinatology* 11 : 227, 1984.

Minde, K., Algieri, A., Hodapp, R., and Young, K. Parental reactions to the birth and development of a premature infant. In press.

Minde, K., Marton, P., Manning, D., and Hines, B. Some determinants of mother-infant interaction in the premature nursery. *J. Am. Acad. Child Psychiatry* 19 : 1, 1980a.

Minde, K., Shosenberg, N., Marton, P., et al. Self-help groups in a premature nursery: A controlled evaluation. *J. Pediatr.* 96 : 933, 1980b.

Shosenberg, N., Minde, K., Swyer, P., and Fitzhardinge, P. *The Premature Infant: A Handbook for Parents.* Toronto: Hospital for Sick Children Foundation, 1980.

Werner, E. E., and Smith, R. S. *Vulnerable but Invincible.* New York: McGraw-Hill, 1982.

Adverse Interactions

Leila Beckwith

I. Parent-infant interaction and its effect on development
The development of high-risk infants as well as normal infants depends on the
environment in which the infants live. The pattern of interactions with the parents exacerbates or attenuates the influence of biologic risk factors in the
child's development. Some family environments are so supportive that they
compensate for risk factors and later developmental problems are avoided;
some family environments have neither emotional, educational, nor economic
resources to adapt to even slight perinatal problems. Children from the latter
environments tend to maintain deficits into later stages of development
(Sameroff and Chandler, 1975).

A. Attachment theory
Attachment theory suggests that because human infants are incapable of
caring for themselves, it is specifically adaptive that they seek to be close to
or have physical contact with adults who can protect them and provide the
care that they need (Ainsworth, 1969; Bowlby, 1969). Evolutionary adapt-
edness has ensured that normal newborns have a behavioral repertoire that
enables them to attain proximity to and contact with others by crying, vocalizing, grasping, sucking, looking, and later by smiling and following.
Infant-adult proximity depends not only on the ability of infants to produce
signals but on a complementary tendency of adults to respond to those signals. Parents are well equipped to be drawn into social interaction with
their infant. Parents find infant cries aversive and seek to terminate them by
holding the infant. Other infant characteristics, such as smiling and vocalizing, attract parents positively to look, smile, vocalize, and touch.

B. Importance of parental responsiveness
Proximity maintenance between infants and parents ensures more than physical survival. In his or her attachment behavior, the parent reassures, con-
soles, and provides comfort as well as reduces stress and anxiety. The parent
does so by tender and long holding, by promptly responding to distress, by
touching, and by interacting affectionately face-to-face. In the process of the
parent's sensitive and contingent responding to the infant's signals, the infant
acquires feelings of security in the parent's presence (Ainsworth et al.,
1978). Securely attached infants are later more enthusiastic and persistent
in tasks, more sociable with adults, and more sociable and competent with
peers (Sroufe, 1983).
Although parental proximity is necessary for responsiveness, it is most
likely that it is sensitive responsiveness that is crucial to infant security. If

the parent, when present, is accessible and responds promptly, lovingly, and appropriately, then the infant develops the belief that he or she can explore the world and interact with others safely and effectively. If the parent fails repeatedly to respond promptly and appropriately, then the infant is likely to develop a chronically anxious or inhibited way of interacting with the environment (Maccoby and Martin, 1983).

C. Parent-infant play

Parent-infant interaction involves more than reassurance and reducing stress. Parents and infants play together, either spontaneously, as in vocal and facial imitation, or in games, such as tickling, "horsie," "I'm gonna get you," "peek-a-boo," or "pat-a-cake." Their play, as is typical of all social play, is characterized by shared rules of behavior and mutual pleasure. When infants and parents play games, they must agree on the game, monitor the partner's rhythms and signals, and act either simultaneously or in turns, as appropriate. Whereas the parents bear the major responsibilities initially to monitor and maintain a level of arousal in which the infant is likely to show positive affect (Stern, 1974) and to set up simple repetitive sequences, the infant quickly begins to learn the game, to anticipate it, and to take initiative in it. The acquisition of game skills amplifies the infant's understanding of rules and promotes turn taking, a skill particularly important for later joint activities such as language conversation. Additionally, both in play and in caretaking, parents facilitate language learning by directing a special kind of speech to their infant, in which the rhythms and inflections are exaggerated (compared with normal speech): The speech is slower, simpler, and more repetitive, and the pitch is higher and more variable (Snow, 1972).

Several studies have indicated that infants are more involved with parents who are fun. The more playful a parent and the more positive affect he or she displays during interaction with the infant, the more socially responsive the infant will be to the parent, and the more positive affect the infant will show (Clarke-Stewart, 1973). Infants who have fun with their parents tend to become securely attached (Blehar et al., 1977). Infants with parents who are tense and irritable during early interactions are likely to become anxiously attached (Egeland and Farber, 1984).

D. Disengagement

The infant's desire for proximity, contact, or play with the parent is not constant. The infant has competing goals that are also essential for development, such as exploring the environment, engaging with peers, and exercising autonomy. Whereas wariness of new people or environments, fatigue, or illness increases the infant's need for proximity and contact, the absence of such conditions allows the infant to turn attention away from the parent and toward other developmental tasks. Infants communicate reluctance to engage in social activity by gaze aversion, head turning, fussiness, drowsiness, and by moving away. The parent's awareness and responsiveness to those signals are as important as their responding to the infant's initiations.

E. How infant and parent contribute to the interaction
Variations in the infant's ability to emit signals and to respond to the parent's interventions and variations in the parent's tendencies to respond promptly, appropriately, and tenderly influence the pattern of parent-infant interaction. Because the characteristics of both the parent and the infant are important, difficulties in parent-infant interactions occur when atypical parents or atypical infants disrupt the reciprocity of the relationship (Brazelton et al., 1975).

F. Factors that interfere with interactions
1. Factors within the parent. Impaired parenting can result from depression, impaired judgment, inability to empathize, or projection of distorted and negative images onto the infant. Parents who have had disrupted and abusive relationships with their own parents; who are stressed because of poverty, immigrant status, or other small children to nurture; who receive little support from others; who have unstable educational, work, and living arrangements; or who are experiencing severe marital conflict are more likely to form deleterious patterns of interaction with their infant (Maccoby and Martin, 1983).
2. Factors specific to high-risk infants. In addition to the factors within the parent's life that may interfere with his or her interaction with the infant, high-risk infants and their parents are especially vulnerable to adverse interactions because of the increased stress, anxiety, grief, disappointment, and guilt associated with the birth, and because the infants themselves may be less rewarding, less predictable, and more difficult to raise (Goldberg and DiVitto, 1983).

Moreover, the infant's stay in the neonatal intensive care unit (NICU) is likely to interfere with the parents' early contact and care of the infant —experiences that facilitate parental bonding, although not essential for most parents (Klaus and Kennell, 1982). Parents of high-risk infants enter the relationship with their infant with a lack of confidence as parents and with many fears about their child's health, welfare, and development. Further adding to the burden is that their high-risk infant is more likely than a normal infant to have disorganized sleep and feeding rhythms and to be more unpredictable, less responsive, and more fussy during social interaction (Field, 1982).

II. Difficulty of differentiating compensatory from adverse interactions
The interactions of high-risk infants with their parents tend to be qualitatively and quantitatively different from those between healthy term infants and their parents. The high-risk group most commonly studied has been the preterm group, and generalizations about this risk group may be relevant to others. In general, parents of preterm infants tend to be more active, more persistent, and more likely to initiate and to continue behavioral exchanges than are parents of full-term infants. Even when the infants grow older and contribute more to the interaction, the responsibility is still disproportionate for parents of high-risk infants compared with parents of term infants. Some high-risk infants may appear more distractible, more fussy, less responsive, and less organized dur-

ing feeding and play, and their mothers stimulate and coax their infants more. Some parents show less pleasure during interactions with high-risk infants throughout the first year of life than do parents of healthy full-term infants. Moreover, the deviation in affect regulation occurs in both the parent and the high-risk infant so that fewer occasions of mutual smiling occur. High-risk infants probably have more difficulty modulating arousal in response to stimulation than do normal infants, creating a more difficult task for their parents in fine-tuning the intensity and amount of social interaction (Field, 1982).

While many studies find that these differences in interaction style have disappeared by the second year of life, some professionals are concerned that the early patterns of increased parental initiative and control may continue and interfere with the infant's taking initiative and asserting independence, which are the developmental tasks of the second year of life. Although it appears normal that parents of high-risk infants work harder, the increased involvement of the parent with the high-risk infant may be somewhat intrusive or overprotective with negative consequences for the infant's development and, at the same time, be somewhat compensatory for the infant's deficits and over time contribute to the infant's well-being. Research findings to date are conflicting. Some investigators have found that parents who make the most effort and succeed in engaging their infants in frequent mutually responsive social interactions promote competence in their children that becomes evident by the end of the first year of life, continuing throughout early childhood (Beckwith and Cohen, 1984). Other investigators have found that parents may interact too actively, overwhelming the infant and impeding the infant's competence (Field, 1982). The latter pattern, while of concern, is less deleterious to the infant's development than decreased parental activity.

A. Decreased parental involvement

There is an indifferent, uninvolved pattern of interaction that is deleterious to most infants but may be particularly so to high-risk infants (Maccoby and Martin, 1983). In a relationship characterized by very low emotional commitment of the parent to the infant and low involvement of the parent in the child's welfare, parents either ignore cues from the infant or respond so as to terminate them. There is a paucity of interaction, and there are few reciprocal exchanges between parent and infant of mutual gazing, vocalizing, touching, or smiling. Children who experience such patterns of interaction are likely to be disturbed in their attachments and show deficits in other areas of emotional and cognitive development.

B. Father-infant interaction

So far, parent-infant interactions have been discussed without discriminating between mothers and fathers. Although the research reported to this time has focused mainly on mothers rather than fathers, the assumption has been that the structure and function of interaction do not depend on the gender of the parent.

Studies specifically of father-infant interaction show that although fathers are engaged in much less interaction with their infants than are mothers, they are capable of being as sensitive and responsive as mothers. It is not clear, however, whether fathers are typically as responsive as mothers.

Rather, mothers and fathers tend to adopt somewhat different parenting roles with their infants and provide somewhat different types of experiences. Mothers tend to be more nurturing and to perform more routine physical care. Fathers tend to play more or to engage in more physically stimulating play (Yogman, 1982). Some, but not all, aspects of these patterns may change when both parents are employed or when the father is the primary caretaker (Campos et al., 1983).

Infants interact with both mothers and fathers and form attachments to both. There may, however, be a hierarchy of attachment relationships that becomes evident when infants are very distressed. Under circumstances of distress, most infants tend to choose their mothers rather than their fathers to console them (Lamb, 1981).

Finally, when the father's interactions with the premature infant are sensitive to the infant's physiologic stability, significant correlations have been found between father-infant play at 5 months and Bayley outcomes at 18 months (Yogman, 1984).

C. Individual variability and change

Although group trends have been emphasized, there are wide individual differences within any high-risk group. Just as low-risk children and their parents are not immune to adverse interactions, many high-risk children and their parents do not develop them. Further, specific parental acts have less of a lasting influence on the child's development than long-term patterns such as sensitivity or insensitivity and responsiveness or emotional unavailability. Yet even when the parents' style of behavior with the infant is unsatisfactory, changes can occur, particularly as family circumstances change. Moreover, just as some infants are less vulnerable to similar perinatal hazards, some children appear to be less vulnerable to the most adverse interactions with their parents. Development proceeds through a series of interactions with many significant others, including grandparents, siblings, teachers, and peers. Attention, responsiveness, and shared pleasure with a significant other can serve as a protective factor in the child's development.

III. Recommendations for management

A. Support parents in interacting and caring for their infant while in the hospital. Frequent contact with the infant as early as possible tends to increase parental confidence.

B. Anticipate with parents the transition from the hospital to home by assisting the parents in the practical aspects of readying the home for the infant, such as clothing, diapers, bathing, feeding, sleeping, and providing information as to resources available for extended medical help.

C. Provide the parents with information as to community resources, including parent support groups, public health home visiting programs, and other professional home visiting programs.

D. Inform the parents that early contact with the infant is only one factor in attachment to the infant and a factor that, in general, does not have long-term consequences. Reassure the parents that the loss of early contact with their infant does not mean that they will not or have not bonded to their infant.

E. Discuss with the parents the infant's biologic rhythms regarding sleep and wakefulness, and anticipate developmental changes. For example, the preterm infant's increased fussiness 1 to 3 months postterm has a positive element: It reflects an advance in an infant who is becoming more alert, more awake, and more sensitive to the environment.

F. Assist the parents in valuing and enjoying noncaretaking activities, such as talking, smiling, and touching the infant.

G. By mutual observation and discussion, help the parents gain skill in observing the infant's motor tone, posture, facial expression, and so forth as signals of the infant's needs. Also, discuss factors that enhance the infant's organization, such as gentle movements, soothing, and sucking.

H. Encourage the parents to put confidence in their infant's ability to communicate needs.

I. Do not prejudge the infant, despite his or her high-risk status. Focus on the infant's individuality and competence and the inherent self-correcting features in the development of most high-risk infants.

J. Because caring for a high-risk infant is more demanding than caring for a normal infant, encourage the parents to seek help from others, even occasionally with the care of the infant so that the parents can get a respite.

REFERENCES

Ainsworth, M. D. S. Object relations, dependency and attachment: A theoretical review of the infant-mother relationship. *Child Dev.* 40 : 969, 1969.

Ainsworth, M. D. S., Blehar, M. C., Waters, E., and Wall, S. *Patterns of Attachment.* Hillsdale, N.J.: Erlbaum, 1978.

Beckwith, L., and Cohen, S. E. Home Environment and Cognitive Competence in Preterm Children During the First Five Years. In A. W. Gottfried (ed.), *Home Environment and Early Cognitive Development: Longitudinal Research.* New York: Academic, 1984.

Blehar, L., Lieberman, A. F., and Ainsworth, M. D. S. Early face-to-face interaction and its relation to later infant-mother attachment. *Child Dev.* 48 : 182, 1977.

Bowlby, J. *Attachment* (Attachment and Loss, vol. 1). London: Hogarth, 1969.

Brazelton, T. B., Tronick, E., Adamson, L., et al. Early Mother-Infant Reciprocity. In M. Hofer (ed.), *Parent-Infant Interaction.* Amsterdam: Excerpta Medica, 1975.

Campos, J. J., Barrett, K. C., Lamb, M. E., et al. Socioemotional Development. In P. H. Mussen (ed.), *Handbook of Child Psychology: Infancy and Developmental Psychobiology* (4th ed.). New York: Wiley, 1983. Vol. 2, pp. 783–916.

Clarke-Stewart, K. A. Interactions between mothers and their young children: Characteristics and consequences. *Monog. Soc. Res. Child Dev.* Vol. 38, Nos. 6, 7, 1973.

Egeland, B., and Farber, E. A. Infant-mother attachment: Factors related to its development and changes over time. *Child Dev.* 55 : 753, 1984.

Field, T. Affective Displays of High-Risk Infants During Early Interactions. In T. Field and A. Fogel (eds.), *Emotion and Early Interaction.* Hillsdale, N.J.: Erlbaum, 1982.

Goldberg, S., and DiVitto, B. *Born Too Soon: Preterm Birth and Early Development.* New York: Freeman, 1983.

Klaus, M., and Kennell, J. *Parent-Infant Bonding.* St. Louis: Mosby, 1982.

Lamb, M. E. (ed.) The Development of Father-Infant Relationships. In *The Role of the Father in Child Development* (2nd ed.). New York: Wiley, 1981.

Maccoby, E. E., and Martin, J. A. Socialization in the Context of the Family: Parent-Child Interaction. In P. H. Mussen (ed.), *Handbook of Child Psychology: Socialization, Personality, and Social Development* (4th ed.). New York: Wiley, 1983. Vol. 4, pp. 1–102.

Sameroff, A., and Chandler, M. Reproductive Risk and the Continuum of Caretaking Casualty. In F. Horowitz (ed.), *Review of Child Development Research.* Chicago: University of Chicago Press, 1975. Vol. 4.

Snow, C. E. Mothers' speech to children learning language. *Child Dev.* 43 : 549, 1972.

Sroufe, L. A. Infant-Caregiver Attachment and Patterns of Adaptation in Preschool: The Roots of Maladaptation and Competence. In M. Perlmutter (ed.), *Minnesota Symposia on Child Psychology.* Hillsdale, N.J.: Erlbaum, 1983. Vol. 16.

Stern, D. N. The goal and structure of mother-infant play. *J. Am. Acad. Child Psychiatry* 13 : 402, 1974.

Yogman, M. W. Development of the Father-Infant Relationship. In H. Fitzgerald, B. Lester, and M. Yogman (eds.), *Theory and Research in Behavioral Pediatrics.* New York: Plenum, 1982. Vol. 1.

Yogman, M. W. The Father's Role with Preterm and Full-term Infants. In J. Call, E. Galenson, and R. Tyson (eds.), *Frontiers of Infant Psychiatry.* New York: Basic Books, 1984. Vol. 2.

Continuing Care: Parents' Retrospective

Barbara B. McCauley and James E. McCauley

Our son was born 10 weeks prematurely and hospitalized for 5 months. His home-coming marked the beginning of an exhilarating and exhausting year, with months of sleepless nights and anxious days. As new parents, we fumbled our way from day to day, sensing that we needed help but not knowing what to ask for or how to get it. As we gradually learned to select and coordinate resources, life became easier and we were able to begin to enjoy our son.

Sean was born on August 29, 1984, at 30 weeks' gestation, weighing 1,840 g. The pregnancy, Barbara's first, was uncomplicated until spontaneous rupture of the membranes 52 hours prior to the birth. Terbutaline was administered to suppress labor; steroids were withheld. Labor occurred despite the terbutaline, and Sean was born by normal spontaneous vaginal delivery. At the time of his birth, we were both 36-year-old clinical social workers and had been married for 14 years. Yet it seemed that life's experiences had not come close to preparing us for the weeks and months that followed.

Sean came out "looking good"; since his Apgar scores were 6 and 8 and he weighed more than 1,800 g, we were optimistic. However, he began to deteriorate rapidly and within hours was intubated and transferred to the neonatal intensive care unit (NICU) at another hospital several blocks away.

Sean's first 3 weeks were marked by extreme instability. He received pancuronium soon after admission and, on the third day, had three pneumothoraxes and a pneumopericardium that required evacuation. He received the first of many blood transfusions, and at 11 days of age a central line was inserted. He had a grade II to III intraventricular hemorrhage, which required serial lumbar punctures. After 3 weeks of instability, his condition became grave once again. He responded well to a trial of dexamethasone (Decadron) and within days was able to be weaned from the pancuronium. A patent ductus arteriosus became evident, and after surgical ligation was performed, Sean began to make good progress. It was at this point that we finally began to believe that he would survive. He was extubated at 7 weeks of age, and we were looking forward to taking him home 4 weeks later, near his term date.

This was not to happen. Sean's progress slowed to a snail's pace, held up by extreme fluid sensitivity, fevers of unknown origin, and difficulty with nippling feeds. When all but the feeding problems were under control, a discharge plan was made. If Sean could be completely on oral feedings within 10 days, he would go home from the NICU. If not, he would be transferred back to the intermediate nursery at the hospital of his birth. It was almost immediately evident to everyone that the transfer would be necessary, and at 3 months of age, Sean returned to the level II nursery, where he would remain for another 2 months.

The transfer from the NICU to the intermediate nursery is said to be difficult for all families, and so it was for us. Our feelings about the NICU staff had ranged from anger and mistrust to admiration and adoration. But after 3 months we had become very attached, and the circumstances of Sean's transfer made it feel more like a failure than a graduation. Every day in the level II nursery felt like overtime and reduced the little confidence we had in our ability to care for Sean at home. He had several setbacks in the next 5 weeks: pneumonia, elevated liver enzymes of unknown cause, and recurrence of acute hydrocephalus, which was managed medically. Congestive heart failure suddenly developed when an attempt was made to wean him from furosemide (Lasix).

As Sean entered his fifth month, poor nippling was again the major holdup. He was not interested in food, tired very quickly, and needed supplementary nasogastric feedings. A gastrostomy in order to allow him to be discharged was suggested, but Sean improved and began to eat well enough to go home.

He was still a frail, scrawny baby with severe bronchopulmonary dysplasia and fluid sensitivity. It was January, and the respiratory syncytial virus was a major threat. The staff expressed considerable ambivalence about whether it was safe to discharge such a fragile baby at that time of year. Although we knew that this ambivalence was no reflection on our competence as parents, it did not enhance our sense of readiness.

We had worked well with the neonatology fellow who had been Sean's primary physician that month and were pleased when she offered to follow him for hospital clinic visits after discharge. We had selected a pediatrician in the third week of Sean's hospitalization, when we were frightened by Sean's deteriorating condition and overwhelmed by the medical procedures and terminology. The hospital staff constantly reassured us that we did not have the responsibility to make medical decisions about Sean. Yet, for our own peace of mind, we needed knowledgeable but objective support. Our pediatrician facilitated our communication with the NICU staff and assured us that we were asking the right questions.

The pediatrician, who had an office near our home but was also on hospital staff, looked in on Sean frequently (at no charge to us) over the course of hospitalization. By discharge, he was very familiar with both Sean's history and the emotional roller coaster we had experienced. This laid the groundwork for mutual trust and understanding in the year to come.

Ten days before discharge, we had a planning conference at the hospital with both the pediatrician and neonatologist. Sean would go home on oxygen, with suction equipment. He would need a cardiac monitor at night, to warn us if bronchospasms caused bradycardia. He would be discharged with six medications and two food supplements.

We began immediately to look for a suitable medical equipment company, because we wanted to be familiar with the equipment in our home well before Sean arrived. Although oxygen services are widely available in this large metropolitan area, cardiac monitors were not; one ambitious salesperson tried to convince Barbara that it would be so much safer to use the apnea monitor he had, although Sean had no history of apnea. All of the companies insisted on being full-service, that is, they would not provide monitor rental if oxygen equipment was obtained elsewhere. The company we selected had a respiratory therapist who would work closely with us if there were problems with any equipment.

As discharge approached, we became increasingly fearful that, once home, Sean would need some medical procedures we could not do. Feeding him was still a struggle, and he was on large doses of diuretics; we feared he would need an occasional nasogastric feeding to prevent dehydration. In addition, mucous secretions sometimes interfered with his feeding, and we thought he might need deep suctioning. We called many nursing agencies and home health agencies. Our local visiting nurse association had no nurses experienced with infants. All other agencies told us that on-call services did not exist: One had to contract, well in advance, for 4 to 8 hours of nursing care, and payment had to be made in advance. Months later we could find out if insurance would reimburse. After 5 months of sharing our baby with nurses around-the-clock, the idea of having one spend 4 to 8 hours in our home was abhorrent. We knew that eventually we would welcome some respite care, but during Sean's first weeks at home, we wanted desperately to be alone, just the three of us, as a family. We decided to hire a favorite nurse, one of Sean's primary team, to be on-call for us that first week; for a flat fee she agreed to be available in her off-work hours, and we would pay her additionally in the event that we actually needed her services. Her availability gave us enormous peace of mind; we needed her only once, to assure us that Sean was not in congestive heart failure.

Although Sean's chronic illness had exhausted us physically and emotionally, we were spared even greater stress because we had excellent insurance coverage and we lived only a half hour from the hospitals. On the negative side, we had only one relative living close enough to help, a cousin who was 30 miles away. Close friends offered comfort and solace, but ultimately we were alone as a couple in facing this crisis.

Like most couples, we felt that the stress of having a critically ill infant tested our marriage. We knew of couples who had broken up after the loss of a child, and in the first weeks of uncertainty, we clung to each other, trying to preserve the bond that had been so strong prior to Sean's birth. As his condition improved, we began to function less as a couple and more as individuals focused on the baby. We usually visited separately, with Barbara spending days by the bedside and Jim coming for several hours in the evening, after work. We found it difficult to share Sean, with each of us needing to be the one standing closest to him in the bedspace and, later, the one to hold him during a visit. During this time we also stopped sharing our grief and fears with each other. We each sensed the other's burden was too great already—we dared not add to that misery. We unconsciously declared a moratorium on conflict and avoided all confrontation. Our focus was on surviving this terrible ordeal and maintaining the homeostasis of our marriage. We imagined that once Sean came home, all would be well, and we could resume the companionship and mutual support we had enjoyed previously.

At discharge, Sean was 151 days old and weighed 3,100 g (7 lbs). In addition to the bronchopulmonary dysplasia, he had a ventricular septal defect, a hydrocele, and alternating esotropia. At follow-up visits, he would need head ultrasonography to monitor his hydrocephalus, and blood work-ups to check his theophylline level, electrolytes, and hematocrit. If weight gain were too slow, a gastrostomy might be necessary.

Sean's actual day of homecoming was not the joyous occasion we had expected it to be. Looking back now at his picture on the day of discharge, it's easy to see why. He was a pale, emaciated, and lethargic baby. He was coming home not because he was well, but because there were no dramatic reasons to support his remaining in the hospital.

For Sean's first few weeks at home, we felt very isolated and alone. Like most families who endure an extended hospital stay, we had grown to depend on the nursery culture for our emotional, social, and medical support. Now we were on our own, and family life was far from how we had dreamed it would be. Each day the tension built. Sean's respiratory rate would soar to 80 per minute for several hours, only to drop as unpredictably as it had risen. He used every ounce of his energy to resist medications: screaming, gagging, vomiting, and refusing to eat afterward. He would often become too congested to eat, prompting us to argue over whether he should be suctioned and whose turn it was to do the much-dreaded procedure. Barbara continued to pump breast milk, in spite of increasing evidence that Sean would never make the transfer to the breast. We faced each day with less and less energy, as Sean never slept longer than 2 hours at a time.

Feeding continued to be a major problem. Insidiously, we found ourselves spending more and more time feeding Sean (up to nine feedings a day) while he was eating less and less. We tried every feeding technique we could think of and looked for reasons why he would not eat. Despite our intense worry, we were still so caught up in trying to prove to our doctors that we were good parents who could handle this infant at home that we were slow to convey how serious the problem was. Instead we felt rebuffed by their suggestions to "stick with it" or call the nurses at the NICU for helpful hints.

Eventually, we accepted a referral for evaluation by a special "feeding team" in the developmental evaluation unit of the hospital. They observed Sean feeding and confirmed the seriousness of the problem. The pressure on us was intensified, however, when the team recommended that we learn to feed Sean with a nasogastric tube. In the months before, however, many of Sean's caretakers had advised us against learning this, and we ultimately decided it was a potentially high-risk medical procedure that we as parents did not want to do. Instead, we agreed to have Sean rehospitalized. There it was determined that the hydrocephalus had recurred and the intracranial pressure had increased dramatically in the 3 weeks Sean had been at home. Sean would need a ventriculoperitoneal shunt. We had been so determined to keep him out of the hospital that we had been unable to see that Sean had lost his ability to suck.

Sean's second hospitalization was for 17 days, long enough for diagnosis, surgery, and recovery. Because no step-down unit was available, he was readmitted to the level II nursery. This was an exception to policy and caused some controversy, although it was generally agreed that this was the safest place for him. He needed protection from the near-epidemic respiratory illnesses of February in the tertiary hospital, and his multisystem problems would have been difficult for any service other than neonatology to follow. For us, the familiarity of the nursery was comforting, and our disappointment at the readmission was tempered by our relief.

In the months after the shunt placement and Sean's return home, we began to see slow but steady improvement in his disposition and energy level. Although his growth rate remained slow, feeding was not the struggle it once was. As his need for medications decreased there was an improvement in his sleep patterns; in particular, when theophylline was discontinued, he began to sleep uninterrupted for

7 hours at night. At 9 months of age, he blossomed socially, smiling often and becoming very visually attuned. We were finally able to really enjoy him. Gradually we were moving away from being an illness-oriented home to achieving some measure of normality. It was quite a milestone when one of Sean's visits to the pediatrician included immunizations—it felt like our first well-baby visit.

Paradoxically, only as Sean improved did we have the energy to pursue respite care and other follow-up services. Prior to Sean's initial discharge, his neonatologist had contacted the state's Department of Social Services on our behalf to document Sean's eligibility for respite-care nursing services. In our state (Massachusetts), each eligible family is entitled to 10 full days (or 20 half-days) of care every 6 months. We began to use the service when Sean returned from his second hospitalization. By that time, we welcomed the nursing assistance and it turned out to be one of our most positive experiences. The nurse we hired had 18 years of pediatric experience, yet she made it clear she was working for us. She adapted to our routines with Sean and was able to free us from many of the medical chores that were required. Ultimately this gave us more time to enjoy and play with Sean.

When we had used all the allotted respite-care hours, we began to look into other home care resources. We contacted a continuing care nurse we had met months before during Sean's hospitalization for shunt surgery. She looked into our insurance coverage and determined that we had missed out on a home health care program, which required approval prior to discharge. Since Sean was still feeding poorly enough for a gastrostomy to remain a possibility, the nurse was able to plead our case successfully with the insurance company. For the next 3 months, we had a nurse's aid twice a week, and the costs of Sean's oxygen and medications were fully covered.

An unexpected but consistent support was the medical equipment company that supplied Sean's oxygen equipment and cardiac monitor. They were on call 24 hours a day and were always patient with our questions about this intimidating equipment. Their respiratory therapist made 2 home visits during Sean's first week at home when we could not stop the monitor's false alarms. The company was also patient when our misjudgments about Sean's oxygen needs resulted in last-minute deliveries.

Sean was almost 8 months old before he was strong enough to really benefit from the services of an early intervention program. Although the program offered services ranging from nutrition education to parent support groups, we were most interested in getting Sean started with physical therapy because of his substantial delay in motor development. He was still quite floppy and could not hold his head up or roll over from back to stomach. The physical therapist came to our home every other week and put Sean through a vigorous pace of exercises that were designed to improve his head and limb control. Through watching the therapist, we were able to replicate the exercises daily. Perhaps more important, we were learning that Sean had more tolerance for exercise than we had given him credit for. The early intervention program also lent us physical therapy equipment and developmental toys to use with Sean.

The most important component of our follow-up care was the successful collaboration between Sean's pediatrician and neonatologist. Each recognized the other's area of expertise and seemed to welcome the shared responsibility for Sean's follow-up care. Their mutual respect made it easy for us to call on both of them freely.

Initially we alternated weekly visits to each. Our pediatrician helped us with normal parenting questions, developmental issues, immunizations, ear examinations, and so on. Visits to the neonatologist at the hospital follow-up clinic were used for such issues as medication adjustments, blood work-ups, and oximeter readings. Both offered us open-ended appointments whenever possible, allowing a lot of time for questions and discussion. The pediatrician often saw us in late afternoon, allowing both of us to attend appointments; he also had a morning call hour. The neonatologist periodically called us between appointments. Telephone contact was especially reassuring during Sean's first cold; we were terrified that he might not be able to fight off this infection, and the neonatologist's calls gave us a measure of relief without undermining our confidence.

Specialists also played a role in Sean's follow-up care. The cardiologist followed him for the ventricular septal defect, which was closing. The neurosurgeon checked the shunt, which had been problem-free, and the neurologist continued to assess Sean for problems related to his intraventricular hemorrhage. The ophthalmologist believed that the esotropia was improving and not in need of intervention.

Sean's hearing had been tested in the NICU when he was 2 months old with a brain-stem auditory evoked response test, which showed no hearing loss. At discharge, he did not orient to sound, but this was assumed to be adaptive behavior for an infant who had spent 5 months in a hospital nursery. After several weeks at home, he was babbling appropriately and becoming socially responsive. When he was 9 months old, our pediatrician suggested another routine hearing evaluation. We were astonished, as were Sean's medical caretakers, to learn that he has a severe to profound bilateral hearing impairment. Without amplification, he heard nothing; and with hearing aids, he heard 45 dB. The quality of what he hears, however, will not be known for years. This news was the hardest of all for us to cope with; it came just as we were beginning to think that Sean might outgrow all of the problems of prematurity.

Sean's second year brought improved medical status but slow growth and ongoing developmental delays. The supplementary oxygen was discontinued at 15 months, but Sean's labored breathing tired him easily and made weight gain difficult. He had no tolerance for textured foods and did not eat table foods until 23 months. His physical therapy sessions were increased to 3 times a week; he sat at 17 months, and by 24 months, he moved around by "seat-scooting," occasionally pulling up and cruising. He developed a good beginning vocabulary in sign language, but made no progress in speech development because he pulled out his hearing aids at every opportunity. On his second birthday, he weighed 20 lbs. The Bayley Scales of Infant Development put him at around the 12- to 14-month level, with some skills at 17 months. In spite of all the obstacles, he continued to be an extremely social, engaging, and good-natured child.

As Sean's parents, we faced the demands of the second year often feeling drained and depleted. We were surprised at how slowly we recovered from the tension and anxiety of the long hospitalization and stressful months that followed. We did not always have the energy to tackle Sean's intensive daily regimen of physical therapy, speech and language exercises, and imaginative feeding techniques. We continued to depend on our respite care nurse, and increasingly turned to Sean's early intervention program team for support and encouragement. Our early worries about Sean's health had shifted to concerns about whether we could provide the intervention and stimulation he would need to catch up.

In summary, the well-noted neonatal roller coaster did not stop with Sean's discharge. The ride just got lonelier. At the critical point of discharge, we did not have the time, energy, and often, the inclination to find our way through the maze of follow-up services and health insurance provisions that would have helped us through the difficult first months at home. Only when we were psychologically ready and Sean was stronger were we able to put together a comprehensive network of medical follow-up, respite care, and early intervention.

The continuing care support system should be in place before discharge. A good case coordinator can provide the necessary expertise as well as relieve parents of the burden of negotiating with insurance companies and agencies. For the first weeks at home, a flexible nursing follow-up service is essential; nurses with neonatal experience should be available by phone and for home visits as needed. The increasing population of complicated and fragile NICU graduates like Sean will demand more specialized and flexible services than have previously been available.

Index

Index

Achievement tests, 162. *See also* Tests
Acoustic reflex thresholds, 109
Acquired immune deficiency syndrome, 78
Acute respiratory insufficiency, 17–18
Adaptation, 105
Adjustment, stages of, 315
Adverse social interactions, 323–328
Affective status, with receptive language disorders, 255
Age
  and communication levels, 263
  corrected, 188
  maternal, 4, 5, 11
Aid to Families with Dependent Children (AFDC), 38, 61
Alopecia areata, 275, 276
Alpha-fetoprotein screening, 79
Alpha-glucosidase, 196
Alpha-thalassemia, 19
Amino acids, 195
Anencephaly, 19
Anger, parental, 318
Anomalies, types of, 265–268. *See also* Congenital anomalies
Anticonvulsants, 235
Apgar scores, 235, 240
Aphonia, psychogenic, 260
Apnea, 298
  incidence and pathogenesis, 205
  management of, 205–207
  in premature infants, 150–151
Articulation disorders, 259–260
Asphyxia, 19, 20
  as cause of death, 17–18
  complications of
    hearing loss, 247
    immunization, 249
    infections, urinary tract, 249
    intellectual disabilities, 244–246
    motor deficits, 246
    nutrition and gastrointestinal problems, 248–249
    prognosis, 249–250
    reflex abnormalities, 243–244
    seizures, 246–247
    speech and language deficits, 248
    vision, 248
  defined, 239

follow-up programs, patient selection for, 86
and hearing loss, 74
management, 239–243
  assessments, 243
  indicators and outcome, 240
  laboratory findings with, 241
  outcomes of, 240, 242
motor behavior screening, 127
Assessment areas. *See also specific assessments*
follow-up clinics. *See* Follow-up clinics
nursing, 103–106
Assessment skills, of parents, 39
Asthma, 160
Asymmetric tonic neck reflex, 243–244
Atrioventricular canal defect, 266
Attachment
  formation of, 168, 169
  hierarchy of, 327
Attachment theory, 323
Attention, 144
Attention deficits, auditory, 255–256
Attentiveness, of infant, 144, 151
Attitudes, family, 318
  assessment of, 102, 105
  and emotional development, 178–179
  with premature infant, 151, 152
  responsiveness, importance of, 323–324
Audiometry, 109, 110–111
Auditory attention deficits, 255–256
Auditory brainstem response audiometry, 110–111
Auditory discrimination disorders, 256
Auditory evoked potentials, 241, 247
Auditory input, in home environment, 152
Auditory processing disorders, 255–257, 278
Auditory Response Cradle, 110
Auditory sequential memory deficits, 257–258
Auditory skills, of premature infant, 151
Auropalpebral reflex, 109

Bayley Scales of Infant Development, 135, 138, 139, 143, 245
  in longitudinal studies, 25–26

341